weber's WAY TO GRILL™

THE STEP-BY-STEP GUIDE TO EXPERT GRILLING

BY JAMIE PURVIANCE

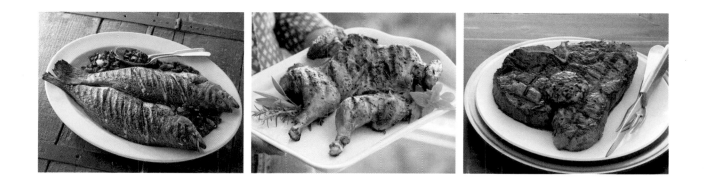

PHOTOGRAPHY BY TIM TURNER

Sunset

weber

Author:	Jamie Purviance
Managing editor:	Marsha Capen
Photographer and photo art direction:	Tim Turner
Food stylist:	Lynn Gagné
Assistant food stylists:	Nina Albazi, Christina Zerkis
Photo assistants:	Christy Clow, David Garcia, Justin Lundquist
Digital guru:	Takamasa Ota
Indexer:	Becky LaBrum
Color imaging and in-house prepress:	Weber Creative Services
Contributors:	Patty Ada, Emily Baird, Gary Bramley, Neal Corman, Jerry DiVecchio, Ryan Gardner, John Gerald Gleeson, Joyce Goldstein, Gary Hafer, Jay Harlow, Rita Held, Susan Hoss, Ellen Jackson, Elaine Johnson, Carolyn Jung, Alison Lewis, James McNair, Andrew Moore, Merrilee Olson, Jeff Parker, David Pazimo, Craig Priebe, Anne-marie Ramo, Justin Roche, Rick Rodgers, James Schend, David Shalleck, and Bob and Coleen Simmons
Photography credit:	Christy Clow, pages 278 and 279, used with permission
Design and production:	Shum Prats, Elaine Chow
Weber-Stephen Products Co.:	Mike Kempster Sr., Executive Vice President Sherry L. Bale, Director, Public Relations Brooke Jones, Marketing Manager
rabble+rouser, inc.:	Christina Schroeder, Chief Rouser Marsha Capen, Content Queen Shum Prats, Creative Director
Sunset Books:	Jim Childs, Vice President and Associate Publisher Bob Doyle, Vice President, Editorial Director Sydney Webber, Director of Marketing

Diamond Crystal® is a registered trademark of Cargill Incorporated, Wayzata, Minnesota; Dr. Pepper® is a registered trademark of Dr. Pepper/Seven Up, Inc., Plano, Texas.

10 9 8 7 6 5 4 3 2 1

ISBN-10: 0-376-02059-8
ISBN-13: 978-0-376-02059-8
Library of Congress Control Number: 2008938334

www.weber.com®

www.sunset.com

ACKNOWLEDGEMENTS

The idea for this book emerged from the agile publishing minds of Mike Kempster, Susan Maruyama, and Christina Schroeder. With the help of Jim Childs and Bob Doyle, they outlined an ambitious project and honored me with the job of tackling it. I am grateful to each of them for their confidence and support.

When it came down to managing all the words and pictures here, Marsha Capen was a thoughtful and remarkably hard-working editor. She always found a gracious way to herd the flock of pigeons involved in this creative process.

The sheer quantity of photographs required for this book would strike fear into the hearts of many photographers, but Tim Turner, who is a master of light and lens (and quite a good griller, too), thrived on the challenge. He was assisted by a particularly talented crew, which included food stylists Lynn Gagné, Nina Albazi, and Christina Zerkis, as well as photo assistants Takamasa Ota, Christy Clow, David Garcia, and Justin Lundquist.

There is another excellent reason why the meat in this book looks so irresistibly fabulous. Almost all of it came from Lobel's of New York (www.lobels.com). Evan, Stanley, Mark, and David Lobel, along with David Richards and all their colleagues, maintain standards so high for meat quality and customer service that whenever I open a box with Lobel's on the label, I am always delighted.

For the recipes, I relied on a sharp team of culinary minds. Many thanks to April Cooper, who handled most of the testing and tweaking, and thank goodness for the many other grillers involved, too. I especially want to acknowledge Patty Ada, Emily Baird, Gary Bramley, Neal Corman, Jerry DiVecchio, Ryan Gardner, John Gerald Gleeson, Joyce Goldstein, Gary Hafer, Jay Harlow, Rita Held, Susan Hoss, Ellen Jackson, Elaine Johnson, Carolyn Jung, Alison Lewis, James McNair, Andrew Moore, Merrilee Olson, Jeff Parker, David Pazimo, Craig Priebe, Anne-marie Ramo, Justin Roche, Rick Rodgers,

James Schend, David Shalleck, and Bob and Coleen Simmons.

I love what Shum Prats and Elaine Chow did with the design of this book, managing to strike a gorgeous balance between clear instructions and imaginative aesthetics.

I want to thank Weber's Creative Services department for improving the look of every last page. Thank you, Becky LaBrum, for a very useful index.

For lots of good advice and generous support all along, I offer special thanks to Sherry Bale, Brooke Jones, Nancy Misch, and Sydney Webber.

While working on this book, I referred to many other books for solid culinary information. I found the following ones very helpful: *The Complete Meat Cookbook*, by Bruce Aidells and Denis Kelly, *The Cook's Illustrated Guide to Grilling and Barbecue*, by the editors of *Cook's Illustrated*, *The New Food Lover's Companion*, by Sharon Tyler Herbst, *The Barbecue Bible*, by Steven Raichlen, and *How to Cook Meat*, by Chris Schlesinger and John Willoughby.

In the final weeks of production, I had impeccable editing help from Sarah Putman Clegg and Carolyn Jung.

This book took me out of town for many days and nights, away from my wife, Fran, and our children, Julia, James, and Peter. I missed some family vacations and quite a few weekends with the people that matter most to me. I owe them a lot for remaining patient and supportive throughout the whole process.

Finally, I want to thank a few mentors who gave a great deal of themselves to me early in my culinary career, Antonia Allegra, Esther McManus, and Becky and David Sinkler. With selfless generosity, each one of them set me on the right course and encouraged me to get going.

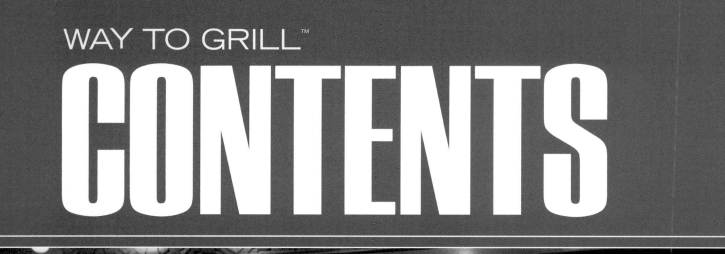

WAY TO GRILL™
CONTENTS

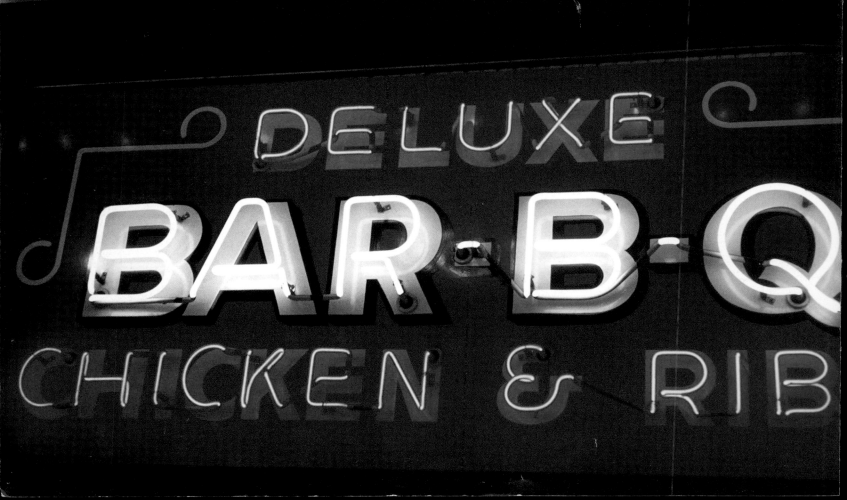

WAY TO GRILL

5

INTRODUCTION

Like you, I wasn't born with a complete understanding and mastery of grilling techniques. As a kid growing up in suburban America, I had to pick up the basics from my dad and other weekend grillers. Eventually, when it was my turn to grill, I had to imitate what I'd seen and I had to develop my own style by doing what so many other grillers do. I had to improvise. I had to experiment. I had to wing it. Sometimes it worked, and other times…well, it did not.

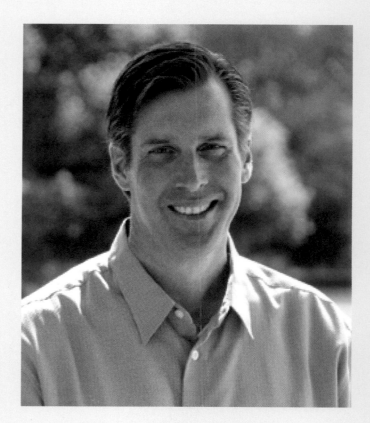

To be honest, I didn't really learn to grill until I was about thirty-years-old. That's when I tackled the subject in a much more methodical way. Obsessed with good food and frustrated by the limitations of winging it, I enrolled at the Culinary Institute of America. There I immersed myself in a rigorous curriculum of the hows and whys of topics like meat butchering, food chemistry, sauce making, and charcuterie. Under the supervision of demanding chefs, I learned serious science-based lessons like how heat affects the structure of meats and fats, how sauces are held together, and how marinades can unravel proteins.

Since my graduation about fifteen years ago, I've focused my attention on how advanced culinary ideas relate specifically to grilling. With the help of many experts at Weber, I've done extensive research on this particular way of cooking and I've written five books on the subject. Each book was an opportunity to learn more about what works on the grill and why some techniques work better than others. This book is a culmination of all the lessons I've learned.

So what is *Weber's Way to Grill?* Well, first of all, it is not just one way to grill. It is not about absolute right

and wrong when it comes to issues like gas versus charcoal, direct versus indirect heat, or grilling with the lid on or off. *Weber's Way to Grill* includes and embraces any way to grill—so long as it works. And what works best, I've learned, is paying attention to culinary details. There is a big difference between winging it and paying attention.

Let me share a couple of examples of what paying attention can do. The first deals with the reason why most steaks turn out beautifully when grilled over direct high heat but most pork chops do not. Why should this be? High heat, of course, can char the surface of meat long before the center is fully cooked. For a steak, that's a fine result, because you are left with a nicely caramelized outer crust and an interior that is dripping with rosy red juices. A pork chop is another matter. We don't like our pork chops raw in the middle, but if we grilled most pork chops over direct high heat until the centers were properly cooked, the surfaces would be badly burned. That's why using medium heat is a better way to grill most pork chops. It allows the centers to reach an ideal degree of doneness without overcooking the surfaces. Simple enough, right? But back in my early days, when I was winging it, I threw every kind of meat over the same high heat. That's one reason things did not always work out.

Weber's Way to Grill is about paying attention to details as basic and significant as salt.

A second example about the importance of paying attention deals with something quite fundamental: salt. Many of you might not give salt much thought, but did you know that, teaspoon for teaspoon, common table salt has about twice the sodium as some types of kosher salt? So if you happened to use common table salt instead of the kosher salt that I call for in almost every recipe in this book, I'm afraid your food would taste awfully salty (and a little metallic

from calcium silicate found in common table salt). To take this topic one step further, I suggest that you pay attention to which brand of kosher salt you use. They are not all the same. I recommend Diamond Crystal® kosher salt, because its salt crystals are hollow diamonds that dissolve easily on the surface of food, meaning the salt is less likely to fall off the food on the grill. On the other hand, there are kosher salts on the market that are made of salt grains mixed with an anti-caking agent, which do not dissolve as well, and are high in sodium to boot. Read the labels carefully.

So, yes, culinary details matter. They explain why you would want to wrap barbecued ribs in foil during the final stages of cooking. They explain why you would grill fish fillets longer on the first side than the second. They explain why you would smoke a turkey with the breast side down.

That's the point of *Weber's Way to Grill*. That's why this book includes so many how-to photographs and explanatory captions and detailed recipes. The emphasis here is on paying close attention. It's about learning how and why certain ways work well, so that you can move beyond the limits of winging it. Great taste lies in the details. Just pay attention and enjoy a new level of grilling success.

Jamie Purviance

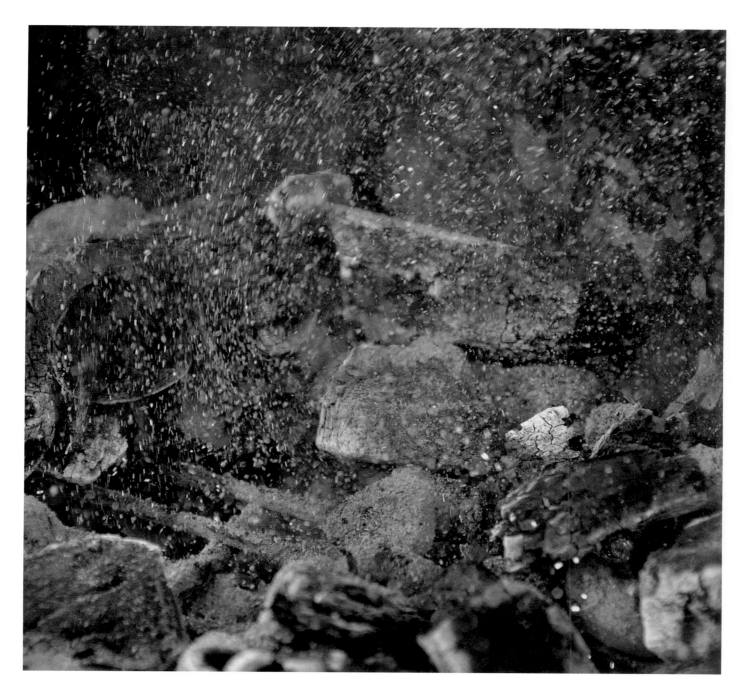

GRILLING BASICS

Grilling is so tightly woven into American culture that almost everyone has something to say about the way to do it. All of us have had experiences that help us to be better grillers. I think what separates the master grillers from the beginners is really an understanding of the fundamentals. What follows here are the questions I hear again and again during my grilling classes around the country. The answers make the biggest difference in anyone's ability to grill.

STARTING A CHARCOAL FIRE

Q: WHAT'S THE DIFFERENCE BETWEEN COOKING OVER A WOOD FIRE VERSUS A CHARCOAL FIRE? IS ONE BETTER THAN THE OTHER?

A: It's all about ease and time management. Barbecuing began over a wood fire, which imparts a wonderful flavor, but it has its drawbacks. A wood-log fire tends to create huge amounts of smoke and often requires waiting up to an hour or more for the flames to settle down and the embers to reach a manageable level of heat. Charcoal is essentially pre-burned wood, which means it reaches ideal grilling temperatures faster than wood and with much less smoke. It is made by slowly burning hardwood logs in an oxygen-deprived environment, like an underground pit or kiln. Over time, the water and resins are burned out of the logs, leaving behind big chunks of combustible carbon. These chunks are then broken into smaller lumps, hence the name lump charcoal. It's also known as "charwood."

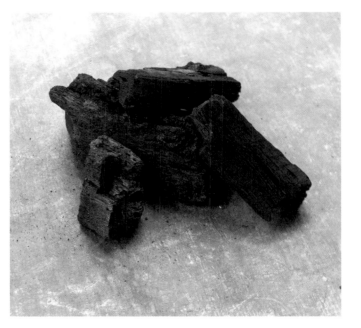

Q: WHAT ABOUT BRIQUETTES? HOW ARE THEY DIFFERENT FROM LUMP CHARCOAL?

A: In North America, briquettes are more popular than lump charcoal. They are inexpensive and available practically everywhere. Most commonly, they are compressed black bundles of sawdust and coal, along with binders and fillers like clay and sodium nitrate. Some are presoaked in lighter fluid so they start easier, but they can impart a chemical taste to food if you don't completely burn off the lighter fluid before you begin cooking.

Standard briquettes don't burn as hot as lump charcoal and the amount of smoke produced is minimal at best. But they do produce predictable, even heat over a long period of time. A batch of 80 to 100 briquettes will last for about an hour, which is plenty of time to grill most foods without having to replenish the fire, whereas a pure lump-charcoal fire may provide only half as much grilling time before it requires more coals.

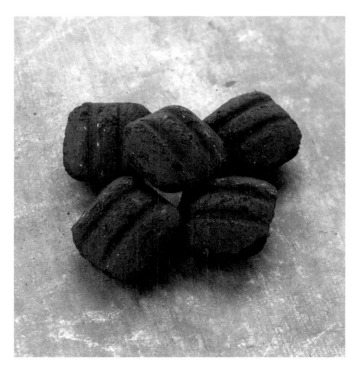

Q: ARE THERE ANY OTHER CHOICES?

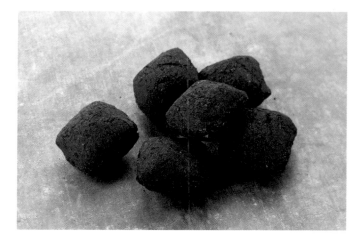

A: Pure hardwood (or "all-natural") briquettes are a great option, if you can find them. They have the same pillow shape of standard briquettes, but they burn at higher temperatures, and with none of the questionable fillers and binders. Usually, they are made of crushed hardwoods bound together with nothing but natural starches. You'll probably pay more for these coals, but many serious grillers and barbecue competitors consider them the gold standard of charcoal.

Q: IF SOMEONE IS ENTIRELY NEW TO CHARCOAL GRILLING (AND MAYBE A LITTLE INTIMIDATED), WHAT'S THE BEST WAY TO GET STARTED?

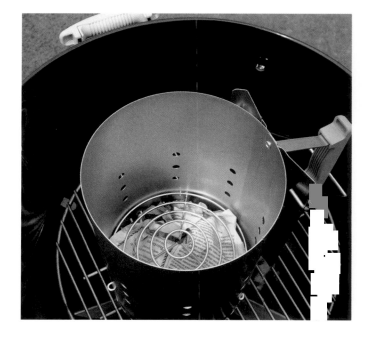

A: My advice is to start by learning to light the charcoal safely and reliably using a chimney starter. This simple device consists of a metal cylinder with holes cut out along the bottom, a wire rack inside, and two handles attached to the outside. Here's how to use the chimney. First, remove the top grate—or cooking grate—from your grill and place the chimney starter on the charcoal grate below. Next, place a couple sheets of wadded-up newspaper under the wire rack, fill the upper chamber of the cylinder with charcoal, and light the newspaper through the holes on the side. (As an alternative, use paraffin cubes in place of the newspaper.) The beauty of this method is that the chimney sucks the hot air up from the bottom and makes it circulate through the coals, lighting them much faster and more evenly than if you spread the coals out.

Lump charcoal will burn strong and be ready for grilling in about 15 minutes. Charcoal briquettes will take a little longer to light fully, generally 20 to 30 minutes.

When the charcoal is lightly coated all over with white ash (or lump charcoal is lit around the edges of all the pieces), it is ready to go. To empty it onto the charcoal grate, put on two insulated barbecue mitts. Grab hold of the heat-proof handle in one hand and the swinging handle in the other. The swinging handle is there to help you lift the chimney and safely aim the contents just where you want them. For safety's sake, always wear insulated barbecue mitts when doing this. And never place a hot, empty chimney starter on the grass or deck. Be sure to put it on a heat-proof surface away from children and pets.

If you don't have a chimney starter, build a pyramid of coals on top of a few paraffin cubes, then light the cubes. When the coals in the middle are lit, use tongs to pile the unlit coals on top. When all the coals are glowing bright orange and covered with ash, arrange them the way you want them on the charcoal grate.

Q: ARE YOU SAYING I SHOULDN'T USE LIGHTER FLUID?

A: That's right. Lighter fluid is a petroleum-based product that can really ruin the flavor of your food. I know there are some people who grew up with the stuff and still think a hamburger is supposed to taste like gasoline, but for the rest of us, we would never think of using it.

Q: HOW DO I KNOW HOW MUCH CHARCOAL TO USE?

A: That depends on the size of your grill and how much food you want to cook. Let's assume you have a classic 22½-inch-diameter kettle grill and you are cooking for four to six people. The simplest way to measure the right amount of coals is to use your chimney starter. (See, aren't you glad you got one?) Use it like a measuring cup for charcoal. Filled to the rim (with 80 to 100 standard briquettes), a chimney starter will provide enough charcoal to spread in a single, tightly packed layer across about two-thirds of the charcoal grate. That's usually enough charcoal to grill a couple of courses for four to six people. If you plan on grilling longer than 45 minutes, you will probably need to add more charcoal.

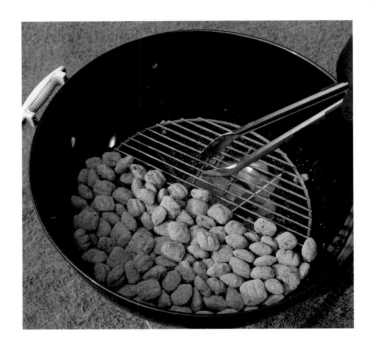

Because lump charcoal comes in irregular shapes and sizes, it is harder to pack tightly in a chimney starter. So do yourself a favor; after you have spread the burning lump charcoal across the charcoal grate, fill in any gaps by adding a few more fist-sized lumps to the fire. The bed of coals should extend at least four inches beyond every piece of food on the cooking grate above, to ensure that every piece of food cooks evenly.

Q: WHY WOULDN'T I FILL THE WHOLE CHARCOAL GRATE WITH BURNING COALS?

A: If you covered the entire grate with coals, then you would have only direct heat available to you. Everything on the cooking grate would be right on top of burning coals. That's fine for some foods like burgers and hot dogs, but a lot of other foods do best grilled over both direct and indirect heat. Bone-in chicken pieces are a prime example. Have you ever seen what happens to them when they cook only over direct heat? They burn. The outside turns black before the meat along the bone has a chance to cook properly. The correct way to grill foods like this is to brown them for a while over direct heat and then move them over indirect heat to finish cooking.

Also, if the food being grilled over direct heat causes flare-ups, you have a convenient place to put the food while you figure out what to do next. At the very least, you can just close the lid and let the food finish cooking over indirect heat.

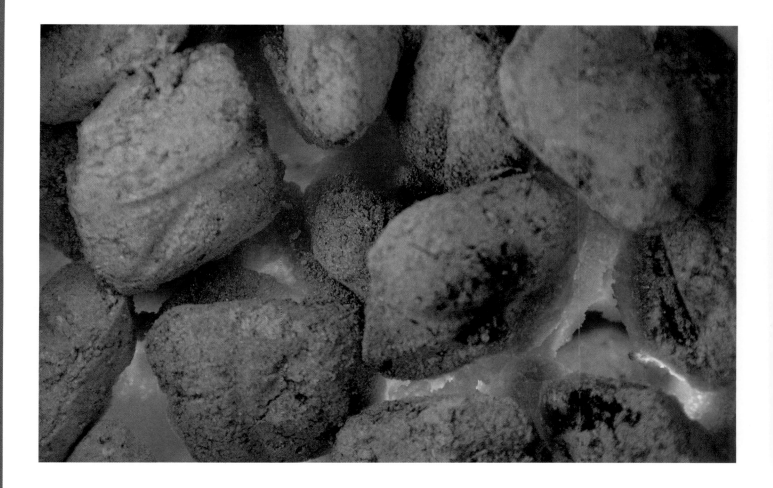

ARRANGING THE COALS

Q: WHAT EXACTLY IS THE DIFFERENCE BETWEEN DIRECT AND INDIRECT HEAT?

A: With direct heat, the fire is right below the food. With indirect heat, the fire is off to one side of the grill, or on both sides of the grill, and the food sits over the unlit part.

Direct heat works great for small, tender pieces of food that cook quickly, such as hamburgers, steaks, chops, boneless chicken pieces, fish fillets, shellfish, and sliced vegetables. It sears the surfaces of these foods, developing flavors, texture, and delicious caramelization while it also cooks the food all the way to the center.

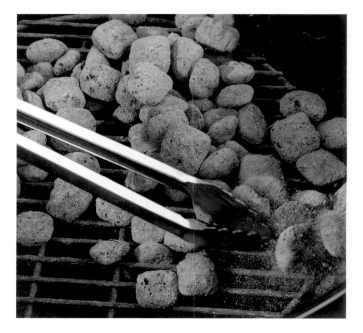

Indirect heat works better for larger, tougher foods that require longer cooking times, such as roasts, whole chickens, and ribs. As I mentioned, it is also just the right method for finishing thicker foods or bone-in cuts that have been seared or browned first over direct heat.

GRILLING BASICS

Q: DOES THE DIRECT METHOD COOK MY FOOD DIFFERENTLY FROM THE INDIRECT METHOD?

A: Yes. A direct fire creates both radiant heat and conductive heat. Radiant heat from the coals quickly cooks the surface of the food closest to it. At the same time, the fire heats the cooking grate rods, which conducts heat directly to the surface of the food and creates those unmistakable and lovely grill marks.

If the food is off to the side of the fire, or over indirect heat, the radiant heat and the conductive heat are still factors, but they are not as intense. However, if the lid of the grill is closed, as it should be, there is another kind of heat generated: convective heat. It radiates off the coals, bounces off the lid, and goes round and round the food. Convection heat doesn't sear the surface of the food the way radiant and conductive heat do. It cooks it more gently all the way to the center, like the heat in an oven, which lets you cook roasts, whole birds, and other large foods to the center without burning them.

Q: ARE THERE ANY OTHER GOOD WAYS TO ARRANGE THE COALS?

A: The basic configuration I've described, with the coals to one side of the grill, is called a two-zone fire because you have one zone of direct heat and one zone of indirect heat. The temperature of a two-zone fire can be high, medium, or low, depending on how much charcoal is burning and how long it has been burning. Remember, charcoal loses heat over time.

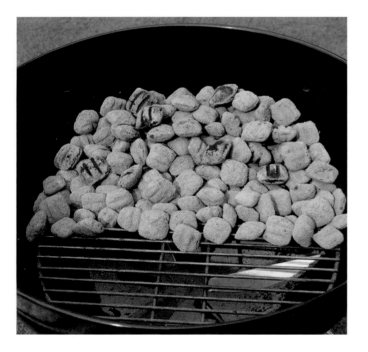 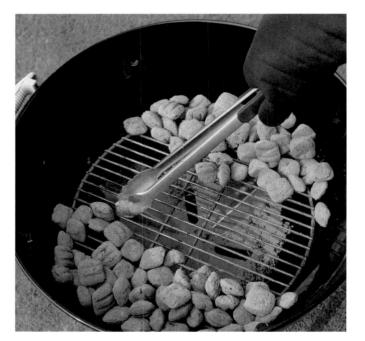

You also can create a three-zone fire, which provides even more flexibility. On one side of the grill, pile coals two or three briquettes deep. Then, slope the coals down to a single layer across the center of the grill, and place no coals on the opposite side. When the coals are completely ashen and have burned down for 10 to 20 minutes more, after being emptied from the chimney—voila!—you have direct high heat on one side, direct medium heat in the center, and indirect heat on the opposite side.

There are also times when you might prefer a three-zone "split" fire, where the coals are separated into two equal piles on opposite sides of the charcoal grate. This gives you two zones for direct heat (high, medium, or low) and one zone between them for indirect heat. This works nicely for cooking a roast over indirect heat, such as pork loin or beef tenderloin, because you have the same level of heat on either side of the roast.

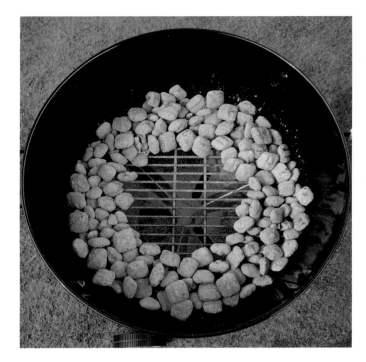
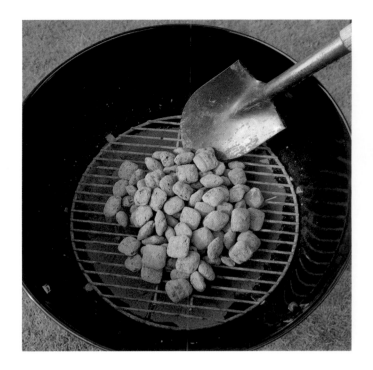

Q: WHAT'S THE RING OF FIRE?

A: It's another way of arranging charcoal for both direct and indirect heat. The ring of coals around the perimeter provides direct heat while the empty center of the ring provides an area of indirect heat.

Q: WHAT'S THE BULL'S-EYE?

A: The bull's-eye is the flip side of the ring of fire. With the coals piled in the center of the charcoal grate, you have a small area of direct heat, but a lot of area around the perimeter for indirect heat. This is a convenient arrangement for slow cooking or warming several small pieces of food, such as bone-in chicken pieces.

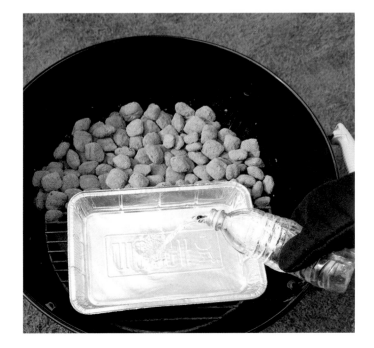

Q: WHAT'S THE PURPOSE OF A DRIP PAN ON A CHARCOAL GRATE?

A: The pan catches drippings, so it extends the life of your grill by keeping it clean. If you fill the pan with water, the water will absorb and release heat slowly, adding a bit of moisture to the cooking process.

JUDGING THE HEAT LEVEL

Q: HOW DO I KNOW I HAVE THE RIGHT LEVEL OF HEAT?

A: As soon as briquettes are lightly covered with gray ash (or lump charcoal is lit around the edges of all the pieces), and you've poured the coals onto the charcoal grate, you have very high heat, actually too high for almost any food to handle without burning quickly.

Spread the coals out the way you like, set the cooking grate in place, and close the lid. It's important now to preheat the grill. You should do this for 10 to 15 minutes, to make the cooking grate hot enough for searing and to make it easier to clean. The heat will loosen all the little bits and pieces clinging to the cooking grate, left over from the last time you grilled, and a grill brush will easily remove them.

There are two reliable ways to judge how hot a charcoal fire is. One is to use the thermometer in the lid of your grill, if there is one. With the lid closed, the temperature should climb past 500°F initially. Then, once it has reached its peak, the temperature will begin to fall. You can begin grilling whenever the temperature has fallen into the desired range.

HEAT	TEMPERATURE RANGE	WHEN YOU WILL NEED TO PULL YOUR HAND AWAY
High	450° to 550°F	2 to 4 seconds
Medium	350° to 450°F	5 to 7 seconds
Low	250° to 350°F	8 to 10 seconds

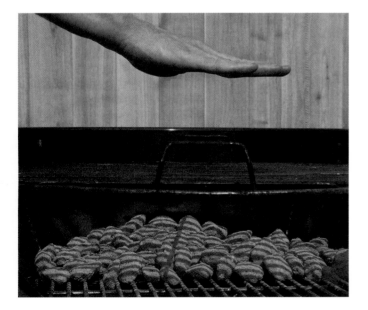

The second way is less technical but surprisingly reliable. It involves extending the palm of your hand over the grill at a safe distance above the charcoal grate. Imagine a soda can standing on the cooking grate, right over the coals. If your palm were resting on top of the can, it would be about five inches from the cooking grate. That's where you should measure the heat of charcoal.

If you need to pull your hand away after 2 to 4 seconds, the heat is high. If you need to pull your hand away after 5 to 7 seconds, the heat is medium. If you need to pull it away after 8 to 10 seconds, the heat is low. Use common sense and always pull your hand away from the heat before it hurts—you don't want to get burned.

Q: WHAT SHOULD I DO TO MAINTAIN THE HEAT FOR A LONG PERIOD OF TIME?

A: Under normal circumstances, a typical charcoal briquette fire will lose about 100 degrees of heat over 40 to 60 minutes. A typical lump charcoal fire will lose heat even faster. To maintain the grill's temperature, you'll need to add new coals during cooking. If you are using standard briquettes, remember that they take 20 minutes or more to reach their highest heat, so plan accordingly. You'll have to add them 20 to 30 minutes before you need them. Alternatively, you can light the briquettes ahead of time in a chimney starter, keep them burning in a safe place, and add them when you need instant results. For me, adding lit coals is a much better way to grill because I find the taste of food suffers when it absorbs the aromas of partially lit (standard) briquettes.

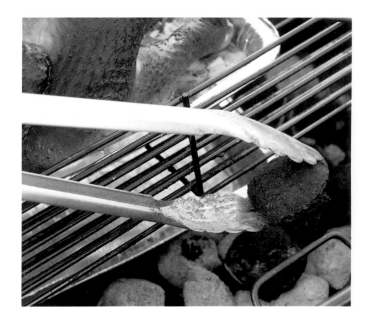

Lump charcoal and all-natural briquettes light faster than most standard briquettes so they require less lead time. Add them just 5 to 10 minutes before you need to raise the heat. Smaller pieces of lump charcoal will burn out quickly, so you will need to add them more often. Larger lumps will take a little more time to get hot, but they will last longer. Fortunately, lump charcoal and all-natural briquettes don't produce any unwanted aromas in the early stages of their burning.

For a fairly even fire, add about 10 to 15 briquettes, or an equivalent amount of lump charcoal, every 45 minutes to an hour.

Q: HOW SHOULD I WORK THE AIR VENTS ON MY GRILL?

A: The vents on the top and bottom of the grill control the airflow inside the grill. The more air flowing into the grill, the hotter the fire will grow and the more frequently you will have to replenish it. To slow the rate of your fire's burn, close the top vent as much as halfway and keep the lid on as much as possible. The bottom vent should be left open whenever you are grilling so you don't kill your fire.

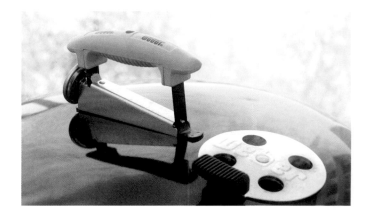

All kinds of charcoal, especially briquettes made with fillers, will leave behind some ash after all the combustible carbon has burned. If you allow the ashes to accumulate on the bottom of the grill, they will cover the vent and starve the coals of air, eventually extinguishing them. So, every hour or so, give the vent a gentle sweep, to clear them of ashes, by opening and closing the bottom vent several times in a row.

STARTING A GAS GRILL

Q: WHAT'S THE PROCESS FOR LIGHTING A GAS GRILL?

A: There's nothing complicated about lighting a gas grill. However, gas grill operation does vary, so be sure to consult the owner's manual that came with your grill. To light a Weber® gas grill, first open the lid so unlit gas fumes don't collect in the cooking box. Next, slowly open the valve on your propane tank (or natural gas line) all the way and wait a minute for the gas to travel through the gas line. Then turn on the burners, setting them all to high. Close the lid and preheat the grill for 10 to 15 minutes.

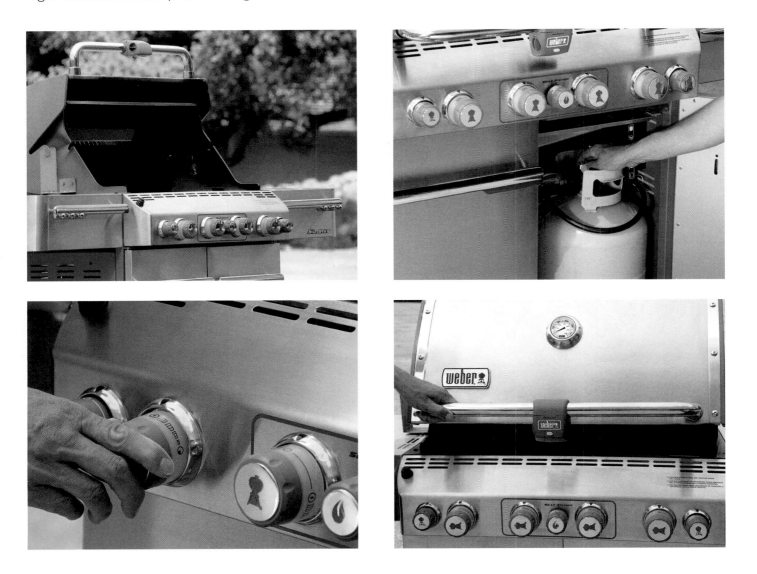

Q: WHAT IF I SMELL GAS?

A: That might indicate a leak around the connection or in the hose. Turn off all the burners. Close the valve on your propane tank (or natural gas line) and disconnect the hose. Wait a few minutes and then reconnect the hose. Try lighting the grill again. If you still smell gas, shut the grill down and call the manufacturer.

DIRECT AND INDIRECT HEAT ON A GAS GRILL

Q: HOW DO I SET UP MY GAS GRILL TO COOK WITH DIRECT HEAT?

A: On a gas grill, simply leave all the burners on and adjust them for the heat level you want. For example, if you want direct medium heat, turn all the burners down to medium, close the lid, and wait until the thermometer indicates that the temperature is in the range of 350° to 450°F. Then set your food on the cooking grate right over the burners. If your gas grill does not have a thermometer, use the "hand test" described on page 15.

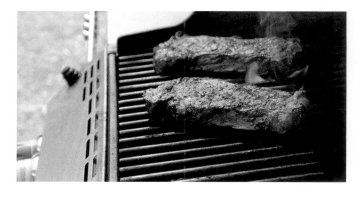

Q: WHAT'S THE SETUP FOR INDIRECT HEAT?

A: On a gas grill, you can switch from direct to indirect heat almost immediately. Just turn off one or more of the burners and place the food over an unlit burner. If your grill has just two burners, turn off the one toward the back of the grill. If your grill has more than two burners, turn off the one(s) in the middle of the grill. The burners that are left on can be set to high, medium, or low heat, as desired. Whenever the food is over an unlit burner and the lid is closed, you're grilling over indirect heat.

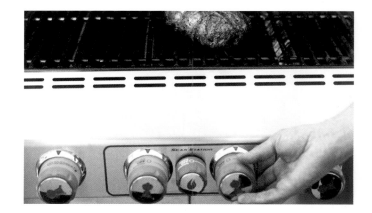

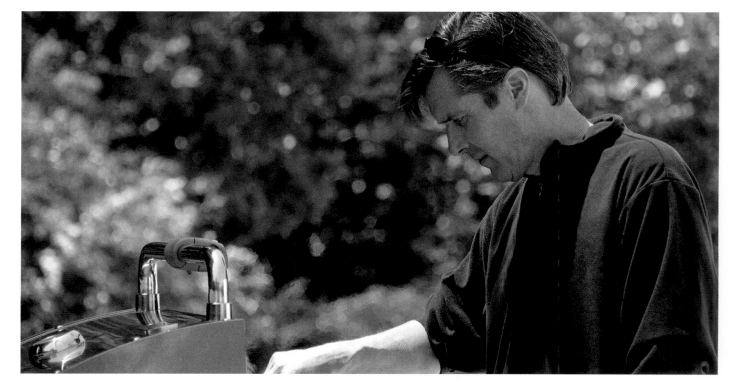

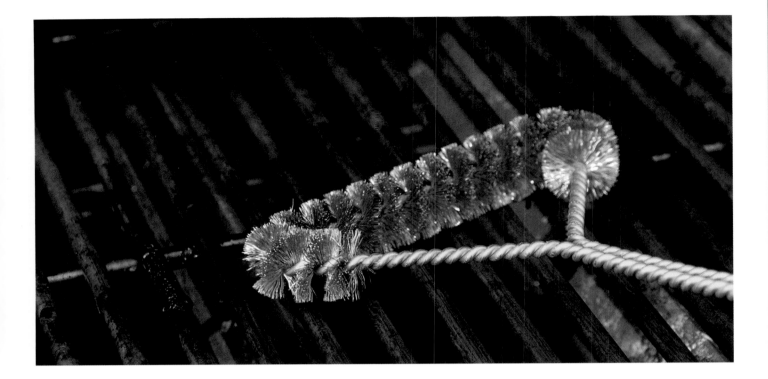

GRILLING KNOW-HOW

Q: DO I NEED TO CLEAN THE COOKING GRATES EVERY TIME I USE THE GRILL?

A: You really should clean the grates every time, not only to be tidy, but also because any residue left on the cooking grates may cause your food to stick. You will find that food releases from the grates much more easily, and with more impressive grill marks, if the cooking grates are clean.

The easiest way to clean your cooking grates is to preheat the grill, with the lid down, to about 500°F. Then, while wearing an insulated barbecue mitt, use a long-handled grill brush to scrape off any bits and pieces that may be stuck to the cooking grates.

Q: WHAT ABOUT CLEANING THE REST OF THE GRILL?

A: Once a month or so, you should do a more thorough cleaning of your grill. Be sure to read the instructions in your owner's manual beforehand. Wipe down the grill with a sponge and warm, soapy water. Scrape off any debris that has accumulated under the lid. Remove the cooking grates, brush the burners, and clean out the bottom of the cooking box and the drip pan. For full care and upkeep instructions, consult your owner's manual. With charcoal grills, remember that ash naturally has a small amount of water in it. Don't leave it sitting in your grill for a long period of time; it can rust some parts of your grill.

Q: DO I NEED TO OIL THE COOKING GRATES BEFORE I GRILL?

A: I do not recommend it. Many grillers do, and that's fine, but keep in mind that oil will drip though the cooking grates and may cause flare-ups on both charcoal and gas grills. You can avoid wasting oil and improve your chances of a food releasing more easily by oiling the food, not the grates.

Q: WHAT SHOULD I DO IF FLARE-UPS HAPPEN?

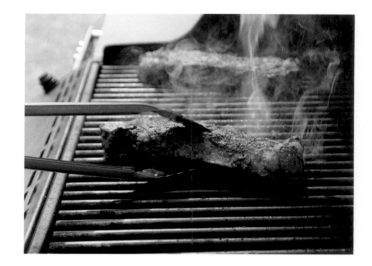

A: A certain number of flare-ups are to be expected. When oil and fat drip into a hot grill, especially a charcoal grill, they tend to produce flames. If the flames are barely reaching the surface of the food and then they subside, don't worry about it. If, however, the flames are rising through the cooking grates and surrounding your food, you need to act quickly. Otherwise, the foods will pick up a sooty taste and color, and could burn.

On a charcoal grill, most flare-ups begin within a few seconds of putting food on the grill, or right after you turn food over. Your first reaction should be to put the lid on the grill and close the top vent about halfway. By decreasing the amount of air getting to the fire, you may extinguish a flare-up. You can check the status of the flare-up by carefully looking through the partially open vent. If the flames are still threatening, open the lid and move the food over indirect heat. That's one very important reason why you should always have an indirect heat zone available. After a few seconds, the oil and fat will usually burn off and the flare-up will subside. When the flare-up dies down, resume cooking your food over direct heat.

You are less likely to have flare-ups with a gas grill because many of them have a system that prevents fat and oil from falling directly onto the burners. For example, most Weber® gas grills have angled steel bars on top of the burners. Not only do they prevent almost all flare-ups, they also transform dripping juices and fat into wonderfully aromatic smoke. The solutions to flare-ups on a gas grill are the same as they are on a charcoal grill. First, make sure the lid is closed. Then, if necessary, move the food over indirect heat.

Q: WHEN SHOULD I GRILL WITH THE LID ON?

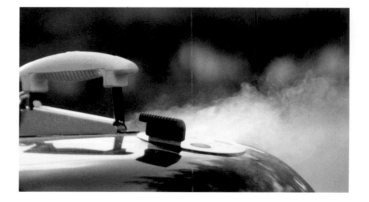

A: As often as possible. Whether using a charcoal grill or a gas grill, the lid is really important. It limits the amount of air getting to the fire, thus preventing flare-ups, and it helps to cook food on the top and bottom simultaneously. While the bottom of the food is almost always exposed to more intense heat, the lid reflects some heat down and speeds up the overall cooking time. Without the lid, the fire would lose heat more quickly and many foods would take much longer to cook, possibly drying out. Plus, using the lid keeps the cooking grate at a higher temperature, giving you more conductive heat, which creates better searing and caramelization. Finally, the lid traps all those good smoky aromas inside the grill and surrounds your food with them. Otherwise, the smoke will drift away and serve no real purpose. One exception to this rule occurs when you are grilling very thin pieces of food, like bread slices and tortillas. They cook (and potentially burn) so quickly that it's wise to leave the lid off and watch them carefully.

Q: IS IT WORTH IT TO GET A ROTISSERIE ATTACHMENT FOR MY GRILL?

A: If you want to cook large hunks of meat—like pork loins, whole chickens, turkey, duck, and prime rib—a rotisserie attachment is a good investment. Any of those meats can be grilled right on the cooking grate over indirect heat, but the advantage of a rotisserie is that the food slowly self-bastes as it rotates and absorbs the flavors of the fire.

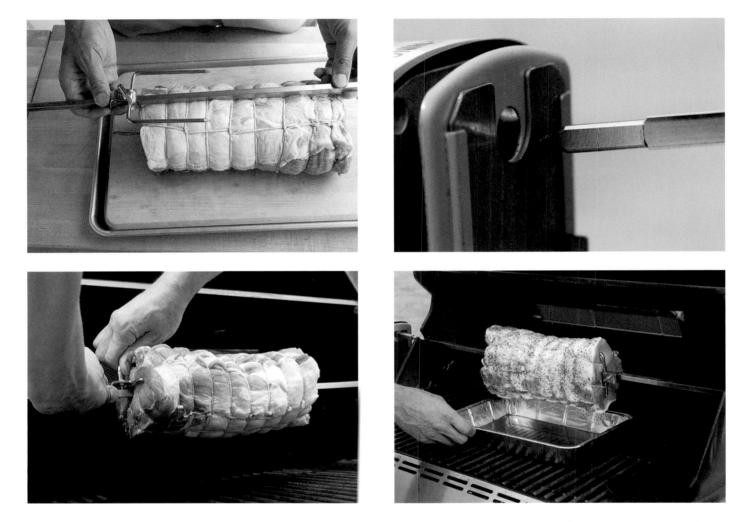

To ensure that the meat stays in place as it turns and cooks uniformly, use butcher's twine to truss your food into a compact shape. Then secure the food on the spit, making sure it is centered as evenly as possible. This will put less strain on the motor. Always preheat the grill first. When ready to cook, set the spit in place, put a disposable foil pan underneath the roast to catch the grease, turn on the motor, and close the lid.

Q: SO WHAT SHOULD I BUY: A CHARCOAL OR GAS GRILL?

A: That decision depends a lot on what kind of griller you are. There are some grillers who put a high priority on enjoying the food as quickly, cleanly, and conveniently as possible. For them, a gas grill makes the most sense. The fire is ready in 10 to 15 minutes. The temperature stays right where you need it for as long as you need it, and cleanup is minimal. Then there are some grillers who relish the opportunity to build their own fires and tend the coals. Glowing embers and wood smoke thrill them so much that charcoal grilling is well worth the extra time and cleanup required. They believe with every last taste bud that the flavor of food cooked over a live fire is better. So, you tell me: which type of griller are you?

SMOKING AND BARBECUING

Q: SUPPOSE I WANT TO TRY SMOKING FOODS. HOW DO I DO THAT?

A: Congratulations, you get a gold star. Every griller ought to try smoking with hardwoods. Done right, it lends food an irresistible flavor.

Smoking on a kettle grill is really easy to do, especially if you are already comfortable grilling with indirect heat. Begin by filling a chimney starter about one-third full with briquettes. When they are fully lit, pour all of the charcoal on one side of the cooking grate (if desired, use a charcoal basket, which holds the coals close together so they burn more slowly) and place an aluminum foil pan on the other side. Then, carefully add about 2 or 3 cups of water to the pan. The water in the pan is important because it helps to maintain a low cooking temperature. It also adds some moisture to the food, which in many cases will cook for hours and hours, so it could dry out otherwise. Allow 30 minutes to 1 hour for the coals to burn down to the correct temperature and

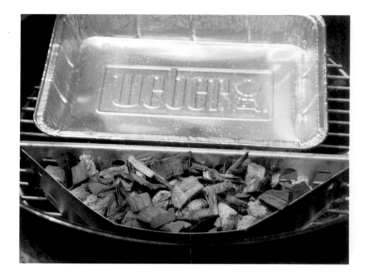

the water to heat up. Next, drop damp wood chips or dry wood chunks directly onto the coals. Then place your food on top of the cooking grate over the water pan and cover your grill. Expect to add more coals every hour or so to maintain the heat.

Wood chips, even when they have been soaked in liquid, will smoke sooner than wood chunks, but they often burn out in a matter of minutes. Wood chunks tend to burn for an hour or more. I suggest using chunks and positioning them on the outer edge of a charcoal fire to prolong and extend smoking times even further.

You've got a lot of options in the hardwoods category, including the most popular ones: oak, hickory, and mesquite. Of those, mesquite has the strongest aroma, so be careful about using too much of it for too long. In fact, be careful about using too much of any kind of wood. A common rookie mistake is to keep adding wood throughout hours and hours of cooking. The aromas of the smoke can eventually overpower the food, so start with just a few handfuls, then stop. Next time, if you want a little more smokiness, add an additional handful or two.

In my opinion, oak and hickory complement beef, lamb, and pork really well. Milder woods pair nicely with milder foods, for example, apple wood, pecan, and alder with chicken and fish. Don't worry about using the "wrong" wood for any kind of food. It's almost impossible to make a mistake here. Some people latch on to a favorite kind of wood and use it to smoke almost anything. That's fine. The differences between the hardwoods are pretty subtle.

But please don't add soft, resinous woods like pine, cedar, and aspen to your fire. They create an acrid (and sometimes toxic) smoke. And never use any wood that has been treated with chemicals.

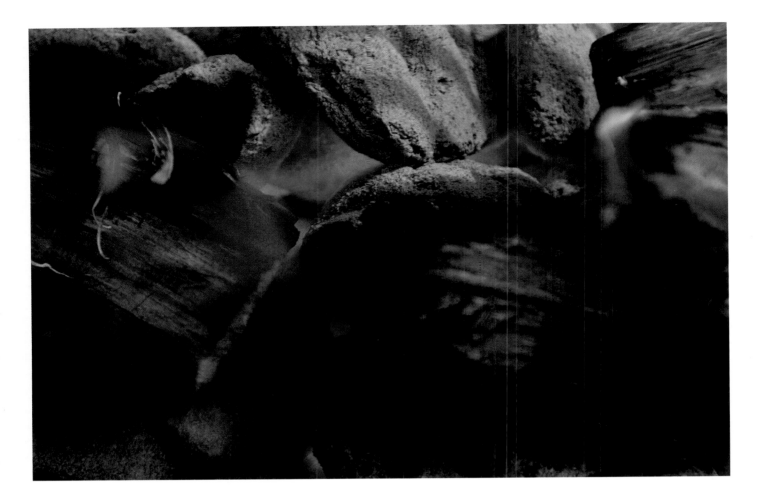

Q: IF SMOKING IS USUALLY DONE WITH LOW TEMPERATURES, HOW DO I GET MY KETTLE GRILL TO DO THAT?

A: Many foods are smoked and simultaneously cooked in the temperature range of 250° to 350°F. You can maintain the correct level of heat by controlling the amount of charcoal and the airflow. This is why you begin the fire with a chimney filled only about one-third full with charcoal (about 30 briquettes). Adding 10 to 15 briquettes (or an equivalent amount of lump charcoal) every hour or so will help to maintain the temperature. So will opening and closing the vents on the lid. Opening the vents will help the fire burn faster and hotter. Closing them partially (not all the way, or you might put out the fire) will restrict the airflow and drop the temperature. Having a thermometer on the lid is very helpful here.

Q: CAN I SMOKE FOOD WITH A GAS GRILL?

A: Yes, some of today's gas grills come equipped with a metal smoker box that sits on top of a dedicated burner. Just turn on the burner and add as many wood chips as you like. You can control how quickly they smoke by turning the knob of the burner higher or lower. Some of the boxes have a separate compartment for water, which will provide a steaming effect on the food, too.

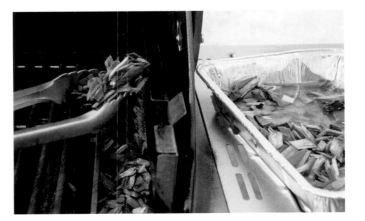

Q: HOW DO I USE A WATER SMOKER?

A: A water smoker allows you to smcke meat at temperatures well below 300°F for many hours. The Weber version is basically an upright bullet-shaped unit with three sections. The charcoal burns in the bottom section. For smoky barbecue aromas, add a few fist-sized chunks of hardwood to the coals right from the beginning. The meat will absorb the smoke best wher it is uncooked.

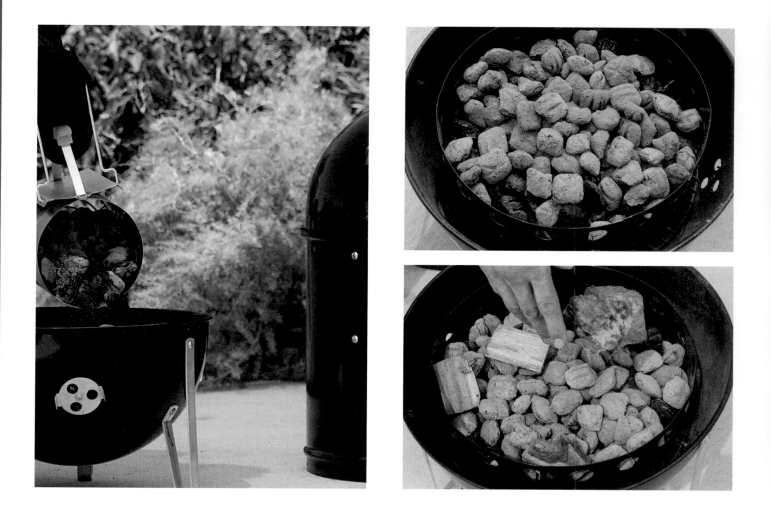

The water sits in a pan in the middle section, preventing any fat from dripping onto the coals and, more importantly, keeping the temperature nice and low. The meat sits on one or two racks in the top section.

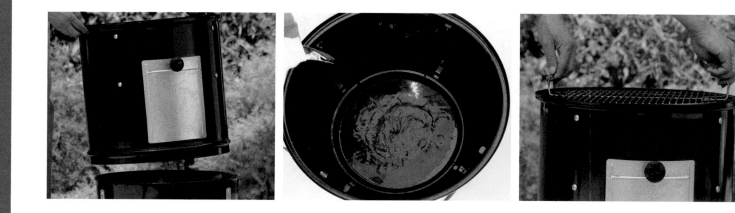

A water smoker has vents on both the bottom and top sections. Generally, it's a good idea to leave the top vent wide open so that smoke can escape. Use the bottom vents as your primary way of regulating the temperature. The less air you allow into the smoker, the lower the temperature will go.

Generally speaking, if the ring in the bottom section of the smoker is filled with lit charcoal, and the water pan is nearly filled, the temperature will stay in the range of 225° to 250°F for 4 to 6 hours. This is an ideal range for barbecuing food like pork ribs, turkeys, and standing rib roasts.

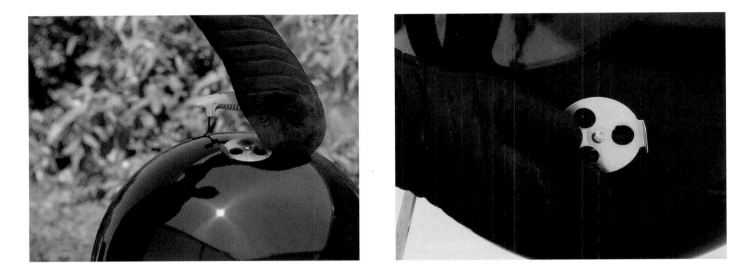

When you see that very little smoke is coming out of the top vent, add another chunk or two through the door on the side. Wood chunks burn slowly and evenly, so they are a better choice than wood chips in this situation. For cooking sessions longer than 6 hours, you will probably need to add more charcoal occasionally. The timing will depend on your type of charcoal and how fast it burns. If you are using charcoal made with unnatural fillers, you may want to light the briquettes in a chimney starter first; some people can taste off flavors in food cooked over unlit briquettes.

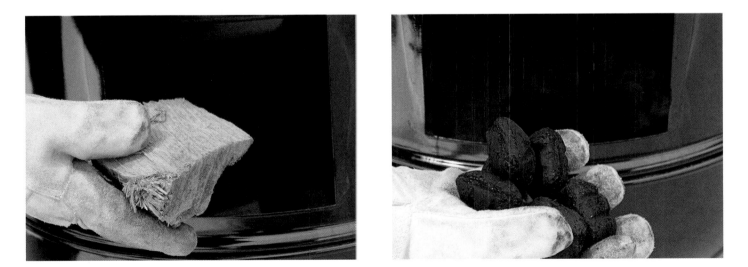

During long cooking times, also be sure to replenish the water pan every few hours with warm water. But keep the lid on the smoker as much as possible. That's critical for maintaining even heat.

MUST-HAVE GRILLING TOOLS

Once you have a good grill that allows you to control the fire easily and cook your food over both direct and indirect heat, it's time to equip yourself with the right tools. I've broken down my recommendations into two groups. The first ten tools are essential for most grilling tasks. The other ten will make many jobs a lot easier.

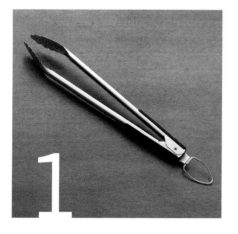

TONGS

Oh, the tongs. Definitely the hardest working tool of all. You will need one pair to load raw food on the grill and move it around. You will need another pair (clean tongs that haven't touched any raw meat, fish, or poultry) to remove the grilled food. Dedicate a third pair for rearranging charcoal.

GRILL BRUSH

Spring for a solid, long-handled model with stainless steel bristles. Use it to clean off the grates before and after grilling, and you will eliminate many problems with food sticking to the grates. And your food won't taste like last night's dinner. Replace the brush when the bristles wear down to about one-half their original length.

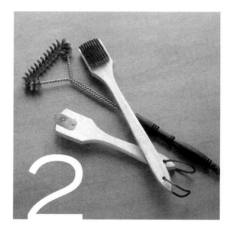

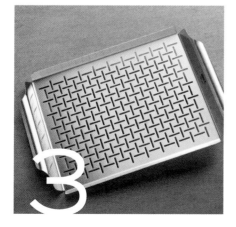

GRILL PAN

At first I didn't see the wisdom of a grill pan, but I came around on the issue when I saw (and tasted) how well a perforated grill pan can handle delicate fish fillets and small foods like chopped vegetables that might otherwise fall through the cooking grate. If you preheat a stainless steel grill pan properly, it will brown the food nicely and allow the smokiness from the grill to flavor the food.

CHIMNEY STARTER

Brilliantly simple, a chimney starter lets you start the coals faster and more evenly than you could with lighter fluid. And who needs all those chemicals in lighter fluid? Look for a chimney starter with a capacity of at least 5 quarts of briquettes roughly 80 to 100 pieces. Also, it should have two handles: a heat-proof side handle for lifting the chimney and a hinged top handle to provide support when dumping hot coals onto the charcoal grate.

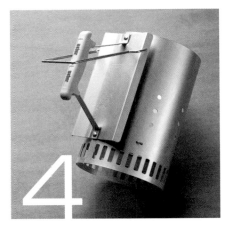

4

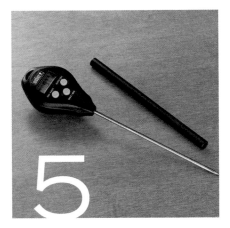

5

INSTANT-READ THERMOMETER

You only have to overcook a fine cut of meat once to learn the importance of a good digital thermometer. Small and relatively inexpensive an instant-read thermometer is essential for quickly gauging the internal temperature of the meat when grilling. To get the most accurate read, insert it into the thickest part of the cut and avoid touching any bone, because the bone conducts heat.

SHEET PAN

I learned the value of a sturdy sheet pan when I was in culinary school, where there were dozens within reach in every kitchen. A half sheet pan, like the one pictured here, is a great portable work surface for oiling and seasoning food, and there's nothing better to use as a landing pad for food coming off the grill

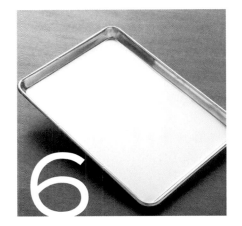

6

7

BASTING BRUSH

In the past, basting brushes were made of wooden/plastic handles and synthetic/natural-boar bristles. Today you can find them made of stainless steel with silicone bristles that have beads at the tips to help load the brush with a sauce or marinade. While most old-style brushes had to be hand washed, this new high-tech style can go right into the dishwasher. Nice.

BARBECUE MITTS

You'll need these to shield your hand and forearm when managing a charcoal fire or reaching toward the back of any hot grill. You will probably put them through the wash a lot, so invest in mitts of good-quality materials and workmanship. Silicone grilling mitts are easy to care for because you can just wipe them off when they get dirty, but insulated cloth mitts will give better dexterity.

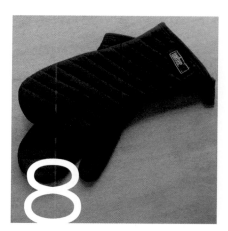

GRILLING SPATULA

Look for a long-handled spatula designed with a bent (offset) neck so that the blade is set lower than the handle. This will make it easier to lift food off of the grill without hitting your knuckles. The blade itself should be at least 4 inches wide; you'll need a longer blade for turning whole fish.

SKEWERS

Bamboo skewers are simple and inexpensive, though they need to be soaked in water for at least 30 minutes prior to loading, in order to keep the wood from burning. If you don't want the hassle, use metal skewers, or freeze bamboo skewers in a bag after soaking them. The flat metal skewers and double-pronged ones are nice because they prevent the food from spinning when you turn the skewers.

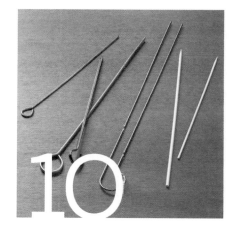

NICE TO HAVE GRILLING TOOLS

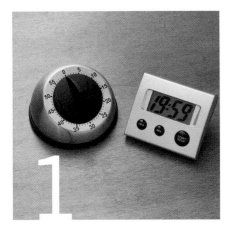

TIMER

As the old saying goes, timing is everything. It's never truer than when you are trying to pull off a perfect meal at the grill. A rotary kitchen timer is adequate, but you can also ante up for a more elaborate digital timer, preferably one that lets you track a couple of grilling times simultaneously.

WIRELESS MEAT THERMOMETER

While an instant-read thermometer is a must-have, a wireless thermometer is a cool little luxury. It's a high-tech gadget that monitors the temperature of meat using a wireless probe. You can walk away from the grill and a remote beeper will tell you when your food is ready.

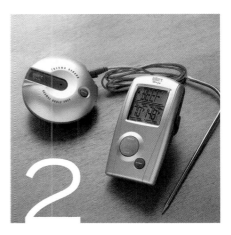

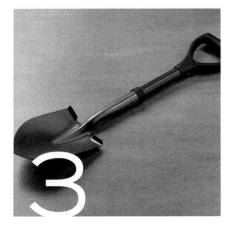

SMALL SHOVEL

Seeing this tool on the list might surprise you, but a small shovel is really helpful for pushing charcoal around. You can buy a shovel specifically for the task at a barbecue retailer, or buy a small shovel (one with no plastic parts) from a hardware store or garden shop.

ROTISSERIE

It's true that you can roast a chicken, turkey, or pork loin on the grill without a rotisserie, but there is something wonderfully medieval about food spinning over a fire. Many people also argue that the rotisserie causes the meat to self-baste while cooking. I agree that food comes out juicier, so I am pro-rotisserie.

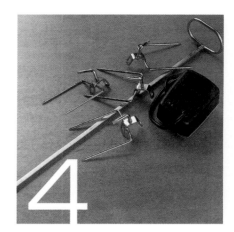

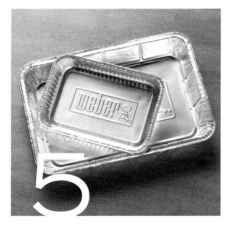

DISPOSABLE PANS

Available in large and small sizes, disposable foil pans offer many conveniences. Use them to move food to and from the grill, keep food warm on the cooking grate, soak wood chunks in them, or set them under the cooking grate to catch drippings and keep a charcoal grill clean.

CAST-IRON SKILLET

A big cast-iron skillet allows you to make favorites in this book, like paella, gingerbread, and a stunning pineapple upside-down cake. Once it gets hot on the grill, you can sauté, stew, or pan-roast just about anything in it without every worrying that the skillet will discolor or deteriorate. It will last you forever.

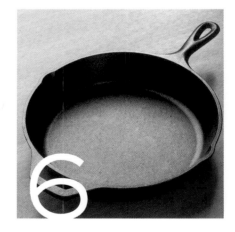

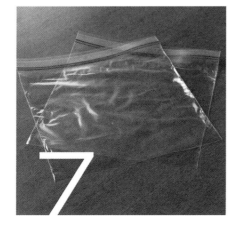

RESEALABLE PLASTIC BAGS

Marinating foods in plastic bags allows you to force some of the marinade up and over the food, particularly when you set a bag snugly in a bowl, giving you better coverage and faster marinating times. Resealable bags also avoid dreaded spills in your refrigerator.

RIB RACK

This wire rack holds multiple slabs of ribs upright so that heat circulates around the ribs, cooking them evenly, and it encourages the pork fat to drip down and away from the ribs. Plus, it frees up real estate on the cooking grates for grilling other food at the same time.

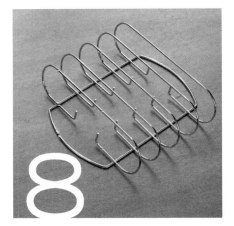

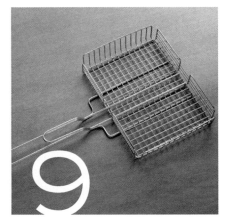

FISH BASKET

Many people resist grilling fish, especially whole fish, for fear that it will stick and fall apart on the cooking grate. For them, there are hinged baskets that provide one degree of separation from the cooking grate, which makes turning a cinch. Sure beats the alternative of cooking the fish inside the house and smelling it for days.

MICROPLANE GRATER

This is terrific at grating garlic, whole nutmeg, and hard cheeses. It's even better used to zest citrus fruits. You'll see microplane graters in several shapes and sizes. I prefer the long, thin one shaped like a paint stick.

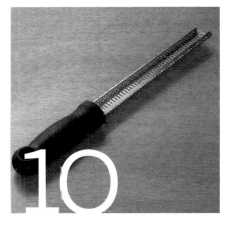

WAY TO GRILL™
RED MEAT

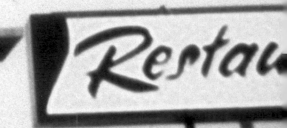

TECHNIQUES

RECIPES

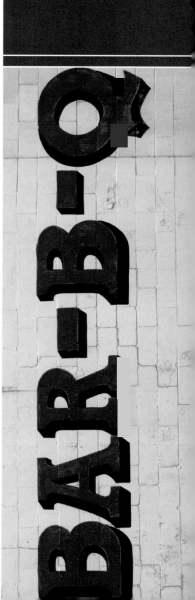

WAY TO GRILL BURGERS
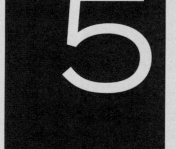 THINGS YOU NEED TO KNOW

1 WHAT MAKES THEM JUICY

Fat makes burgers juicy. That's a big reason why ground chuck (from the shoulder) is better for burgers than ground round (from the rump). Chuck is typically about 18 percent fat, whereas round is often down around 12 percent fat. The reality is that most ground beef in supermarkets comes from all kinds of parts of the animal, but that shouldn't stop you from asking the person behind the counter to grind some chuck just for you, maybe mixing in some sirloin for extra flavor.

2 SEASONING WORKS

Ground beef alone makes a pretty dull-tasting hamburger, so make sure that the meat is mixed throughout with at least salt and pepper. Other ingredients, like Worcestershire sauce, hot sauce, or grated onions, will improve not only the taste but also the juiciness of your hamburgers.

3 SHAPING UP

The ideal thickness for a raw patty is ¾ inch. If it's any thinner, it's likely to overcook and dry out before a nice crust develops on the outside. If it's much thicker, the crust might turn black and unappetizing before the center reaches the safe internal doneness level of medium.

4 LEVELING OFF

Burgers tend to puff up in the middle as they cook, making the tops rounded and awkward for piling on the toppings. A good trick for avoiding this problem is pressing a little indentation into the top of each raw patty with your thumb or the back of a spoon. Then, when the center pushes up, the top of each burger will be relatively level.

5 FLIPPING ONLY ONCE

You should flip each burger only once, and only when it's ready to flip. You'll know when by slipping the edge of a spatula underneath the edge of the burger and lifting up very gently. If the meat is sticking to the cooking grate, back off and try again a minute later. When you can lift the edge of the burger without sticking, it's ready to flip.

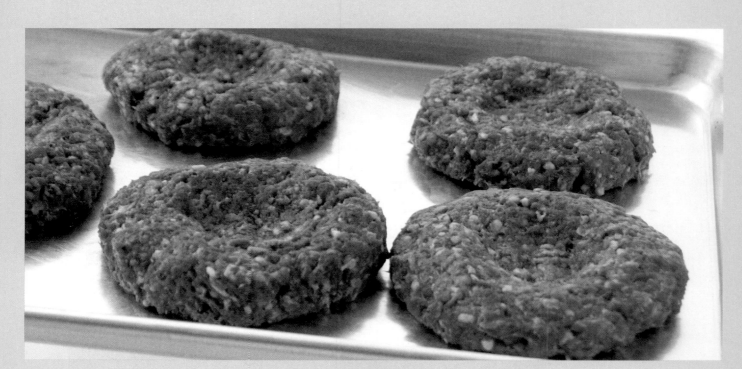

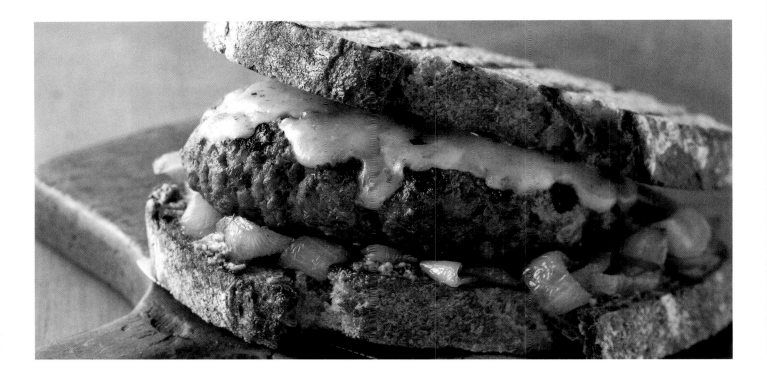

CLASSIC PATTY MELTS ON RYE

SERVES: 6
PREP TIME: 25 MINUTES

WAY TO GRILL: DIRECT HIGH HEAT (450° TO 550°F)
   AND DIRECT MEDIUM HEAT (350° TO 450°F)
GRILLING TIME: 11 TO 13 MINUTES

   3 tablespoons vegetable oil
   2 large yellow onions, halved and thinly sliced
   ½ teaspoon granulated sugar
      Kosher salt
   ¼ cup (½ stick) unsalted butter, softened
   12 slices crusty rye bread, each about ⅓ inch thick
   2 pounds ground chuck (80% lean)
   2 tablespoons Worcestershire sauce
   ½ teaspoon freshly ground black pepper
   1½ cups (about 4 ounces) grated Havarti or Swiss cheese
      Dijon or spicy brown mustard, optional

1. In a large skillet over medium heat, warm the oil. Add the onions, sprinkle with the sugar, cover, and cook until the onions are tender and golden brown, 15 to 20 minutes, stirring occasionally. Season to taste with salt. Remove from the heat.

2. Butter the bread on each side and set aside.

3. Prepare the grill for direct cooking over high heat. In a large bowl gently mix the ground chuck with the Worcestershire sauce, 1 teaspoon of salt, and the pepper, incorporating the spices evenly. Gently shape into 6 patties of equal size and thickness, about ¾ inch thick. With your thumb or the back of a spoon, make a shallow indentation about 1 inch wide in the center of each patty.

4. Brush the cooking grates clean. Grill the patties over **direct high heat**, with the lid closed as much as possible, until cooked to medium, 8 to 10 minutes, turning once. Transfer the patties to a work surface.

5. Lower the temperature of the grill to medium heat. Grill the bread slices over **direct medium heat** until toasted on one side only, about 1 minute. Transfer the bread, toasted sides up, to a work surface.

6. Evenly divide the caramelized onions on 6 of the toasted bread slices and top each with a patty. Scatter the cheese over the patties. Place the remaining bread slices, toasted sides down, on top of the patties. Using a wide spatula, carefully place the patty melts back onto the cooking grate and grill over **direct medium heat** until the bread on the bottom is toasted, about 1 minute, and then carefully turn the sandwiches and toast the other side. Serve the patty melts warm with mustard, if desired.

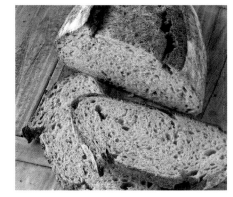

The sturdy texture of crusty rye bread holds up well under the weight of all the wonderfully messy ingredients in a patty melt.

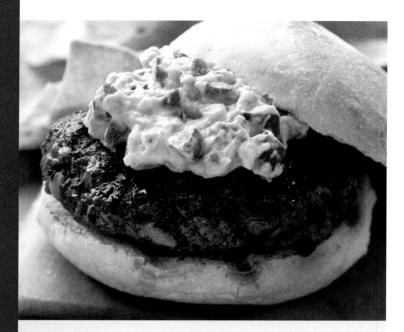

CALIFORNIA BURGERS WITH GUACAMOLE MAYONNAISE

SERVES: 4
PREP TIME: 25 MINUTES

WAY TO GRILL: DIRECT HIGH HEAT (450° TO 550°F)
GRILLING TIME: 18 TO 20 MINUTES

MAYONNAISE
2 tablespoons grated white onion
1 ripe Haas avocado, pitted and peeled
2 tablespoons mayonnaise
2 plum tomatoes, cored, seeded, and chopped
1 tablespoon finely chopped fresh cilantro
2 teaspoons fresh lime juice
1 small garlic clove, grated
  Kosher salt

2 poblano chile peppers
1½ pounds ground chuck (80% lean)
1½ teaspoons kosher salt
1 teaspoon freshly ground black pepper

4 hamburger buns

1. Using a sieve, rinse the grated onion under cold water and let the excess water drain off. In a medium bowl mash the avocado and mayonnaise together with a fork. Stir in the onion, tomatoes, cilantro, lime juice, and garlic. Season generously with salt. Cover with plastic wrap, pressing the wrap directly onto the surface, and set aside. (The mayonnaise can be prepared up to 8 hours ahead.)

2. Prepare the grill for direct cooking over high heat. Brush the cooking grates clean. Grill the chiles over **direct high heat**, with the lid closed as much as possible, until the skin is blackened on all sides, about 10 minutes, turning occasionally. Remove from the grill and allow to cool completely. Peel off and discard the blackened skin, and then remove and discard the stem, seeds, and ribs. Chop the chiles into ½-inch dice.

3. In a large bowl gently mix the ground chuck, chiles, salt, and pepper, and shape into 4 patties of equal size and thickness, about ¾ inch thick. With your thumb or the back of a spoon, make a shallow indentation about 1 inch wide in the center of each patty so the centers are about ½ inch thick. This will help the patties cook evenly and prevent them from puffing on the grill.

4. Grill the patties over **direct high heat,** with the lid closed as much as possible, until cooked to medium, 8 to 10 minutes, turning once when the patties release easily from the grate without sticking. During the last minute of cooking time, toast the buns, cut sides down, over direct heat. Top the burgers with the mayonnaise and serve warm.

WAY TO SPICE UP MAYONNAISE

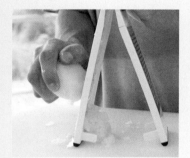

1. Tame the sharp flavor and crunch of raw onion in your mayonnaise by grating the onion on the medium-sized holes of a grater. Then rinse the grated onion in a sieve for a sweet, mild taste.

2. A microplane grater with tiny holes will quickly make a paste out of fresh garlic.

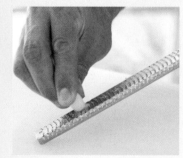

3. Swipe the paste right off the back side of the grater and into your mayonnaise.

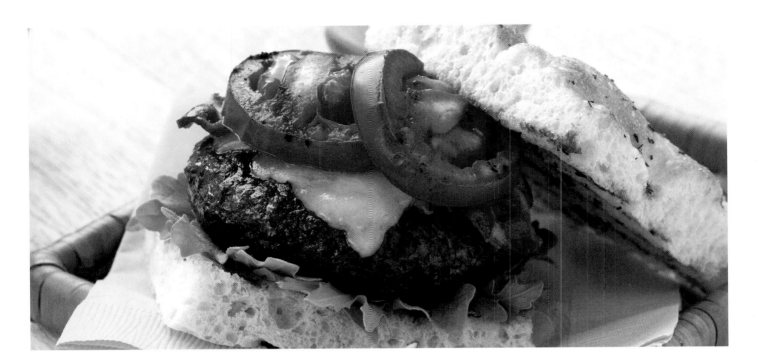

CABERNET BURGERS WITH ROSEMARY FOCACCIA

SERVES: 4

PREP TIME: 25 MINUTES

WAY TO GRILL: DIRECT HIGH HEAT (450° TO 550°F) AND
   DIRECT MEDIUM HEAT (350° TO 450°F)

GRILLING TIME: 10 TO 14 MINUTES

GLAZE

- 2 cups Cabernet Sauvignon wine
- 1 tablespoon brown sugar

BUTTER

- ¼ cup unsalted butter (½ stick), softened
- 1 tablespoon minced fresh rosemary leaves

PATTIES

- 1½ pounds ground chuck (80% lean)
- ¼ cup Cabernet glaze (above)
- 2 teaspoons kosher salt
- ½ teaspoon freshly ground black pepper

- 4 slices white cheddar cheese
- 8 slices ripe tomato, each about ½ inch thick
  Extra-virgin olive oil
  Kosher salt
- 4 focaccia squares, each about 4½ inches,
  sliced in half horizontally, or 4 focaccia buns, split
- 2 cups baby arugula

- 4 thick slices crisp bacon

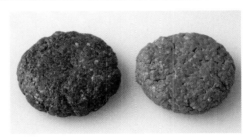

Thanks to a red wine reduction, the patty on the left has improved dramatically in flavor, moisture, and appearance.

1. In a heavy, non-reactive saucepan over medium heat, combine the wine and brown sugar. Cook until reduced to ½ cup, 20 to 25 minutes. Set aside to cool.

2. In a small bowl mix the butter and rosemary.

3. Prepare the grill for direct cooking over high heat. In a large bowl gently combine the patty ingredients and shape into 4 patties of equal size and thickness, about ¾ inch thick. With your thumb or the back of a spoon, make a shallow indentation about 1 inch wide in the center of each patty.

4. Brush the cooking grates clean. Grill the patties over ***direct high heat***, with the lid closed as much as possible, until cooked to medium, 8 to 10 minutes, brushing with the glaze every 2 minutes and turning them once when the patties release easily from the grate without sticking. During the last minute of cooking, place a slice of cheese on each patty to melt.

5. Lower the temperature of the grill to medium heat. Brush the tomato slices with oil, season to taste with salt, and grill over ***direct medium heat*** until soft, 2 to 4 minutes, turning once. Spread the cut sides of the focaccia with the rosemary butter and grill over ***direct medium heat***, cut sides down, until lightly toasted, about 1 minute. Build each burger with arugula, a patty, a slice of bacon, and 2 slices of tomato. Serve warm.

BRIE AND SHALLOT PARISIAN BURGERS

SERVES: 4
PREP TIME: 30 MINUTES

WAY TO GRILL: DIRECT HIGH HEAT (450° TO 550°F)
GRILLING TIME: 8 TO 10 MINUTES

   1 cup thinly sliced shallots
   2 tablespoons extra-virgin olive oil

PATTIES
  1½ pounds ground chuck (80% lean)
   3 tablespoons fine dry bread crumbs
   3 tablespoons beef or chicken broth
   1 teaspoon kosher salt
   ½ teaspoon freshly ground black pepper

   2 ounces brie cheese (not the triple cream variety)
   4 round crusty rolls, each about 4 inches in diameter
   ⅓ cup whole-grain mustard
   2 cups baby arugula

1. In a medium skillet over low heat, combine the shallots with the oil and cook until they are browned but not scorched, about 20 minutes, stirring often. Let cool to room temperature.

2. Prepare the grill for direct cooking over high heat. In a large bowl gently mix the patty ingredients and shape into 4 patties of equal size and thickness. Make a hole in the center of each patty for the cheese.

3. Trim away the rind of the brie and bury the cheese, about ¼ ounce for each patty, into the hole of each patty. Close the opening to seal the cheese inside. It's important that there is one-third of an inch of meat on the top and bottom of the cheese so it doesn't seep out.

4. Brush the cooking grates clean. Grill the patties over **direct high heat,** with the lid closed as much as possible, until cooked to medium, 8 to 10 minutes, turning once when the patties release easily from the grate without sticking. During the last minute of cooking time, toast the buns, cut sides down, over direct heat.

5. Assemble the burgers with shallots, mustard, and arugula. Serve warm.

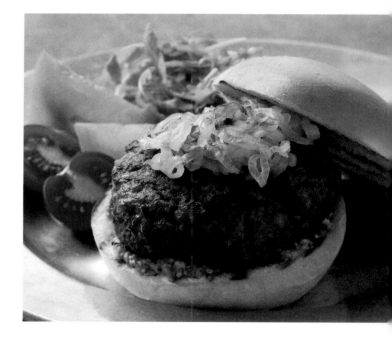

WAY TO MAKE "OUTSIDE IN" BURGERS

A fun way to turn a cheeseburger outside in is by nestling a little knob of cheese in the center and letting it soften slowly while the burger grills.

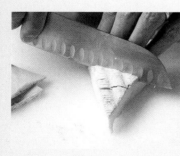 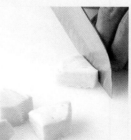 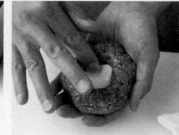 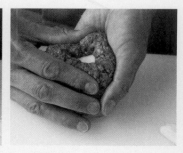

1. Trim off any unwanted rind.

2. Cut the pieces small enough so that the cheese won't seep out of the burger.

3. Nestle each piece right in the center of each burger.

4. Seal each burger tightly to enclose the cheese completely.

RED MEAT

KOFTA IN PITA POCKETS WITH CUCUMBER AND TOMATO SALAD

SERVES: 6
PREP TIME: 25 MINUTES

WAY TO GRILL: DIRECT AND INDIRECT HIGH HEAT
   (450° TO 550°F)
GRILLING TIME: 8 TO 10 MINUTES

DRESSING
- ½ cup plain Greek-style yogurt
- ½ cup sesame tahini
- ¼ cup finely chopped fresh cilantro or mint leaves, or a combination
- 3 tablespoons fresh lemon juice
- 2 tablespoons extra-virgin olive oil
- ½ teaspoon kosher salt

SALAD
- 1 cup chopped English cucumber
- 1 cup quartered cherry tomatoes
- ¼ cup finely chopped red onion
  Kosher salt

KOFTA
- 1½ pounds ground chuck (80% lean)
- ½ cup minced fresh Italian parsley
- 1 tablespoon minced garlic
- 2 teaspoons ground coriander
- 1½ teaspoons ground cumin
- 1½ teaspoons kosher salt
- ½ teaspoon freshly ground black pepper
- ½ teaspoon ground allspice
- ¼ teaspoon ground cardamom
- ¼ teaspoon ground turmeric

  Extra-virgin olive oil
- 3 whole-wheat pitas

1. In a small bowl combine the dressing ingredients. If the dressing is too thick, whisk in up to 3 tablespoons of water until your desired consistency is reached.

2. In a medium bowl combine the salad ingredients, including salt to taste.

3. Prepare the grill for direct and indirect cooking over high heat. In a large bowl gently combine the *kofta* ingredients. Shape into 6 patties of equal size and thickness, about ¾ inch thick. With your thumb or the back of a spoon, make a shallow indentation about 1 inch wide in the center of each patty. Brush the patties with oil.

4. Sprinkle the pitas with water and wrap them in foil.

5. Brush the cooking grates clean. Grill the patties over **direct high heat**, with the lid closed as much as possible, until cooked to medium, 8 to 10 minutes, turning once when the patties

release easily from the grate without sticking. While they cook, warm the pita packet over **indirect high heat** for 4 to 5 minutes, turning once.

6. Cut each pita in half. Scoop about 3 tablespoons of the salad into each pita. Spoon some of the dressing over the salad. Place a patty into each pita pocket and spoon in more dressing, if desired. Serve warm.

WAY TO SEASON KOFTA

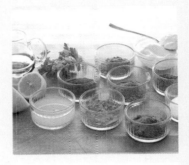

1. The bold flavors of this dish rely on a panoply of international ingredients.

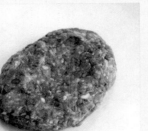

2. *Kofta* refers to any kind of ground meat mixed with grains, vegetables, or spices.

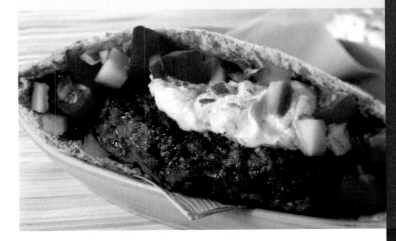

3. Pressing a shallow indentation in each patty prevents the meat from puffing up like a meatball.

WAY TO GRILL

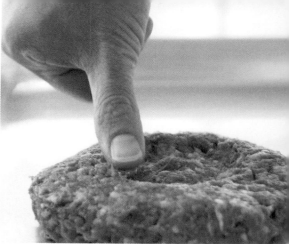

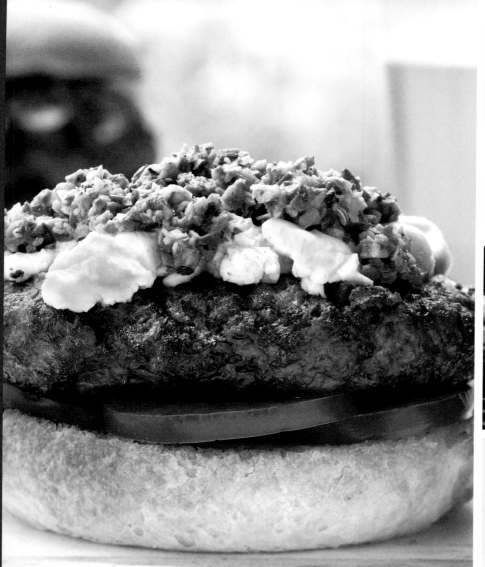

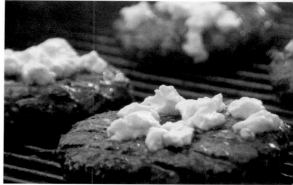

As with any type of burger, the key to keeping this one flat instead of puffed up is to make a shallow indentation in the meat while it is raw. During the last minute of grilling, scatter crumbled goat cheese on top so that it oozes a little into the burger.

LAMB BURGERS WITH TAPENADE AND GOAT CHEESE

SERVES: 6
PREP TIME: 25 MINUTES

WAY TO GRILL: DIRECT HIGH HEAT (450° TO 550°F)
GRILLING TIME: 8 TO 10 MINUTES

TAPENADE
  1   medium garlic clove
  ½   cup pitted kalamata olives
  ½   cup pitted green olives
  2   tablespoons nonpareil capers, rinsed
  2   tablespoons extra-virgin olive oil
  ½   teaspoon Dijon mustard
  ½   teaspoon herbes de Provence

2¼   pounds ground lamb
  ½   teaspoon herbes de Provence
  ½   teaspoon kosher salt
  ½   teaspoon freshly ground black pepper
  5   ounces goat cheese, crumbled
  6   hamburger buns
  3   plum tomatoes, thinly sliced

1. Fit a food processor with the metal chopping blade. With the machine running, drop the garlic through the feed tube and mince. Add the rest of the tapenade ingredients and pulse until coarsely chopped. (The tapenade can be made, and then covered and refrigerated, up to 1 week ahead. Bring to room temperature before serving.)

2. Prepare the grill for direct cooking over high heat. In a large bowl, using your hands, gently mix the lamb, herbs, salt, and pepper. Shape the meat into 6 patties of equal size and thickness, about 4 inches in diameter and ¾ inch thick. With your thumb or the back of a spoon, make a shallow indentation about 1 inch wide in the center of each patty.

3. Brush the cooking grates clean. Grill the patties over **direct high heat**, with the lid closed as much as possible, until cooked to medium, 8 to 10 minutes, turning once. During the last minute of grilling, top each burger with the cheese to allow the cheese to soften, and toast the buns.

4. Build the burgers with tomato slices and tapenade. Serve warm.

LAMB MEATBALLS WITH CHOPPED SALAD AND MINTED YOGURT

SERVES: 6
PREP TIME: 30 MINUTES

WAY TO GRILL: DIRECT MEDIUM-HIGH HEAT
  (ABOUT 400°F)
GRILLING TIME: 4 TO 6 MINUTES
SPECIAL EQUIPMENT: METAL OR BAMBOO SKEWERS (IF
  BAMBOO, SOAK IN WATER FOR AT LEAST 30 MINUTES)

SALAD
- ¼ cup extra-virgin olive oil
- 2 tablespoons red wine vinegar
- 1 teaspoon finely grated lemon zest
- 2 teaspoons minced garlic
- 3 large plum tomatoes, seeded and cut into ½-inch cubes
- ½ English cucumber, cut into ½-inch cubes
- ½ small red onion, finely diced
- ⅓ cup crumbled feta cheese
- ¼ cup chopped fresh Italian parsley
- ½ teaspoon kosher salt
- ¼ teaspoon freshly ground black pepper

MEATBALLS
- 1½ pounds ground lamb
- 1 tablespoon minced garlic
- 2 teaspoons ground cumin
- 1 teaspoon kosher salt
- ½ teaspoon freshly ground black pepper

  Extra-virgin olive oil

SAUCE
- 1½ cups plain Greek-style yogurt
- 2 tablespoons fresh lemon juice
- ¼ cup loosely packed fresh mint leaves, coarsely chopped
- ½ teaspoon kosher salt

4–6 pieces naan

1. In a large, non-reactive bowl whisk the oil, vinegar, lemon zest, and garlic. Add in the rest of the salad ingredients and gently toss with the dressing.

2. In a medium bowl, using your hands, gently mix the meatball ingredients. Do not overwork the mixture or the meatballs will be tough. Make about 24 meatballs. Thread 4 meatballs onto each skewer. Lightly brush with oil.

3. Prepare the grill for direct cooking over medium-high heat.

4. In a small bowl mix the yogurt and lemon juice. Fold in the mint and season with the salt

5. Brush the cooking grates clean. Grill the meatballs over **direct medium-high heat**, with the lid closed as much as possible, until they have browned but are still slightly pink in the center, 4 to 6 minutes, turning occasionally. During the last 30 seconds of grilling time, heat the naan over direct heat.

6. Cut the naan in half, or into pieces large enough to hold 4 meatballs. Top with a generous spoonful of sauce and some salad.

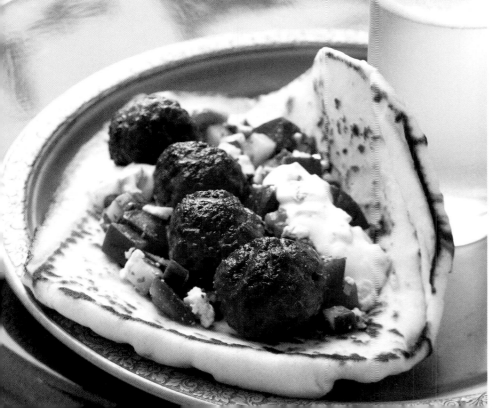

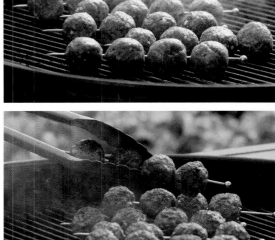

Skewering these meatballs allows you to turn 4 of them at a time, rather than having to turn them individually. Skewers are ready to turn only when the meat releases from the cooking grate without any sticking.

WAY TO BARBECUE MEAT LOAF

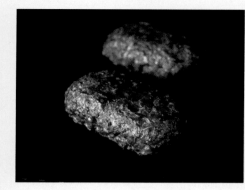 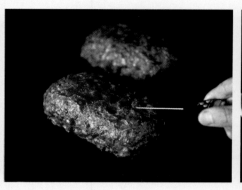 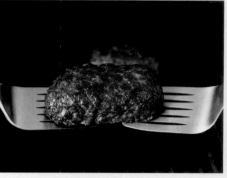

1. Light panko bread crumbs hold these meat loaves together without making them dense.

2. Check the internal temperature near the top because that part takes the longest to cook.

3. To remove each meat loaf in one whole piece, support both ends with spatulas.

BARBECUED MEAT LOAF

SERVES: 8 TO 10
PREP TIME: 20 MINUTES

WAY TO GRILL: INDIRECT MEDIUM-LOW HEAT
   (ABOUT 300°F)
GRILLING TIME: 50 TO 60 MINUTES
SPECIAL EQUIPMENT: INSTANT-READ THERMOMETER

MEAT LOAF
1¼ pounds ground beef (80% lean)
1¼ pounds ground pork
  2 cups panko bread crumbs
  1 cup finely chopped yellow onion
  1 large egg
  1 teaspoon Worcestershire sauce
  1 teaspoon granulated garlic
  1 teaspoon dried tarragon
  1 teaspoon kosher salt
  1 teaspoon freshly ground black pepper

SAUCE
  ½ cup bottled barbecue sauce
  ¼ cup ketchup

1. In a large bowl, using your hands, gently combine the meat loaf ingredients.

2. Divide the meat loaf mixture in half and form into 2 loaves, each about 4 inches wide and 6 to 7 inches long. Place the loaves on a sheet pan. Prepare the grill for indirect cooking over medium-low heat.

3. In a small bowl mix the sauce ingredients. Set aside half of the sauce to serve with the meat loaf. Top each meat loaf with 3 tablespoons of the remaining sauce and coat thoroughly.

4. Brush the cooking grates clean. Using a metal spatula, gently

pick up each loaf from the sheet pan and place directly on the cooking grate. Grill the meat loaves over *indirect medium-low heat*, with the lid closed, until a thermometer inserted horizontally through the top of each loaf registers 155°F, 50 to 60 minutes. Remove the loaves from the grill and let rest 10 to 15 minutes. Once removed from the grill, the loaves will continue to cook, allowing them to reach the recommended 160°F for ground beef and pork. Cut the loaves into ½-inch slices and serve with the reserved sauce.

TO MAKE MEAT LOAF SANDWICHES
Cut the meat loaf into ½-inch-thick slices and slather both sides with some of the reserved sauce. Grill over *direct low heat* (250° to 350°F), with the lid closed as much as possible, for 4 to 6 minutes, turning once. Serve on sourdough bread. Also great with melted provolone cheese.

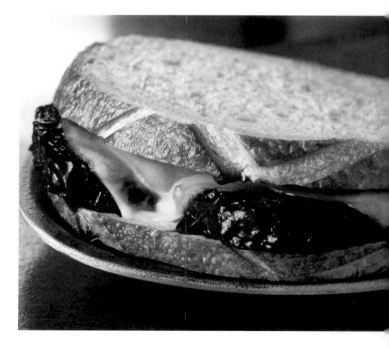

TUBE STEAKS WITH PICKLED ONIONS

SERVES: 8
PREP TIME: 15 MINUTES
MARINATING TIME: 2 TO 3 HOURS

WAY TO GRILL: DIRECT MEDIUM HEAT (350° TO 450°F)
GRILLING TIME: 5 TO 7 MINUTES

ONIONS
- 1 small white or yellow onion
- 1 small red onion
- ½ cup cider vinegar
- ½ cup distilled white vinegar
- ½ cup granulated sugar
- 1 tablespoon kosher salt
- 2 teaspoons celery seed
- 1 teaspoon crushed red pepper flakes

- 8 all-beef hot dogs, about ¼ pound each
- 8 hot dog buns
  Yellow mustard
  Ketchup

1. Trim off the ends of the onions. Cut each onion in half lengthwise. With a very sharp knife, cut the onions into paper-thin slices and place in a shallow, non-reactive dish, such as a glass pie plate. In a medium bowl combine the remaining onion ingredients. Whisk thoroughly to dissolve the sugar and salt. Pour the vinegar mixture over the onions and stir to coat them evenly. Set aside at room temperature for about 3 hours, stirring the onions occasionally. Drain the pickled onions and set aside.

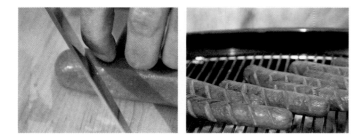

2. Using a sharp knife, cut a few shallow slashes in each hot dog.

3. Prepare the grill for direct cooking over medium heat. Brush the cooking grates clean. Grill the hot dogs over **direct medium heat**, with the lid closed as much as possible, until lightly marked on the outside and hot all the way to the center, 5 to 7 minutes, turning occasionally.

4. Place the hot dogs in buns. Squeeze your condiment of choice alongside each hot dog and top with pickled onions. Serve warm.

WAY TO PICKLE ONIONS

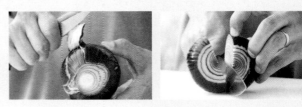

1. Peel and halve the onions, and make sure the root and stem ends are completely removed.

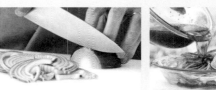
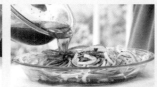

2. Cut the onions into paper-thin slices, place them in a shallow glass dish, and pour the pickling liquid over them.

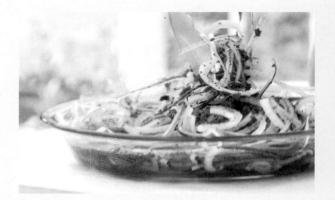

3. Stir to coat them evenly and set aside to marinate for about 3 hours.

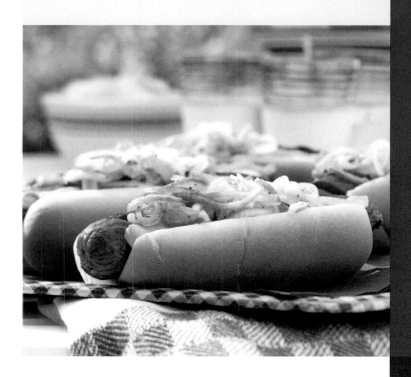

WAY TO GRILL STEAK

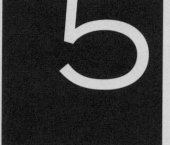

5 THINGS YOU NEED TO KNOW

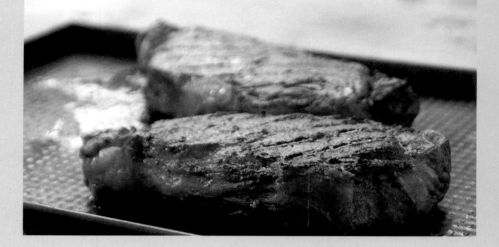

1 SALTING EARLY PAYS OFF

You might have heard the warning that you shouldn't salt meat too far ahead of cooking because it can draw out moisture. It's true that salt draws moisture toward itself, but over the course of 20 to 30 minutes that's a good thing, because the salt begins to dissolve into that little bit of moisture. When the steak hits the hot cooking grate, the sugars and proteins in the moisture combine with the salt and other seasonings to create a delicious crust. Any moisture you might lose is well worth the flavor of that crust.

2 TAKING OFF THE CHILL SPEEDS UP COOKING

The goal of grilling a steak is to brown and lightly char the surface while also cooking the interior to a perfectly juicy doneness, right? If the steak is too cold, the interior might require so much cooking time to reach that perfect doneness that the steak overcooks deep below the surface, turning gray and dry. Let your steaks stand at room temperature for 20 to 30 minutes before grilling. They will cook faster all the way to the center and stay juicer.

3 SEARING EQUALS FLAVOR

One good habit that separates professional chefs from many home cooks is that chefs spend more time searing their steaks. They understand that searing develops literally hundreds of flavors and aromas on the surface of steak, so they let their steaks sizzle over direct heat until the surfaces are dark, dark brown. Don't let anyone tell you that searing "locks in the juices." That's a myth. But searing sure does make steak tasty.

4 THICKER STEAKS SHOULD SLIDE OVER

Most steaks grill beautifully over direct high heat alone. The only time you might need to move them is if/when they cause flare-ups. However, some steaks are so thick that if you left them over direct heat alone, they would burn on the outside before they reached the internal doneness you like. If your steaks are much thicker than about an inch, consider the sear and slide approach. After you have seared both sides nicely over direct high heat, slide the steaks to a part of the grill that is not so hot, perhaps over indirect heat, and finish cooking them safely there.

5 YOU CAN'T PUT MOISTURE BACK INSIDE A STEAK

As steaks grill over high heat, they lose moisture. Fat and juices are literally pushed out of the meat. That's the price we pay for making the steaks easier to digest. Perhaps the most important part of grilling a steak is taking it off the heat before it has lost too much moisture. There is a short window of time, usually just a minute or two, when steaks go from medium rare to medium, or from medium to medium well. Catching that window requires vigilance. Don't walk away from a steak on the grill. And remember, it's always better to take it off when it's underdone and then return it to the grill than it is to let a steak overcook.

WAY TO BUTCHER A STRIP LOIN

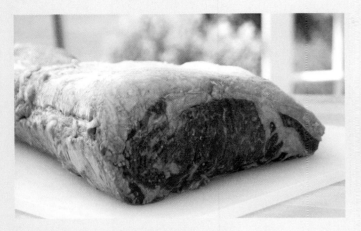

1. Buying a whole strip loin is a great way to save money on strip steaks.

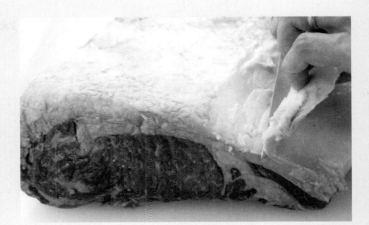

2. You'll need to trim away most of the thick "fat cap" on the top side.

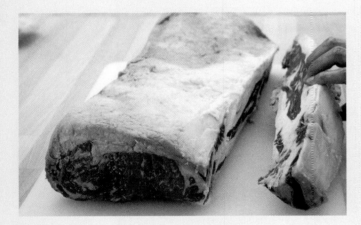

3. Next, remove the long section of scraggy meat and fat on the thinnest edge.

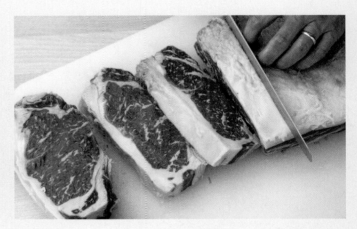

4. Cutting the loin yourself allows you to make the steaks just the right thickness.

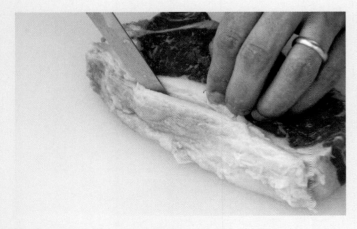

5. After cutting the steaks, go back and trim the fat around the outer edges to about ¼ inch.

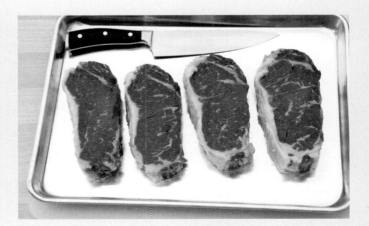

6. Grill some of the steaks now and freeze the remaining ones for another day (for the way to freeze steaks, see page 296).

WAY TO GRILL

WAY TO PREP AND GRILL STRIP STEAKS

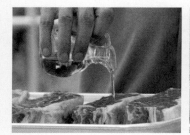

1. Lean strip steaks benefit from the rich flavor and slickness of extra-virgin olive oil.

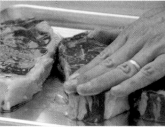

2. Rub the oil evenly all over the steaks to prevent them from sticking to the cooking grate.

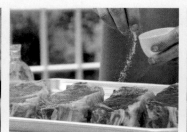

3. The oil also helps the seasonings adhere to the meat.

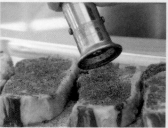

4. Sometimes coarse salt and freshly ground pepper are all you need for a great-tasting steak.

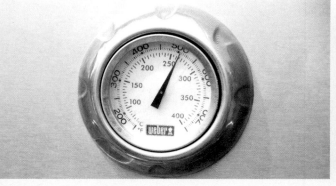

5. Bring the grill temperature to 500°F. A hot cooking grate will sear the steaks quickly.

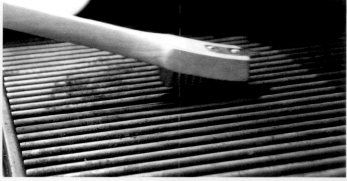

6. Once the cooking grates are smoking hot, they are easy to clean with a stainless steel-bristle brush.

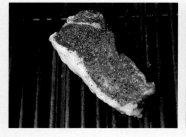

7. Lay each steak on the cooking grate over high heat as if it were the small hand of a clock pointing to ten o'clock. Then close the lid.

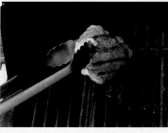

8. After a couple of minutes, lift each steak with tongs—not a fork! Piercing the steaks means losing delicious juices.

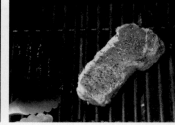

9. Rotate the steaks so they point to two o'clock, close the lid, and let them sear for another minute or two.

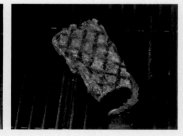

10. Flip each steak and check out those handsome crosshatch grill marks.

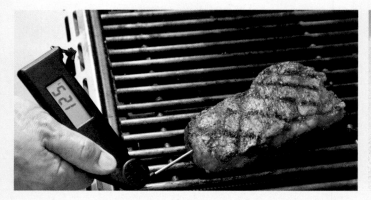

11. Putting crosshatches on the second side is optional. The key now is to finish the steaks, with the lid down, without overcooking them. An internal doneness of 125°F will give you a medium-rare steak.

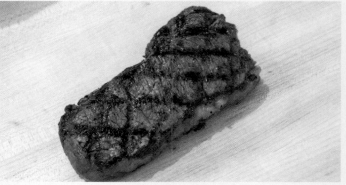

12. As the steaks rest for a few minutes after grilling, the internal temperature will climb about 5°F and the juices will redistribute evenly.

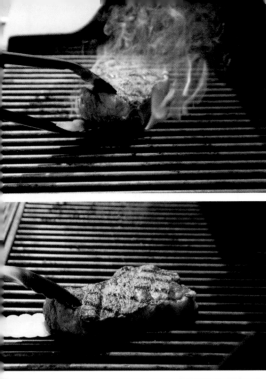

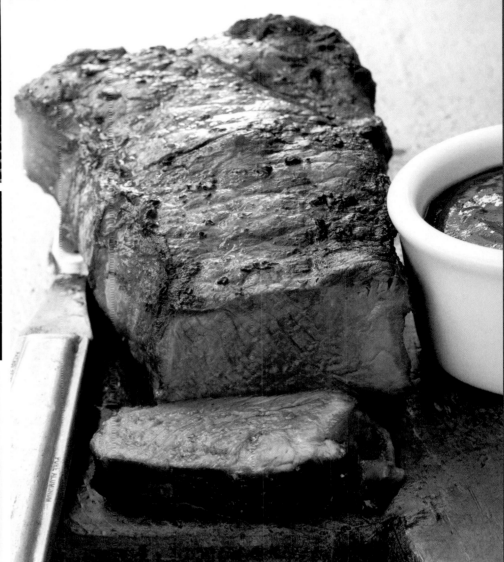

Occasionally the fat and juices dripping from a steak will cause flare-ups on the grill. Don't panic. Simply slide the steak to a cooler area of the grate. If your steak already has good charring on both sides, finish cooking it over indirect heat, with the lid closed. If you want more charring, slide the steak back over high heat once the flare-ups have died out.

STRIP STEAKS WITH RED-EYE BARBECUE SAUCE

SERVES: 4
PREP TIME: 20 MINUTES

WAY TO GRILL: DIRECT HIGH HEAT (450° TO 550°F)
GRILLING TIME: 6 TO 8 MINUTES

SAUCE
- 1 tablespoon unsalted butter
- 2 teaspoons minced shallot
- 1 teaspoon minced garlic
- ½ cup ketchup
- ¼ cup brewed dark-roast coffee or espresso
- 1 tablespoon balsamic vinegar
- 1 tablespoon brown sugar
- 2 teaspoons ground ancho chile powder

- 4 New York strip steaks, each 10 to 12 ounces and about 1 inch thick, trimmed of excess fat
- 2 tablespoons extra-virgin olive oil
- ¾ teaspoon kosher salt
- ¾ teaspoon freshly ground black pepper

1. In a medium saucepan over medium heat, melt the butter. Add the shallot and cook, stirring often, until it begins to brown, about 3 minutes. Add the garlic and cook until fragrant, about 1 minute. Stir in the rest of the sauce ingredients, bring to a simmer and reduce the heat to low. Simmer, stirring often, until slightly reduced, about 10 minutes. Transfer to a bowl to cool.

2. Lightly brush the steaks on both sides with the oil. Season evenly with the salt and pepper. Let the steaks stand at room temperature for 20 to 30 minutes before grilling. Prepare the grill for direct cooking over high heat.

3. Brush the cooking grates clean. Grill the steaks over **direct high heat**, with the lid closed as much as possible, until cooked to your desired doneness, 6 to 8 minutes for medium rare, turning once. Remove from the grill and let the steaks rest for 3 to 5 minutes. Serve the steaks warm with the sauce on the side.

Grilled red onions make a great addition to a steak sandwich, and here they benefit from soaking twice in a bold sweet-and-sour marinade: once before grilling and once afterwards.

STEAK SANDWICHES WITH GRILLED ONIONS AND CREAMY HORSERADISH SAUCE

SERVES: 4
PREP TIME: 15 MINUTES
MARINATING TIME: 30 MINUTES

WAY TO GRILL: DIRECT HIGH HEAT (450° TO 550°F)
AND DIRECT MEDIUM HEAT (350° TO 450°F)
GRILLING TIME: 7 TO 9 MINUTES

MARINADE
2 cups red wine
1 cup soy sauce
¼ cup balsamic vinegar
3 tablespoons brown sugar
1 tablespoon finely chopped garlic
1 teaspoon freshly ground black pepper
½ cup extra-virgin olive oil

½ teaspoon baking soda

4 New York strip steaks, each about 12 ounces and 1 inch thick
2 red onions, sliced into ¼-inch rings

½ cup sour cream
¼ cup prepared horseradish
1 teaspoon finely chopped fresh thyme
Kosher salt
Freshly ground black pepper

4 French rolls
2 bunches watercress, trimmed and rinsed

1. In a large bowl combine the marinade ingredients, whisking in the oil until blended. Divide the marinade, pouring 3 cups into a non-reactive baking dish and leaving the other 1 cup in the bowl. Add the baking soda to the marinade in the baking dish for a tenderizing effect (the mixture may fizz a little).

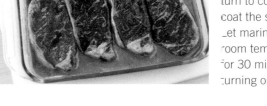

2. Put the steaks into the dish with the marinade and turn to completely coat the steaks. Let marinate at room temperature for 30 minutes, turning once.

3. Place the sliced onions in the bowl with the marinade and gently stir to coat them evenly. Set aside and let them marinate alongside the steaks.

4. In a medium bowl mix the sour cream and horseradish. Stir in the thyme, and season to taste with salt and pepper. Cover and refrigerate until ready to use.

5. Prepare the grill for direct cooking over high heat on one side of the grill and medium heat on the other. Brush the cooking grates clean. Remove the steaks from the dish, allowing most of the marinade to drip back into the dish. Discard the marinade. Grill the steaks over ***direct high heat***, with the lid closed as much as possible, until cooked to your desired doneness, 6 to 8 minutes for medium rare, turning once. While the steaks are grilling, carefully remove the onions from the marinade, keeping the bowl of marinade close by, and grill the onions over ***direct medium heat*** for 6 to 8 minutes, turning once. Remove the onions from the grill and plunge back into the bowl of marinade. Toss to coat and let the onions soak up the marinade while the steaks rest for 3 to 5 minutes. Slice and toast the cut sides of the rolls over ***direct medium heat***, about 1 minute.

6. To assemble the sandwiches, slice the steaks on the bias into thin strips. Pile the bottom of a French roll with onions and layer with strips of steak. Top with horseradish sauce and watercress.

WAY TO CHECK STEAKS FOR DONENESS

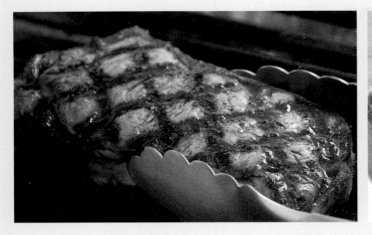

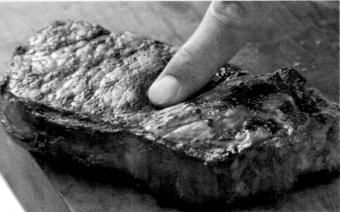

1. Because steaks get firmer as they grill, one way to judge their doneness is by lightly squeezing the sides with tongs. It takes time to learn just how firm each type of steak will feel at each level of doneness, but this is how many restaurant chefs work, and it's a technique worth practicing.

2. Another popular method is to press the surface of a steak with your fingertip. When the meat is no longer soft, but is not yet firm either, you know a steak has reached medium-rare doneness. See below for more hints on judging doneness by touch.

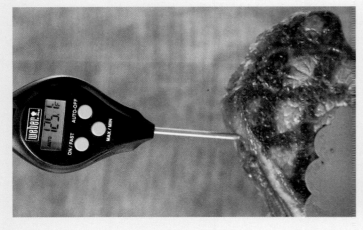

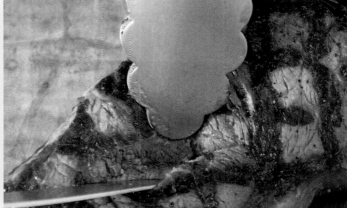

3. A more scientific approach is to use an instant-read thermometer. If you are sure to position the thermometer sensor right in the middle of the steak, you'll have a perfectly accurate reading of doneness.

4. Perhaps the most straightforward approach is to have a look at the color of the meat inside the steak. On the underside of the steak (the side that will face the plate), cut a little slit down to the center of the meat and peek inside. When it's cooked just the way you want it, turn the steak over and press the surface with your fingertip. Note how it feels so that next time you won't need to cut into your steak.

WAY TO CHECK DONENESS BY TOUCH

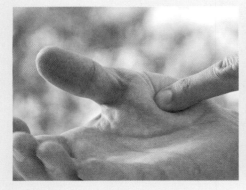

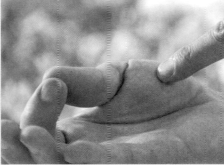

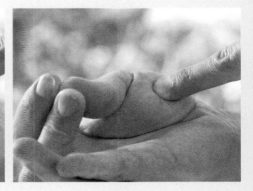

1. Most raw steaks are as soft as the base of your thumb when your hand is relaxed.

2. If you touch your index finger and thumb together, and then press the base of your thumb, that's how most steaks feel when they are rare.

3. If you touch your middle finger and thumb together, and then press the base of your thumb, that's how most steaks feel when they are medium rare.

PANZANELLA STEAK SALAD

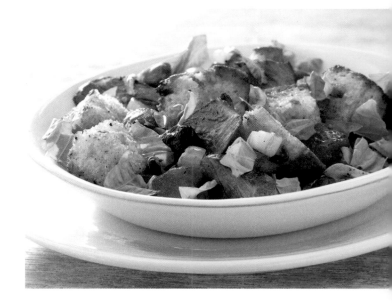

SERVES: 4 TO 6
PREP TIME: 20 MINUTES

WAY TO GRILL: DIRECT AND INDIRECT HIGH HEAT
   (450° TO 550°F)
GRILLING TIME: 12 TO 16 MINUTES
SPECIAL EQUIPMENT: BAMBOO SKEWERS,
   SOAKED IN WATER FOR AT LEAST 30 MINUTES

DRESSING
   3 tablespoons red wine vinegar
   1 teaspoon kosher salt
   1 teaspoon freshly ground black pepper
   2 teaspoons minced garlic
   ½ cup extra-virgin olive oil

   2 New York strip steaks, each about 12 ounces and 1 inch
      thick, trimmed of excess fat
   8 ounces dense, crusty bread, cut into 1½-inch cubes
   6 plum tomatoes, about 1½ pounds, cut in half
      lengthwise, seeds removed
   1 medium yellow onion, cut crosswise into ½-inch slices
   1 cup oil-cured black olives, drained and pitted
   1 cup lightly packed fresh basil leaves, torn into pieces

1. In a small bowl combine the dressing ingredients, gradually
whisking in the oil until emulsified.

2. Put the steaks in a shallow dish, pour 3 tablespoons of the
dressing on top, and turn to coat them evenly. Let stand at room
temperature for 20 to 30 minutes before grilling. Set aside the
remaining dressing.

3. Put the bread cubes into a large bowl, add 2 tablespoons of
the dressing, and toss to coat them evenly. Thread the bread
cubes onto skewers. Brush the cut sides of the tomatoes and
the onion slices with 2 tablespoons of the dressing.

4. Prepare the grill for direct and indirect cooking over high heat.

5. Brush the cooking grates clean. Grill the tomatoes and onions
over **direct high heat** and the bread skewers over **indirect
high heat**, with the lid closed as much as possible, until the
tomatoes are lightly charred, the onions are browned, and the
bread is toasted, turning as needed. The tomatoes will take
2 to 4 minutes and the onions and bread skewers will take
6 to 8 minutes. Remove the food from the grill as it is done.

6. Brush the cooking grates clean. Grill the steaks over **direct
high heat**, with the lid closed as much as possible, until cooked
to your desired doneness, 6 to 8 minutes for medium rare,
turning once. Remove from the grill and let rest 3 to 5 minutes.

7. Pull off and discard the tomato skins. Cut the onion,
tomatoes, and steak into bite-sized chunks, and then place in
a large serving bowl. Add the remaining dressing, olives, bread
cubes, and basil and gently mix. Serve immediately.

WAY TO PREP PANZANELLA STEAK SALAD

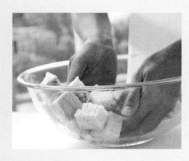
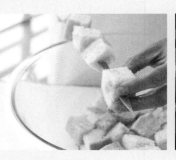
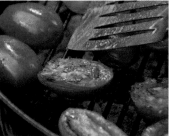
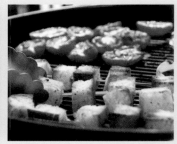

1. Toss big cubes of dense bread in salad dressing for flavor and even browning.

2. Skewer the bread cubes to make them easier to handle on the grill.

3. Firm but ripe plum tomatoes maintain their shape even when you lightly char them.

4. Grilling the bread cubes over indirect heat allows you to brown them slowly, with little risk of burning.

STRIP STEAK PAILLARDS

SERVES: 4
PREP TIME: 20 MINUTES

WAY TO GRILL: DIRECT HIGH HEAT (450° TO 550°F)
GRILLING TIME: ABOUT 3 MINUTES

4 New York strip steaks, each 7 to 8 ounces and
½ to ¾ inch thick, trimmed of all fat and silver skin
Extra-virgin olive oil
Kosher salt
Freshly ground black pepper

DRESSING
¼ cup sour cream
¼ cup mayonnaise
2 tablespoons Dijon mustard
½ teaspoon Worcestershire sauce

1 beefsteak tomato, about 12 ounces, cut into
4 even slices
4 thin slices red onion
2 ounces triple cream cheese, cut into thin wedges
at room temperature

1. One at a time, place each steak between 2 sheets of plastic wrap and pound to an even ¼-inch thickness. Lightly brush the paillards with oil and season them evenly with salt and pepper.

2. In a small bowl combine the dressing ingredients, including salt to taste.

3. Prepare the grill for direct cooking over high heat.

4. Lightly brush each tomato slice with oil and season to taste with salt and pepper. Brush the cooking grates clean. Grill the tomatoes over **direct high heat** until slightly charred on one side, 2 to 3 minutes. Transfer to a sheet pan, grilled sides up.

5. Grill the paillards over **direct high heat**, with the lid open, 1½ to 2 minutes, turning when the first side is nicely marked. The second side will only take 10 to 15 seconds for medium-rare doneness (the paillards will continue to cook as they rest).

6. Transfer the paillards, with the first grilled sides facing up, to a serving platter or individual plates. Place a slice of tomato in the center of each paillard.

7. Evenly divide the dressing over the tomatoes. Separate the slices of onion into rings and place a small mound on the tomatoes. Finish with a piece of cheese and a grinding of pepper on top of each.

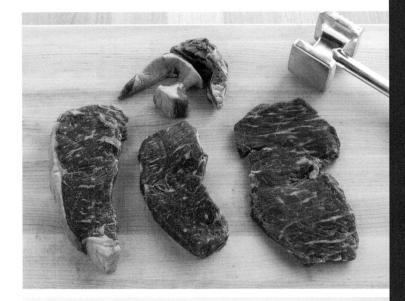

Three stages of a steak paillard. On the left, a strip steak just as you find it at the market. In the middle, a steak trimmed of all the fat around the edges, to make it easier to pound. On the right, an evenly pounded paillard ready for oiling, seasoning, and grilling.

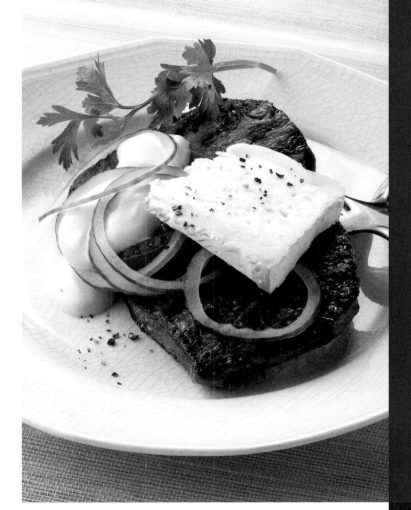

WAY TO BUTCHER A BONE-IN RIB ROAST

Many chefs and carnivores will tell you that their favorite steak for grilling is a rib-eye. The meat is magnificently tender and flavorful, due in large part to the generous interior marbling of milky white fat. Sadly, though, many mega-marts cut rib-eyes too thin, so the steaks tend to overcook rather quickly, squandering some of their magnificence. One solution is to cut your own rib-eyes from a bone-in rib roast, also known as a prime rib.

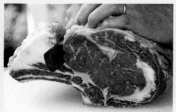

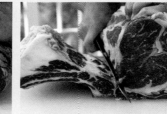

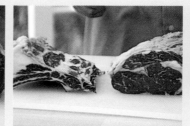

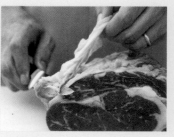

1. Use a long, sharp knife to cut right along the ribs, separating them from the meat.

2. Now cut along the bone at the base of the roast to separate the meat from the bones completely.

3. Don't throw away those ribs. Barbecue them! See page 85.

4. Trim off most of the surface fat from your boneless rib roast.

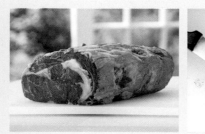

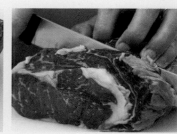

5. At this point, you could grill the whole boneless roast in one piece for a big event (see page 91), or you can slice it into thick steaks and freeze the ones you don't use right away (for the way to freeze steaks, see page 296).

6. Use the blade of a carving knife to measure a consistent thickness for each steak.

7. Make a shallow slit at each point where you plan to slice.

8. Slice the steaks as evenly as possible. Avoid sawing back and forth, which tears the surface of the meat and gives the steaks a ragged appearance.

WAY TO PREP RIB-EYE STEAKS

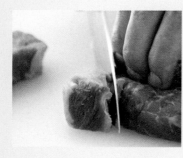

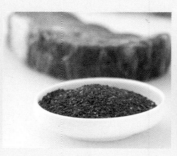

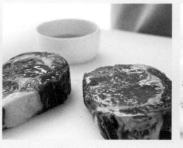

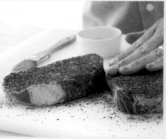

1. As with any steak, trim off any sections along the edges that include more fat than meat.

2. A flavorful cut like rib-eye requires no marinade or elaborate sauce, but consider using a bold blend of dry seasonings as a complement to the meat's richness.

3. With so much marbling in the steak, just a light coating of oil is all you'll need to prevent sticking on the grill.

4. Once your steaks are seasoned, let them stand at room temperature for 20 to 30 minutes before grilling to take the chill off. They will cook a little faster and stay juicier.

RIB-EYE STEAKS
WITH ESPRESSO-CHILE RUB

SERVES: 4
PREP TIME: 10 MINUTES

WAY TO GRILL: DIRECT HIGH HEAT (450° TO 550°F)
GRILLING TIME: 6 TO 8 MINUTES
SPECIAL EQUIPMENT: SPICE MILL

RUB

- 2 teaspoons cumin seed, toasted
- 2 tablespoons dark-roast coffee or espresso beans
- 1 tablespoon ground ancho chile pepper
- 1 teaspoon sweet paprika
- 1 teaspoon kosher salt
- 1 teaspoon freshly ground black pepper

- 4 rib-eye steaks, each about 8 ounces and 1 inch thick
  Extra-virgin olive oil

1. In a spice mill, pulse the cumin seed and coffee beans until finely ground. Transfer to a small bowl, add the remaining rub ingredients, and stir to combine.

2. Lightly brush the steaks with oil and season evenly with the rub, pressing the rub into the meat. Cover and let stand at room temperature for 20 to 30 minutes before grilling. Prepare the grill for direct cooking over high heat.

3. Brush the cooking grates clean. Grill the steaks over **direct high heat**, with the lid closed as much as possible, until cooked to your desired doneness, 6 to 8 minutes for medium rare, turning once (if flare-ups occur, move the steaks temporarily over *indirect high heat*). Remove from the grill and let rest for 3 to 5 minutes. Serve warm.

WAY TO PREP ESPRESSO-CHILE RUB

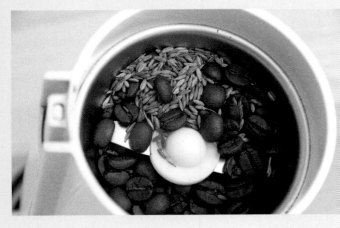

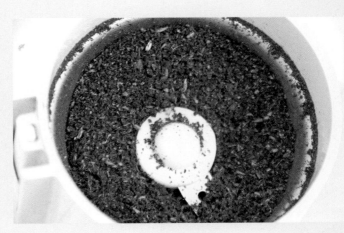

1. A coffee grinder works well for grinding spices, too. Clean it out later by whirling raw white rice in it to absorb the spice residue.

2. Grind your cumin and coffee to a coarse texture, similar to that of kosher salt.

WAY TO MAKE PAN-ROASTED CHILE SALSA

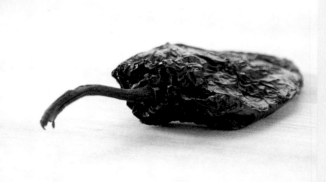

1. The distinctive flavor of the salsa on the opposite page comes mostly from an ancho chile pepper, which is a dried poblano chile pepper. It is not terribly spicy, but it has a brilliant sweet heat, especially when it is toasted first.

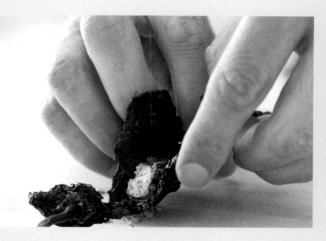

2. Cut off and discard the stem of the chile, then slice open the chile so that you can lay it flat like a book.

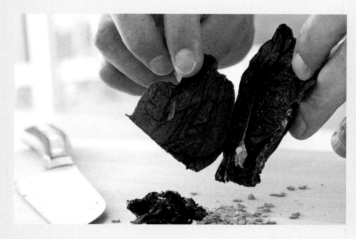

3. A lot of the spiciness is in the seeds, so tap the chile on a board or use a knife to remove them, if you like.

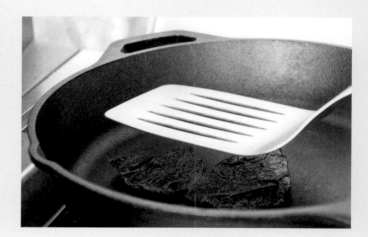

4. Use a spatula to flatten the chile in a hot, dry skillet. This step brings out big flavor. Next, soak the chile in hot water for 20 to 30 minutes.

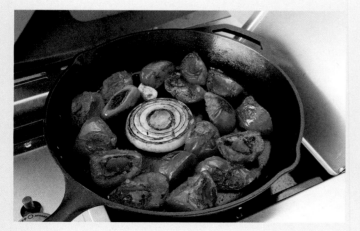

5. You can blacken and blister tomatoes, onions, a jalapeño chile pepper, and garlic in the same skillet. Don't be afraid to get them dark and caramelized.

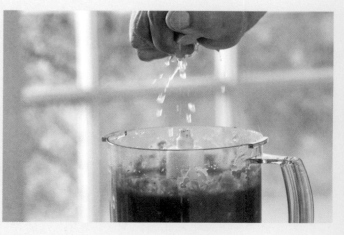

6. Pureeing all the ingredients with some fresh lime juice, salt, and oregano gives you an exciting salsa to serve with steaks. If it seems a little thick, thin it out with a touch of the water used to soak the ancho chile pepper.

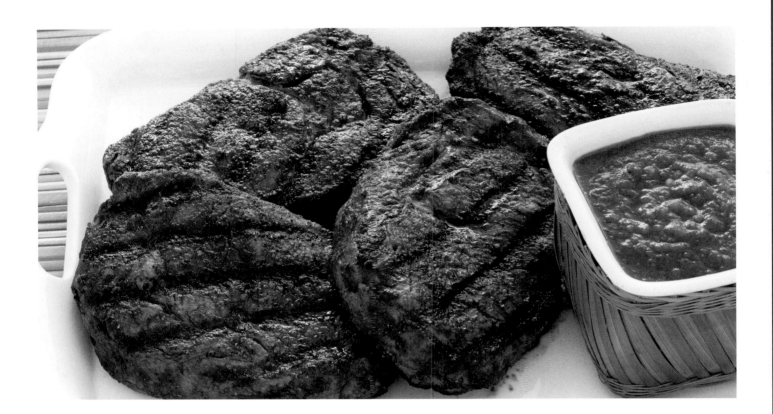

RIB-EYE STEAKS WITH PAN-ROASTED CHILE SALSA

SERVES: 4
PREP TIME: 20 MINUTES

WAY TO GRILL: DIRECT HIGH HEAT (450° TO 550°F)
GRILLING TIME: 6 TO 8 MINUTES
SPECIAL EQUIPMENT: 12-INCH CAST-IRON SKILLET

SALSA
- 1 medium dried ancho chile pepper
- 1 tablespoon extra-virgin olive oil
- 4 medium, ripe tomatoes, quartered, stems and seeds removed
- 1 slice white onion, about ¾ inch thick
- 1 medium jalapeño chile pepper, stem removed
- 1 large garlic clove (do not peel)
- 1 teaspoon fresh lime juice
- ½ teaspoon kosher salt
- ¼ teaspoon dried oregano

RUB
- 1 tablespoon kosher salt
- 2 teaspoons paprika
- 1 teaspoon granulated onion
- 1 teaspoon freshly ground black pepper

- 4 rib-eye steaks, each about 8 ounces and 1 inch thick
  Extra-virgin olive oil

1. In a small saucepan bring 2 cups of water to a simmer. Preheat a 12-inch cast-iron or ovenproof skillet over medium heat on your side burner or stove top.

2. Remove and discard the stem from the ancho chile, open up the chile like a book, and discard the seeds. Flatten the chile and place it in the hot, dry skillet. Press down on the chile with a spatula to flatten it. Toast the chile until the aroma is obvious and you begin to see wisps of smoke. Transfer the chile to the saucepan of hot water and soak it until very soft, 20 to 30 minutes. Reserve the water; you may need a little to thin out the salsa.

3. Meanwhile add the oil, tomatoes, onion, jalapeño, and garlic to the skillet. Cook over medium heat until the vegetables have blackened and blistered in spots, 10 to 15 minutes, turning occasionally. Remove the vegetables as they are finished cooking (they may not finish cooking at the same time). Let cool until you can handle the garlic, and then squeeze the garlic out of its skin into a blender or food processor. Add the ancho chile, tomatoes, onion, jalapeño, lime juice, salt, and oregano. Process to make a salsa. For a thinner consistency, add a little of the water used to soak the ancho chile pepper.

4. In a small bowl mix the rub ingredients. Lightly brush or spray the steaks on both sides with oil. Season evenly with the rub. Let the steaks stand at room temperature for 20 to 30 minutes before grilling. Prepare the grill for direct cooking over high heat.

5. Brush the cooking grates clean. Grill the steaks over **direct high heat**, with the lid closed as much as possible, until cooked to your desired doneness, 6 to 8 minutes for medium rare, turning once (if flare-ups occur, move the steaks temporarily over *indirect high heat*). Remove from the grill and let rest for 3 to 5 minutes. Serve warm with the salsa.

WAY TO GRILL PIADINI

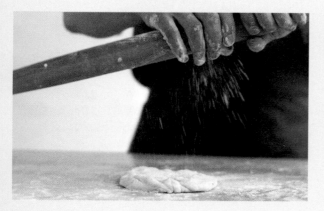

1. Your dough should be at room temperature and you should have flour on both your board and your rolling pin.

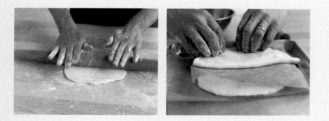

2. Roll each piece of dough to a diameter of 8 to 10 inches and a thickness of about ⅓ inch. Stack the dough rounds between sheets of parchment paper.

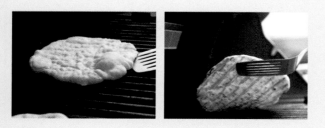

3. Grill the dough rounds over direct medium heat, with the lid closed, until they bubble on top and turn gold brown on the bottom. Then turn them over with a spatula to tcast the other side.

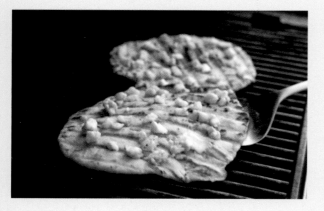

4. While the second side grills, distribute the cheese on top so that it begins to melt. Rotate each dough round and move it around the grill as needed for even cooking.

STEAK AND GORGONZOLA PIADINI

SERVES: 4
PREP TIME: 30 MINUTES
RISING TIME: 1½ TO 2 HOURS

WAY TO GRILL: DIRECT HIGH HEAT (450° TO 550°F)
   AND DIRECT MEDIUM HEAT (350° TO 450°F)
GRILLING TIME: 14 TO 18 MINUTES
SPECIAL EQUIPMENT: ELECTRIC STAND MIXER

DOUGH
- 1½ cups warm water (100° to 110°F)
- 1 package rapid-rise active dry yeast
- ½ teaspoon granulated sugar
- 4½ cups all-purpose flour, plus more for rolling the dough
- 3 tablespoons extra-virgin olive oil
- 2 teaspoons kosher salt

DRESSING
- 2 tablespoons extra-virgin olive oil
- 2 teaspoons balsamic vinegar
- ½ teaspoon minced garlic
- ½ teaspoon Dijon mustard
- ¼ teaspoon kosher salt
- ⅛ teaspoon freshly ground black pepper

- 2 rib-eye steaks, each 6 to 8 ounces and about 1 inch thick
  Extra-virgin olive oil
  Kosher salt
  Freshly ground black pepper
- 8 ounces Gorgonzola dolce or other soft, mild blue cheese, broken into small pieces
- 4 cups baby arugula or spinach, about 3 ounces

1. In the bowl of an electric stand mixer, combine the water, yeast, and sugar. Stir briefly and let stand for 5 minutes or until the top surface has a thin, frothy layer (this incicates that the yeast is active). Add 4½ cups of the flour, the oil, and salt. Fit the mixer with the dough hook and mix on low speed for about 1 minute or until the dough begins to come together. Increase the speed to medium. Continue to mix until the dough is slightly sticky, smooth, and elastic, about 10 minutes. Form the dough into a ball and place in a lightly oiled bowl. Turn it over to coat all sides and tightly cover the bowl with plastic wrap. Allow the dough to rise in a warm place until it has doub ed in size, 1½ to 2 hours.

2. In a small bowl whisk the dressing ingredients.

3. Trim most of the exterior fat from the steaks. Allow to stand at room temperature for 20 to 30 minutes before grilling. Prepare the grill for direct cooking over high heat.

4. Punch down the dough in the bowl. Transfer to a lightly floured surface and cut into 4 equal pieces. Cut parchment

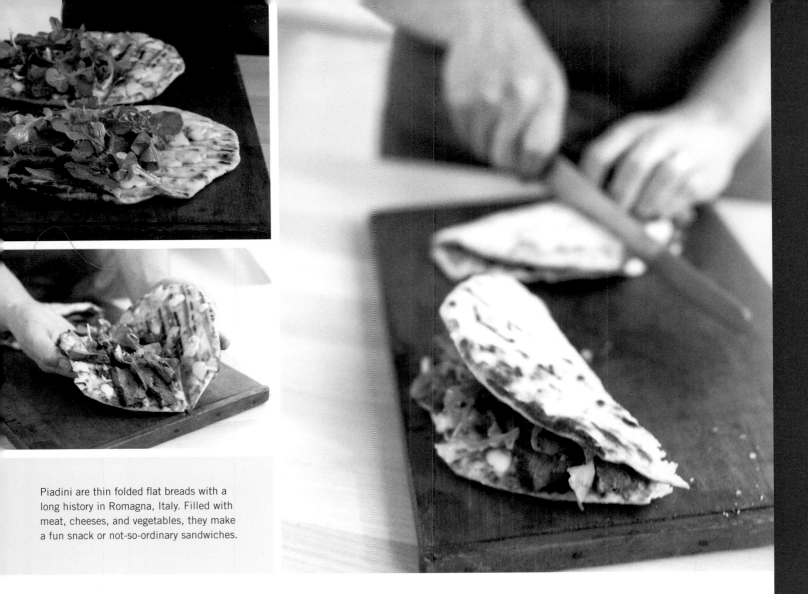

Piadini are thin folded flat breads with a long history in Romagna, Italy. Filled with meat, cheeses, and vegetables, they make a fun snack or not-so-ordinary sandwiches.

paper into 10-inch squares and lightly oil each sheet of paper on one side. Roll each piece of dough flat into rounds 8 to 10 inches in diameter. Lay each dough round on an oiled sheet of parchment paper and lightly oil the top of each round. Stack the dough rounds between the sheets of parchment paper and set aside on a sheet pan.

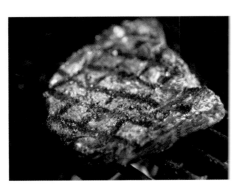

5. Lightly brush or spray both sides of the steaks with oil and season them evenly with salt and pepper. Brush the cooking grates clean. Grill the steaks over **direct high heat**, with the lid closed as much as possible, until cooked to your desired doneness, 6 to 8 minutes for medium rare, turning once (if flare-ups occur, move the steaks temporarily over *indirect high heat*). Remove from the grill, cover, and keep warm.

6. Reduce the temperature of the grill to medium heat. Lay 2 dough rounds over **direct medium heat**, with the paper sides facing up. Grab one corner of the paper with tongs and peel it off. Grill until the rounds are golden and marked on the underside, 2 to 3 minutes, rotating them occasionally for even cooking.

7. Turn the crusts over and distribute one quarter of the cheese over each crust, leaving a ½-inch border around the edges. Continue grilling over **direct medium heat** until the crusts are crisp and the cheese is melted, about 2 minutes, rotating the crusts occasionally for even cooking. Transfer the grilled crusts to a work surface. Repeat with the remaining crusts.

8. Place the greens in a salad bowl, pour the dressing over the greens, and toss to combine.

9. Cut the steaks into thin slices, removing any pockets of fat, and distribute evenly over the crusts, then top with equal portions of the salad. Fold each piadini in half and eat it like a sandwich or, for easier eating or sharing, cut each piadini in half with a serrated knife after folding.

WAY TO CUT BONE-IN STEAKS FROM A RIB ROAST

You can tell a lot about the taste and tenderness of a cut of meat by where it comes from on the animal. The parts of the animal that get a lot of exercise, like the shoulder and the back end (the round), develop more tough connective tissue than the parts of the animal that don't work so hard, like the loin and rib sections. From the loin, we get tender steaks like the porterhouse, the T-bone, and the New York strip. The rib section, pictured below, is where you'll find incredibly tender and succulent rib steaks.

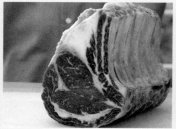 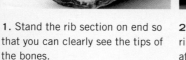 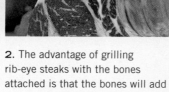 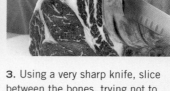 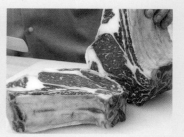

1. Stand the rib section on end so that you can clearly see the tips of the bones.

2. The advantage of grilling rib-eye steaks with the bones attached is that the bones will add mouthwatering flavor to the steaks and help keep the meat moist during cooking.

3. Using a very sharp knife, slice between the bones, trying not to saw back and forth too much. A hollow-ground knife will give the cleanest cut and best appearance.

4. What you have now is a big, brawny masterpiece called a bone-in rib-eye steak or, more simply, a rib steak.

WAY TO MAKE GARLIC PASTE

Fresh garlic on a steak lights up all the endorphins in my brain. When time is short and I'm craving a full-throttled steak experience, I always turn to chopped garlic. The only problem is, I often grill my steak over very high heat, and so the bits and pieces of garlic sometimes burn, turning them bitter. I avoid this problem by making a garlic paste instead. The paste melts into the surface of the meat, and all the fat and juices collected there prevent it from burning.

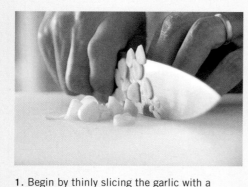 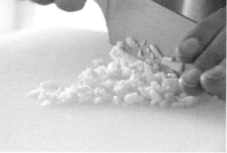 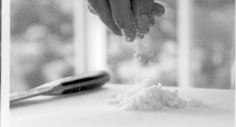

1. Begin by thinly slicing the garlic with a chef's knife.

2. Finely chop the garlic, keeping the knife tip on the board and moving the blade from side to side.

3. Add some kosher salt for flavor, crumbling it between your fingers if it is very coarse.

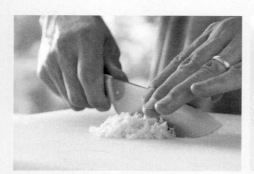 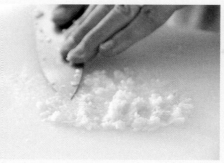 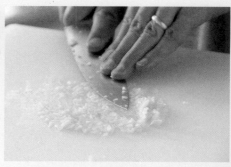

4. The salt will also hold the garlic together while you mince it.

5. Now, drag the side of the knife over the garlic, putting extra pressure near the tip, to smash the garlic into a paste.

6. Keep swishing the knife back and forth until the garlic is so thin it's almost transparent. Now it's ready to smear on your steaks.

RED MEAT

GARLIC-CRUSTED RIB-EYE STEAKS WITH GRILLED BROCCOLINI

SERVES: 4
PREP TIME: 15 MINUTES

WAY TO GRILL: DIRECT AND INDIRECT HIGH HEAT
(450° TO 550°F)
GRILLING TIME: 11 TO 15 MINUTES

PASTE

- 4 large garlic cloves
- 1 tablespoon kosher salt
- ¼ cup finely chopped fresh Italian parsley
- ¼ cup extra-virgin olive oil
- 2 teaspoons balsamic vinegar
- 1 teaspoon freshly ground black pepper

- 4 bone-in rib-eye steaks, 10 to 12 ounces each and about 1 inch thick, trimmed of excess fat
- ¾ pound broccolini, with stalks no wider than ½ inch
  Extra-virgin olive oil
  Kosher salt

1. On a cutting board finely chop the garlic, then sprinkle with the salt. Use the side of a knife to smash the garlic into a paste. Put the garlic paste into a small bowl and add the remaining paste ingredients.

2. Smear the paste evenly over both sides of each steak. Let the steaks stand at room temperature for 20 to 30 minutes before grilling. Meanwhile soak the broccolini.

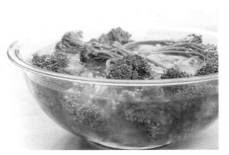

3. In a large bowl of water submerge the broccolini for 20 to 30 minutes so that they absorb water. This will help them steam a little on the grill.

4. Prepare your grill for direct and indirect cooking over high heat.

5. Pour off the water from the bowl of broccolini. Lightly drizzle some oil over the broccolini and season with ½ teaspoon salt. Toss to coat them evenly with oil and salt.

6. Brush the cooking grates clean. Grill the steaks over ***direct high heat***, with the lid closed as much as possible, until cooked to your desired doneness, 6 to 8 minutes for medium rare, turning once (if flare-ups occur, move the steaks temporarily over *indirect high heat*). Remove from the grill and let rest while you grill the broccolini.

7. Using tongs, lift the broccolini and allow any excess oil to drip back into the bowl. Grill the broccolini over ***direct high heat***, with the lid closed as much as possible, until lightly charred, 3 to 4 minutes, turning occasionally. Finish cooking the broccolini over ***indirect high heat*** for 2 to 3 minutes. Serve warm with the steaks.

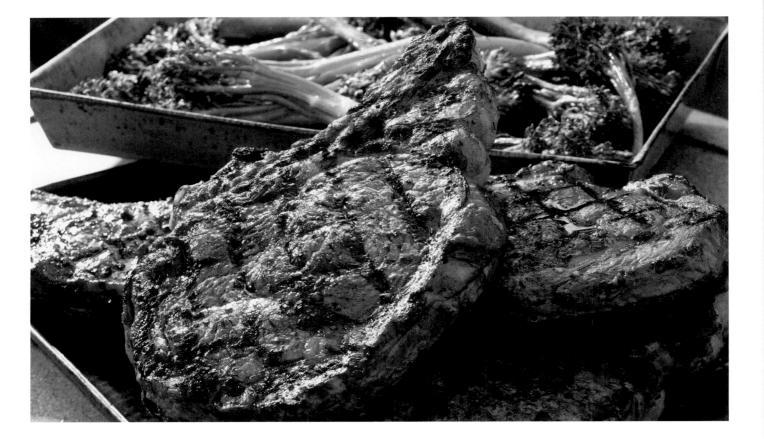

WAY TO MAKE TEA PASTE

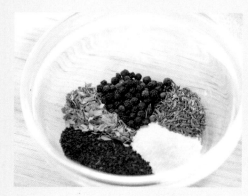 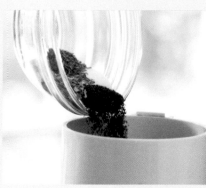 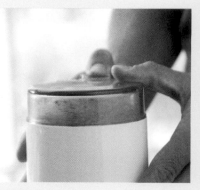

1. A bit of Earl Grey tea leaves adds a deep, unexpected fragrance to this spice rub.

2. To get the best peppery zing, grind whole black peppercorns in a spice mill with the other seasonings. As with other spices, whole peppercorns retain more aromatic flavor than pre-ground pepper.

3. Pulse all the seasonings into a coarse blend to release their flavors, then mix them in a bowl with oil to make a paste.

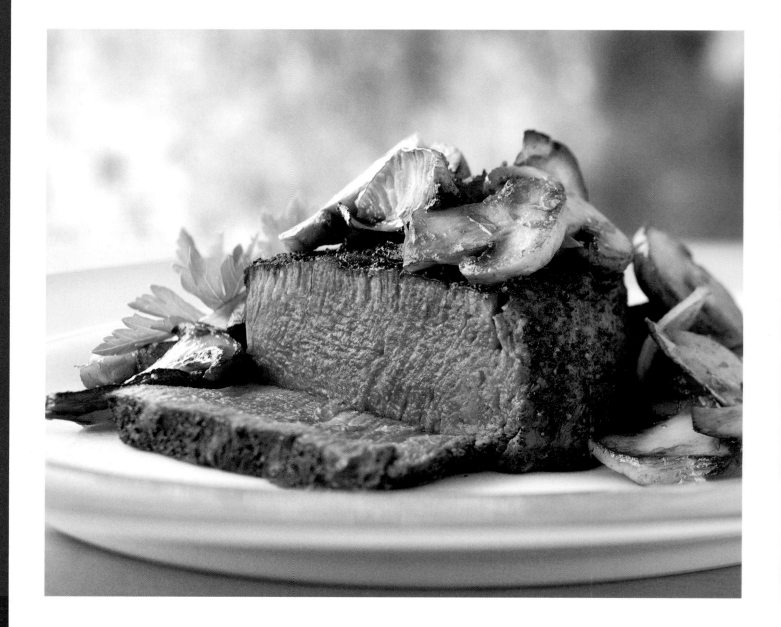

TEA-RUBBED FILET MIGNON STEAKS WITH BUTTERY MUSHROOMS

SERVES: 4
PREP TIME: 25 MINUTES

WAY TO GRILL: DIRECT MEDIUM HEAT (350° TO 450°F)
GRILLING TIME: ABOUT 8 MINUTES
SPECIAL EQUIPMENT: SPICE MILL, 12-INCH
    CAST-IRON SKILLET

PASTE
- 2 teaspoons (about 2 tea bags) Earl Grey tea leaves
- 1 teaspoon whole black peppercorns
- 1 teaspoon dried tarragon
- 1 teaspoon kosher salt
- ½ teaspoon dried thyme
- 3 tablespoons extra-virgin olive oil

- 4 filet mignon steaks, each about 8 ounces and 1½ inches thick

MUSHROOMS
- ½ pound button mushrooms
- 2 tablespoons unsalted butter
- 2 tablespoons extra-virgin olive oil
- 4 large garlic cloves, thinly sliced
- ¼ teaspoon kosher salt
- ⅛ teaspoon freshly ground black pepper
- ¼ cup roughly chopped fresh Italian parsley
- 1 teaspoon sherry or red wine vinegar

1. In a spice mill, whirl the tea leaves, peppercorns, tarragon, salt, and thyme until finely ground. Pour the spice mix into a bowl, add the oil, and stir to make a paste.

2. Brush all sides of each filet with the paste. Let stand at room temperature for 20 to 30 minutes before grilling.

3. Before you grill the steaks, prepare the mushrooms and have all the other ingredients in place. Lay the mushrooms on their sides. Cut off a ¼-inch slice lengthwise, and then roll the mushrooms over so the flat sides are on your cutting board and the mushrooms no longer roll around. Then cut the mushrooms lengthwise into ¼-inch slices.

4. Prepare the grill for direct cooking over medium heat.

5. Brush the cooking grates clean. Grill the steaks over *direct medium heat*, with the lid closed as much as possible, until cooked to your desired doneness, about 8 minutes for medium rare, turning once. Remove from the grill and let rest while you sauté the mushrooms.

6. In a 12-inch cast-iron skillet over high heat (on your grill's side burner or on your stove top), melt the butter with the olive oil. Add the mushrooms and spread them out in a single layer so that most of them are touching the bottom of the skillet. Cook the mushrooms without moving them for 2 minutes. Stir the mushrooms, and then add the garlic, salt, and pepper. Cook until the mushrooms are barely tender, 2 to 3 minutes, stirring 2 or 3 times. Add the parsley and vinegar. Mix well. Season to taste with salt and pepper, if needed. Spoon the hot mushrooms over the steaks.

WAY TO BROWN MUSHROOMS

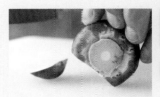
1. Cut off one round edge to make a flat, stable surface.

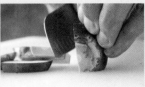
2. Then cut ¼-inch slices.

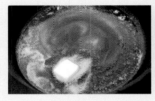
3. Melt the butter with a little oil, which helps to prevent the butter from burning.

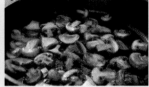
4. Spread the mushrooms in a single layer and don't touch them for 2 minutes.

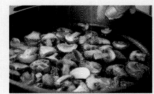
5. Add the salt toward the end of cooking because it draws moisture out of the mushrooms and hinders browning.

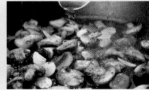
6. A little sherry vinegar near the end of cooking cuts the richness of the butter.

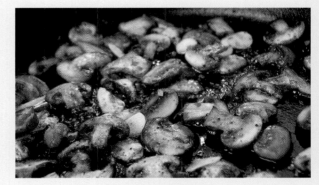
7. By resisting the urge to stir the mushrooms often, you will brown them better and create deeper flavors.

WAY TO MAKE FLAVORED BUTTER

If you like to grill steaks—or any kind of meat, fish, or poultry, for that matter—I think you should have at least one flavored butter waiting for you at all times in the refrigerator or freezer. One of the surest ways to please your palate and delight your guests is to crown each grilled steak with a savory slice of butter blended with the flavors of your choice. The heat of the steak will melt the butter and send the flavors running to mingle with the meat juices for a luxurious sauce.

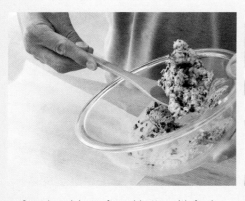

1. Start by mixing softened butter with fresh herbs and other seasonings, along with shallots that have been simmered in red wine.

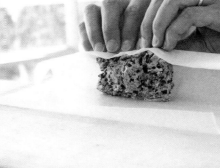

2. Shape the butter into a little log on parchment paper.

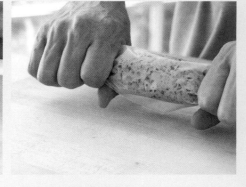

3. Wrap the log tightly in the paper and squeeze both ends to compact it.

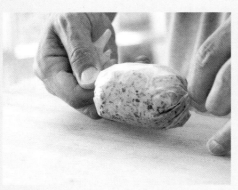

4. Twist the ends of the parchment wrapper in opposite directions and store the flavored butter in the refrigerator.

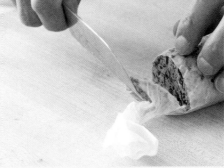

5. When it's time to serve, trim off one end.

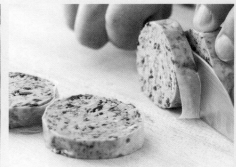

6. Cut as many rounds as you need and pull off the paper.

WAY TO MAKE CROSSHATCH MARKS

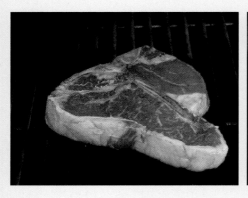

1. For a nice diamond pattern on your steaks, position them at a 45-degree angle to the bars of the cooking grate.

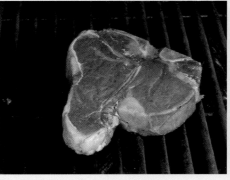

2. After searing for a couple of minutes, rotate your steaks 90 degrees.

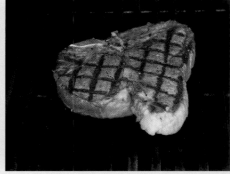

3. Turn the steaks over and, if you like, mark the other side in the same way.

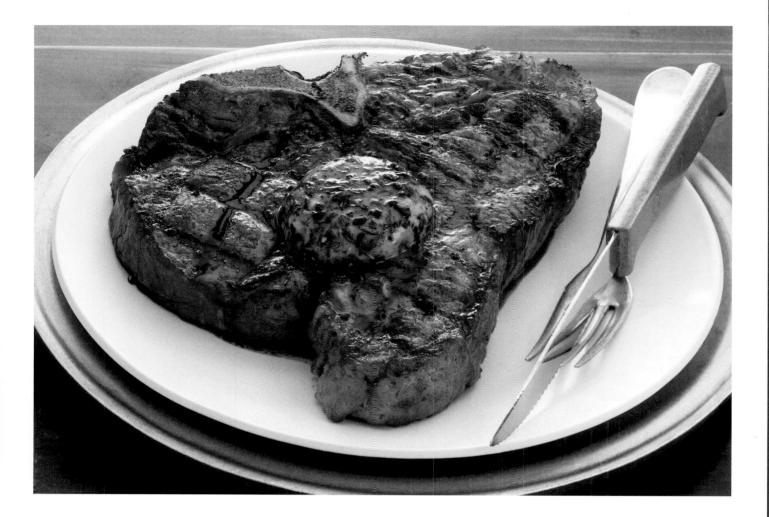

PORTERHOUSE STEAKS WITH RED WINE-SHALLOT BUTTER

SERVES: 4 TO 6
PREP TIME: 15 MINUTES

WAY TO GRILL: DIRECT HIGH HEAT (450° TO 550°F)
GRILLING TIME: 8 TO 10 MINUTES

BUTTER
   3 tablespoons hearty red wine
   2 tablespoons minced shallot
  ½ cup (1 stick) unsalted butter, softened
   1 tablespoon minced fresh Italian parsley
   1 tablespoon minced fresh tarragon
  ½ teaspoon kosher salt
  ¼ teaspoon freshly ground black pepper

   4 porterhouse steaks, each about 1 pound
     and 1 inch thick
   2 tablespoons extra-virgin olive oil
   2 teaspoons kosher salt
  ½ teaspoon freshly ground black pepper

1. In a small, heavy-bottomed saucepan over high heat, bring the wine and shallot to a boil. Boil until the wine is reduced to a glaze and is absorbed mostly by the shallots, 3 to 5 minutes. Transfer to a bowl and let cool completely.

2. Add the butter, parsley, tarragon, salt, and pepper to the shallot wine reduction and mix to combine. Scoop the mixture out of the bowl onto a sheet of parchment or wax paper. Loosely shape the mixture into a log about 1 inch in diameter. Roll the log in the paper and twist the ends in opposite directions to form an even cylinder. Refrigerate until about 1 hour before serving. (The butter can be made up to 1 week ahead.)

3. Allow the steaks to stand at room temperature for 20 to 30 minutes before grilling. Prepare the grill for direct cooking over high heat.

4. Lightly brush the steaks with the oil and season evenly with the salt and pepper. Brush the cooking grates clean. Grill the steaks over *direct high heat* with the lid closed as much as possible, until cooked to your desired doneness, 8 to 10 minutes for medium rare, turning once (if flare-ups occur, move the steaks temporarily over *indirect high heat*). Remove the steaks from the grill and let rest for 3 to 5 minutes. Serve the steaks hot with the butter smeared over the top.

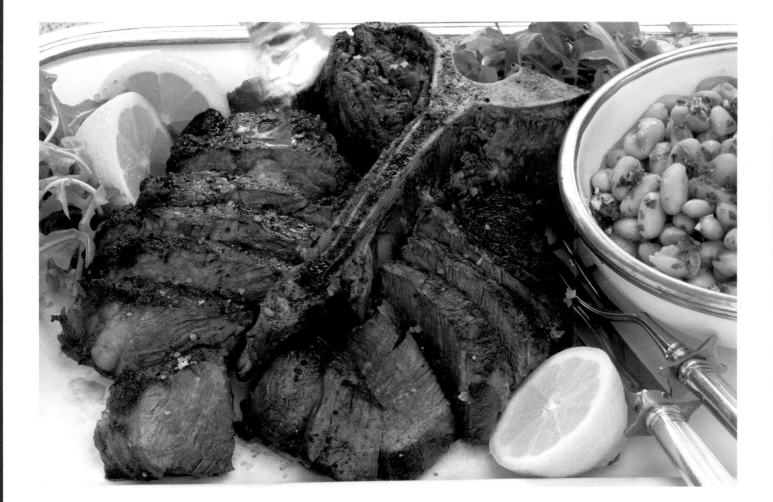

WAY TO GRILL REALLY THICK STEAKS

One of the noblest dishes in the pantheon of international grilled steaks is Bistecca alla Fiorentina, an enormous porterhouse steak jockeyed over and beside the hot coals until the outside is crisply charred and the interior is just rosy red and deliciously tender. The seasonings are pure and simple—nothing more than coarse salt, preferably sea salt, and freshly ground black pepper. The finishing touches are a squeeze of lemon juice and a drizzle of the best olive oil in the house.

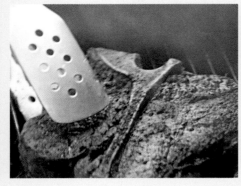

1. Whereas most steaks do best when you don't fiddle with them on the grill, this one is so thick and monstrous that you will need to move it every few minutes.

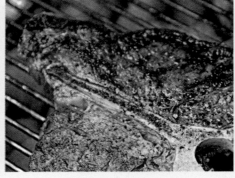

2. Charcoal fires are inherently uneven, so don't be surprised if one part of the steak browns faster than another. Move the steak around to compensate for the unevenness.

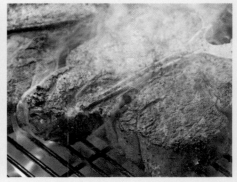

3. This is a case where the charcoal is as much an ingredient in the recipe as the seasonings. The smokiness permeates the meat and delivers great primordial flavors.

BISTECCA ALLA FIORENTINA

SERVES: 4
PREP TIME: 5 MINUTES

WAY TO GRILL: DIRECT AND INDIRECT MEDIUM HEAT
   (350° TO 450°F)
GRILLING TIME: 25 TO 27 MINUTES

  1 porterhouse steak, about 2½ pounds and
     2¼ inches thick
     Gray or coarse sea salt
     Freshly ground black pepper
  2 lemons
     Extra-virgin olive oil

1. Let the steak rest at room temperature for 1 hour before grilling. During this hour, you can prepare and cook the grill-baked beans, and then keep them warm.

2. Prepare the grill for direct and indirect cooking over medium heat.

3. Liberally season the steak on both sides with salt and pepper. Rub the seasoning into the meat.

4. Grill the steak over **direct medium heat** for 10 to 12 minutes, rotating the steak 45 degrees about every 3 minutes to create a nice crust, turning once. Move the steak over **indirect medium heat** and continue to cook until the internal temperature reaches 125°F for rare, about 15 minutes, rotating the steak as needed for even cooking. Let the steak rest for about 10 minutes before carving.

5. To carve the steak, cut the filet side first as close to the bone as possible. Repeat the procedure for the strip steak. Slice each piece crosswise into ½-inch slices, keeping the slices intact. Transfer to a serving platter and reassemble the steak with the bone. Drizzle some extra-virgin olive oil over the slices and serve with fresh lemon and grill-baked beans.

GRILL-BAKED BEANS ALLA CONTADINA

PREP TIME: 10 MINUTES

WAY TO GRILL: INDIRECT MEDIUM HEAT (350° TO 450°F)
GRILLING TIME: ABOUT 15 MINUTES

  2 cans (14 ounces each) cannellini beans, rinsed
 ¾ cup low-sodium vegetable stock
 ¼ cup tomato sauce
  1 tablespoon extra-virgin olive oil
  1 teaspoon minced fresh thyme
 ½ teaspoon kosher salt
  1 teaspoon minced garlic
  1 tablespoon plus 1 teaspoon minced fresh Italian parsley

1. Prepare the grill for indirect cooking over medium heat.

2. Place the beans in a 9-inch square ovenproof baking dish.

3. In a small bowl combine the stock, tomato sauce, oil, thyme, and salt. Pour over the beans. Lightly press the beans so they are all immersed in the liquid. Bake the beans over **indirect medium heat**, with the lid closed, until they are bubbling and most of the liquid has reduced, about 15 minutes.

4. Blend the garlic with the parsley and scatter over the beans. Serve with the steak.

■■■

This steak dish hails from the culinary epicenter of Tuscany, so it is more than appropriate to serve it with another famed dish from that region of Italy: white beans simmered with stock, tomatoes, and herbs.

■■■

WAY TO CARVE BISTECCA

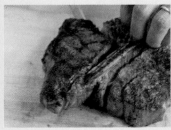 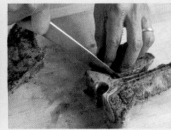 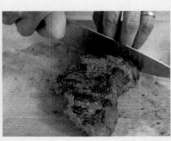 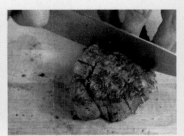

1. The porterhouse is a large cut that includes a T-shaped bone, with meat from the strip loin on one side and the tenderloin on the other.

2. The traditional way to serve it is to cut all the meat from the bone in two big sections, then slice it.

3. Cut the strip loin crosswise in nice thick slices.

4. Also cut the tenderloin section in thick slices, and then arrange all the slices back along the bone.

SKIRT STEAKS WITH RED POTATOES AND FETA

SERVES: 4
PREP TIME: 15 MINUTES

WAY TO GRILL: INDIRECT AND DIRECT HIGH HEAT
   (450° TO 550°F)
GRILLING TIME: 34 TO 46 MINUTES
SPECIAL EQUIPMENT: PERFORATED GRILL PAN, LARGE
   DISPOSABLE FOIL PAN

RUB
   1 teaspoon kosher salt
   1 teaspoon ground cumin
  ½ teaspoon granulated garlic
  ¼ teaspoon freshly ground black pepper

1½ pounds small red-skinned potatoes,
     1½ to 2 inches in diameter, cut into quarters
   2 tablespoons extra-virgin olive oil
  ½ teaspoon kosher salt

   2 skirt steaks, about 12 ounces each,
     trimmed of excess surface fat

  ½ cup crumbled feta cheese
   2 tablespoons chopped fresh Italian parsley
     Kosher salt
     Freshly ground black pepper

1. Prepare the grill for indirect and direct cooking over high heat.

2. In a small bowl combine the rub ingredients.

3. In a large bowl combine the potatoes, oil, and salt and stir to coat them evenly.

4. Preheat a grill pan over **_indirect high heat_** for about 10 minutes. Add the potatoes to the pan and grill them, with the lid closed as much as possible, until they are golden brown and tender, 30 to 40 minutes, turning 2 or 3 times.

5. After the potatoes have cooked for about 10 minutes, season the steaks evenly with the rub, pressing the spices into the meat. Let the meat stand at room temperature for 20 to 30 minutes before grilling.

6. When the potatoes are fully cooked, transfer them to a large disposable foil pan. Add the cheese and parsley. Mix well and then season to taste with salt and pepper. To keep the potatoes warm, place the pan over indirect heat while the steaks cook.

7. Grill the steaks over **_direct high heat_**, with the lid closed as much as possible, until cooked to your desired doneness, 4 to 6 minutes for medium rare, turning once. Transfer the steaks to a cutting board and let rest for 3 to 5 minutes. Keep the potatoes warm on the grill. Cut the meat across the grain into thin slices. Serve warm with the potatoes.

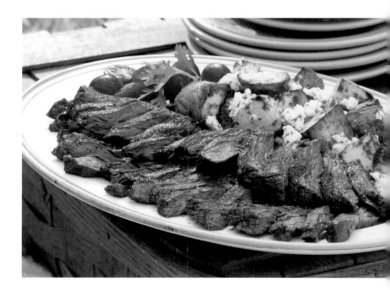

WAY TO PREP SKIRT STEAK

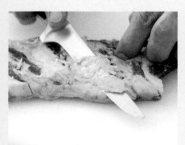

1. With a sharp knife, trim away most of the fat that clings to both sides of the skirt steaks.

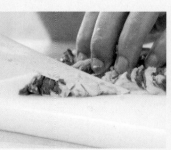

2. Thoroughly trimming the fat will help prevent flare-ups.

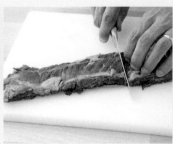

3. Cutting the steaks into lengths of about 1 foot will make them easier to handle on the grill.

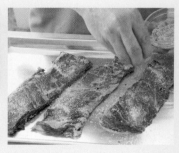

4. Season the meat generously with the rub, patting and massaging it in with your fingertips so it won't fall off during grilling.

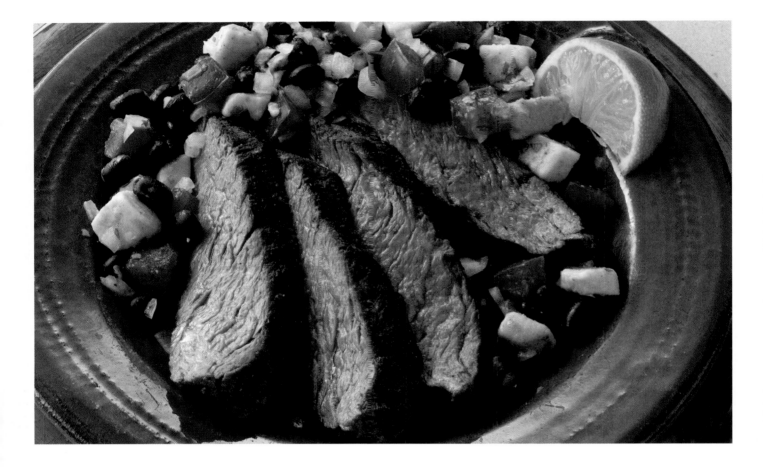

CARNE ASADA WITH BLACK BEAN AND AVOCADO SALSA

SERVES: 4 TO 6
PREP TIME: 20 MINUTES

WAY TO GRILL: DIRECT HIGH HEAT (450° TO 550°F)
GRILLING TIME: 4 TO 6 MINUTES

SALSA
- 1 can (15 ounces) black beans, rinsed
- 1 ripe Haas avocado, finely chopped
- 1 cup finely chopped white onion, rinsed in a sieve
- 1 cup finely chopped ripe tomato
- 2 tablespoons roughly chopped fresh cilantro
- 1 tablespoon fresh lime juice
- ½ teaspoon kosher salt
- ¼ teaspoon chipotle chile powder
- ¼ teaspoon ground cumin
- ⅛ teaspoon freshly ground black pepper

RUB
- 1 teaspoon chipotle chile powder
- 1 teaspoon kosher salt
- ½ teaspoon ground cumin
- ¼ teaspoon freshly ground black pepper

- 1½ pounds skirt steak, trimmed of excess fat
  Extra-virgin olive oil

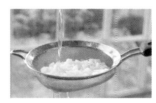

Raw onions can taste a little harsh in a salsa, but a good rinse will take the edge off.

1. In a medium, non-reactive bowl combine the salsa ingredients. Cover with plastic wrap, pressing the wrap directly onto the surface, and set aside at room temperature for as long as 2 hours before serving.

2. In a small bowl mix the rub ingredients. Cut the steak into foot-long pieces to make them easier to handle on the grill. Lightly coat both sides of the steaks with oil. Season evenly with the rub. Let stand at room temperature for 20 to 30 minutes before grilling. Prepare the grill for direct cooking over high heat.

3. Brush the cooking grates clean. Grill the steaks over ***direct high heat***, with the lid closed as much as possible, until cooked to your desired doneness, 4 to 6 minutes for medium rare, turning once or twice. Remove the steaks from the grill and let rest for 3 to 5 minutes.

4. Cut the steaks across the grain into ½-inch-thick slices. Serve warm with the salsa.

WAY TO PREP SHALLOTS

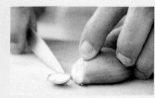 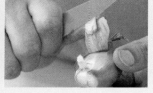

1. Trim off most of each root end.

2. Peel off the papery skin.

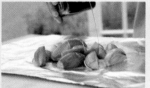 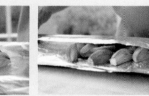

3. Spread the shallots on foil and drizzle with oil.

4. Wrap the foil over the shallots to make a neat packet.

WAY TO PREP FLATIRON STEAKS

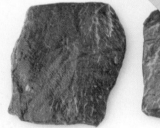 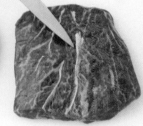

1. Some flatiron steaks, like the one on the right, have a tough streak running down the middle.

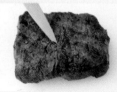 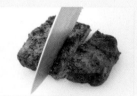

2. It's harder to see it after the steak is cooked.

3. To ensure that every slice is tender, cut away that tough streak before serving.

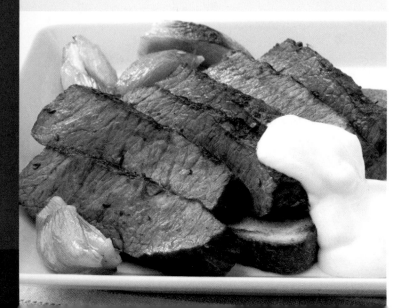

BISTRO STEAKS WITH MUSTARD CREAM SAUCE

SERVES: 4
PREP TIME: 15 MINUTES

WAY TO GRILL: INDIRECT AND DIRECT MEDIUM HEAT (350° TO 450°F)
GRILLING TIME: ABOUT 1 HOUR

- 8 large shallots, about 12 ounces total
  Extra-virgin olive oil
- 1¾ teaspoons kosher salt, divided
- 1 teaspoon dried thyme
- 1 teaspoon paprika
- ¾ teaspoon freshly ground black pepper
- 4 flatiron steaks, each 6 to 8 ounces and about 1 inch thick
- ½ cup sour cream
- 1 tablespoon Dijon mustard

1. Prepare the grill for indirect and direct cooking over medium heat.

2. Peel and trim the shallots, removing most of each root end. Cut the larger shallots in half lengthwise or pull apart the distinct halves. Pile the shallots in the middle of a large square of aluminum foil. Drizzle with 1 tablespoon of oil and season with ¼ teaspoon of the salt. Fold up the sides and seal to make a packet. Grill over **indirect medium heat**, with the lid closed as much as possible, until a knife slides easily in and out of the shallots, 20 to 30 minutes, turning once or twice. Open the packet and continue to cook the shallots in the foil until nicely browned, 20 to 30 minutes more, turning the shallots very gently once or twice. Remove the packet from the grill.

3. In a small bowl mix the remaining 1½ teaspoons of salt with the thyme, paprika, and pepper. Lightly coat the steaks on both sides with oil. Season evenly with the spices. Let the steaks stand at room temperature for 20 to 30 minutes before grilling.

4. In a small bowl combine the sour cream and mustard.

5. Brush the cooking grates clean. Grill the steaks over **direct medium heat**, with the lid closed as much as possible, until cooked to your desired doneness, 8 to 10 minutes for medium rare, turning once. At the same time reheat the packet of shallots over **indirect medium heat**. Remove the steaks from the grill and let rest for 3 to 5 minutes before slicing. While the steaks rest, remove any charred outer layers from the shallots.

6. Cut each steak lengthwise on either side of the gristle that runs down the middle. Thinly slice the steak against the grain and shingle the slices on serving dishes. Serve the steaks warm with the shallots and sauce.

SESAME-GINGER FLANK STEAK WITH ASPARAGUS AND GOMASHIO

SERVES: 4 TO 6
PREP TIME: 25 MINUTES
MARINATING TIME: 3 TO 4 HOURS

WAY TO GRILL: DIRECT MEDIUM HEAT (350° TO 450°F)
GRILLING TIME: 12 TO 16 MINUTES
SPECIAL EQUIPMENT: MORTAR AND PESTLE

MARINADE
- 5 tablespoons soy sauce
- 2 tablespoons granulated sugar
- 3 tablespoons rice wine vinegar
- 2 tablespoons toasted sesame oil
- 1 tablespoon minced garlic
- 1½ tablespoons grated ginger
- 1½ teaspoons sambal oelek or other ground fresh chili paste
- 1 cup finely chopped scallions, white and light green parts
- ¼ cup coarsely chopped fresh cilantro

- 1 flank steak, 1½ to 2 pounds and about ¾ inch thick

GOMASHIO
- ¼ cup sesame seed
- 1 teaspoon sea salt

ASPARAGUS
- 1 large bunch asparagus, about 1 pound
- 1 tablespoon extra-virgin olive oil
- ½ teaspoon kosher salt

- 2 tablespoons finely chopped fresh cilantro or Italian parsley

1. In a small bowl whisk the soy sauce, sugar, vinegar, oil, garlic, ginger, and chili paste. Add the scallions and cilantro. Place the steak in a non-reactive (glass or stainless steel) dish and pour in the marinade, turning the steak to coat both sides. Cover and refrigerate for 3 to 4 hours, turning the steak once or twice.

2. Toast the sesame seeds in a clean, dry nonstick skillet over low heat. Shake and stir until the seeds are golden brown, but before they begin to pop, 2 to 3 minutes. Turn out onto a plate and allow to cool for 10 minutes. Add the sea salt and combine in a mortar and pestle. Lightly crush the seeds so that some texture remains; do not make a fine powder. (The unused portion can be stored in a glass jar in the refrigerator for up to 2 months.)

3. Snap or cut off the dry, woody ends from the asparagus spears. Lightly coat them with the oil and season with the salt.

4. Prepare the grill for direct cooking over medium heat.

5. Remove the steak from the refrigerator and allow to stand at room temperature for 20 to 30 minutes before grilling. Brush

WAY TO MAKE GOMASHIO

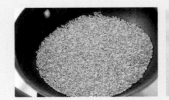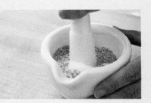

1. Toast the sesame seeds just until they start to color.

2. Grind coarsely with sea salt to make a delicious seasoning.

WAY TO SLICE FLANK STEAK

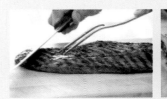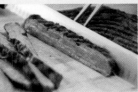

1. For the sake of tenderness, cut flank steak crosswise, or against the grain.

2. Keep the slices no thicker than about ⅓ inch.

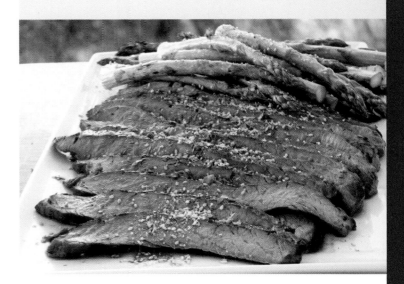

the cooking grates clean. Grill the steak over **direct medium heat**, with the lid closed as much as possible, until cooked to your desired doneness, 8 to 10 minutes for medium rare, turning once. Transfer to a cutting board and let rest while you grill the asparagus.

6. Arrange the asparagus perpendicular to the bars on the cooking grate. Grill over **direct medium heat**, with the lid closed as much as possible, until lightly charred and crisp-tender, 4 to 6 minutes, rolling the spears a couple of times. Remove the spears from the grill and arrange on one side of a large platter.

7. Thinly slice the steak on the bias and arrange on the platter with the asparagus. Sprinkle the gomashio and cilantro all over. Serve warm.

WAY TO STUFF AND ROLL FLANK STEAK

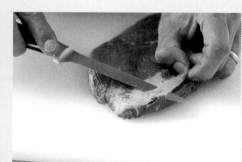

1. Trim the silver skin and most of the fat from the surface of the meat.

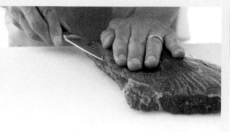

2. Holding your knife parallel to the board, make a shallow cut along the length of the steak.

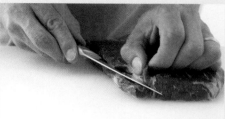

3. Slice again, making the cut a little deeper.

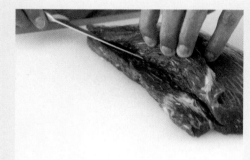

4. Keep making strokes with the tip of your knife as you open up the meat with your other hand.

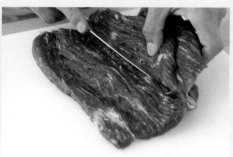

5. Continue cutting until you come within about ½ inch from the opposite edge.

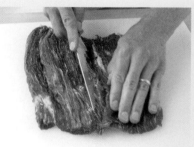

6. Now open the steak like a book, laying it flat.

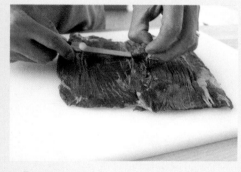

7. Turn the steak over and carefully trim off the seam that sticks up.

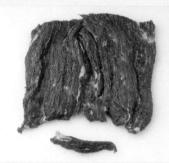

8. Turn the steak back over so the cut side is facing up.

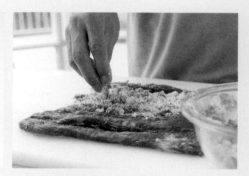

9. With the grain of the meat running horizontally, spread the stuffing mixture to within an inch of the outer edges and a few inches from the top.

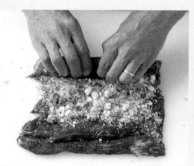

10. Roll up the meat from the bottom edge to the top.

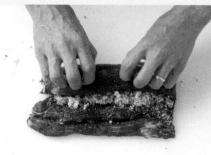

11. With no stuffing at the top of the meat, all the ingredients will stay nicely inside the roll.

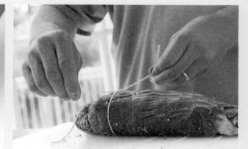

12. Tie the roll every couple of inches with lengths of butcher's twine.

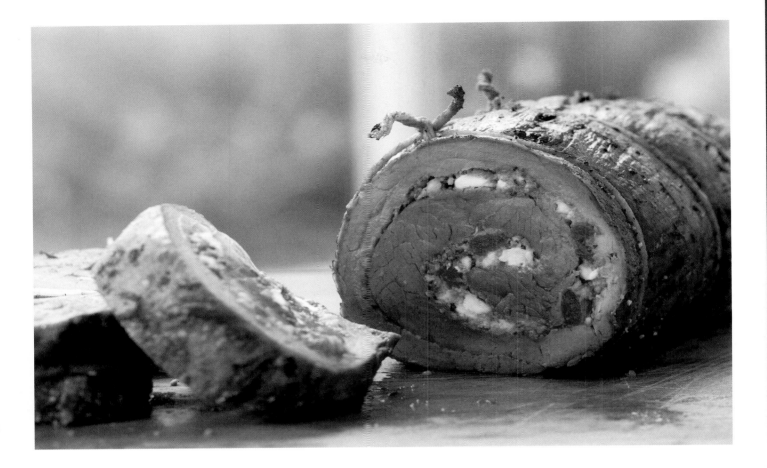

FLANK STEAK WITH ROASTED PEPPER AND FETA STUFFING

SERVES: 6
PREP TIME: 40 MINUTES

WAY TO GRILL: INDIRECT MEDIUM HEAT (350° TO 450°F)
GRILLING TIME: 20 TO 30 MINUTES
SPECIAL EQUIPMENT: BUTCHER'S TWINE

- 3 ounces feta cheese, drained and crumbled
- ½ cup dried bread crumbs
- 1 small red bell pepper, roasted, peeled, seeded, and diced
- 1 large garlic clove
- ⅓ cup loosely packed fresh Italian parsley
- 1 tablespoon fresh thyme
- ½ teaspoon kosher salt
- ¼ teaspoon freshly ground black pepper

- 2 flank steaks, about 1½ pounds each
- 1 tablespoon extra-virgin olive oil
  Kosher salt
  Freshly ground black pepper

1. In a medium bowl combine the cheese, bread crumbs, and diced pepper. Finely chop the garlic and fresh herbs together and add to the bowl. Blend thoroughly with a fork. Season with the salt and pepper.

2. Lay out the flank steak on a cutting board. Starting near one end of the steak, carefully insert a boning knife horizontally into one long edge (the edge parallel to the grain), splitting the steak evenly top to bottom. Continue this cut until the entire steak can be opened up like a book (see directions at left). Repeat with the other flank steak.

3. Prepare your grill for indirect cooking over medium heat.

4. Evenly spread the stuffing mixture over the inside of the butterflied steaks to within an inch of the edges and a few inches from the top (you may not need all of it). Be careful not to overstuff or it will just fall out and make it harder to roll. Roll up the steaks around the filling, with the grain running the length of the roll. Tie the rolls every few inches with butcher's twine. Brush the outside of the rolls with oil and lightly season with salt and pepper.

5. Brush the cooking grates clean. Grill over **indirect medium heat**, with the lid closed as much as possible, until cooked to your desired doneness, 20 to 30 minutes for medium rare, turning once. Transfer to a carving board, lightly cover with foil, and let rest for 10 minutes before slicing.

6. To serve, cut the rolls into ½- to ¾-inch slices. Serve warm.

ARGENTINE BEEF SKEWERS WITH CHIMICHURRI SAUCE

SERVES: 4 TO 6
PREP TIME: 20 MINUTES

WAY TO GRILL: DIRECT HIGH HEAT (450° TO 550°F)
GRILLING TIME: 6 TO 8 MINUTES
SPECIAL EQUIPMENT: BAMBOO SKEWERS,
  SOAKED IN WATER FOR AT LEAST 30 MINUTES

SAUCE
    1 cup fresh Italian parsley leaves and tender stems
    ½ cup fresh basil leaves
    ¼ cup finely chopped white onion, rinsed
    ¼ cup finely chopped carrot
    1 medium garlic clove
    ½ teaspoon kosher salt
    6 tablespoons extra-virgin olive oil
    2 tablespoons rice vinegar

RUB
    1½ teaspoons kosher salt
    ½ teaspoon paprika
    ½ teaspoon ground coriander
    ½ teaspoon ground cumin
    ¼ teaspoon freshly ground black pepper

    2 pounds top sirloin, 1 to 1¼ inches thick,
       cut into 1-inch cubes
       Extra-virgin olive oil
   18 large cherry tomatoes

1. In a food processor or blender, finely chop the parsley, basil, onion, carrot, garlic, and salt. With the machine running, add the oil and vinegar in a steady stream, using just enough oil to create a fairly thick sauce.

2. In a small bowl mix the rub ingredients.

3. Place the meat cubes in a large bowl. Lightly coat the meat with oil and then season with the rub, stirring to coat the meat evenly. Allow the meat to stand at room temperature for 20 to 30 minutes before grilling. Prepare the grill for direct cooking over high heat.

4. Thread the meat and tomatoes alternately onto skewers. Brush the cooking grates clean. Grill the skewers over **direct high heat,** with the lid closed as much as possible, until cooked to your desired doneness, 6 to 8 minutes for medium rare, turning occasionally. Serve warm with the sauce on the side or drizzled over the top.

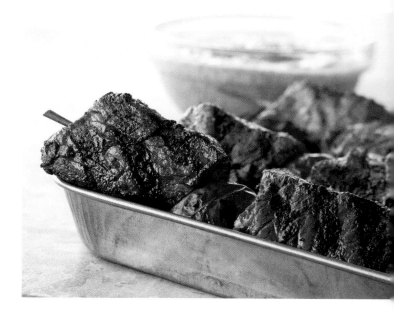

WAY TO CUBE TOP SIRLOIN

When making kabobs, the goal is to create cubes of the same size and thickness so they all cook at the same rate.

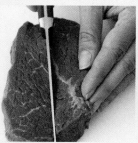

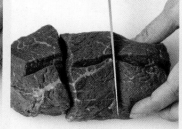

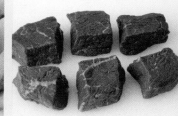

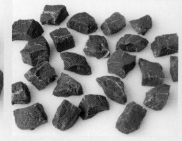

1. Start with a nice even piece of sirloin at least 1 inch thick.

2. Cut it down the center and side to side in whichever way leaves you with 1-inch cubes.

3. With so many flat sides, you now have plenty of opportunities to lightly char and flavor the surface of the meat.

4. If some cubes end up a little smaller than most, combine all the small ones on a skewer or two of their own and grill them for a shorter time.

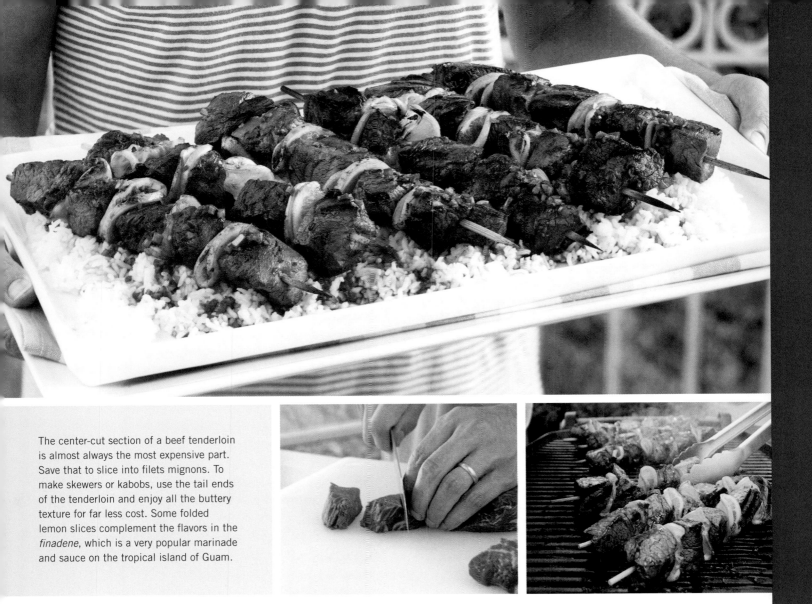

The center-cut section of a beef tenderloin is almost always the most expensive part. Save that to slice into filets mignons. To make skewers or kabobs, use the tail ends of the tenderloin and enjoy all the buttery texture for far less cost. Some folded lemon slices complement the flavors in the *finadene*, which is a very popular marinade and sauce on the tropical island of Guam.

BEEF TENDERLOIN KABOBS WITH FINADENE

SERVES: 4 TO 6
PREP TIME: 20 MINUTES
MARINATING TIME: 1 TO 2 HOURS

WAY TO GRILL: DIRECT HIGH HEAT (450° TO 550°F)
GRILLING TIME: 4 TO 6 MINUTES
SPECIAL EQUIPMENT: BAMBOO SKEWERS,
    SOAKED IN WATER FOR AT LEAST 30 MINUTES

SAUCE
  ½ cup soy sauce
  ¼ cup finely minced white onion
  3 tablespoons fresh lemon juice
  3 tablespoons water
  1 teaspoon minced jalapeño chile

  1 beef tenderloin roast, about 2½ pounds
  ¼ cup extra-virgin olive oil
  2 lemons, thinly sliced

1. In a medium bowl mix the sauce ingredients. In a small bowl reserve ⅓ cup of the sauce to spoon over the grilled meat.

2. Trim any excess fat and sinew from the surface of the roast. Cut the roast crosswise into steaks about 1¼ inches thick. Then cut each steak into pieces 1 to 1½ inches thick, cutting away and discarding any clumps of fat and sinew. Place the meat into a large, resealable plastic bag and pour in the remaining sauce. Add the oil. Press the air out of the bag, seal tightly, and turn the bag several times to incorporate the oil and evenly coat the meat. Refrigerate for 1 to 2 hours.

3. Thread the meat onto skewers, placing a folded slice of lemon between each piece so that the meat cooks evenly. Let stand at room temperature for 20 to 30 minutes before grilling. Prepare the grill for direct cooking over high heat.

4. Brush the cooking grates clean. Grill the skewers over **direct high heat**, with the lid closed as much as possible, until the meat is cooked to your desired doneness, 4 to 6 minutes for medium rare, turning 2 or 3 times. Serve warm with the reserved sauce spooned over the top.

WAY TO PREP CUCUMBER

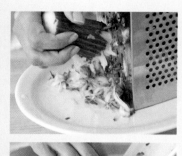

1. Grate the cucumber coarsely on the side of a box grater.

2. Arrange the pieces in the middle of a sturdy paper towel.

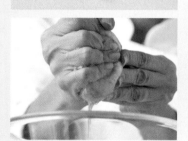

3. Squeeze gently to remove the water. Then mix the cucumbers into the sauce.

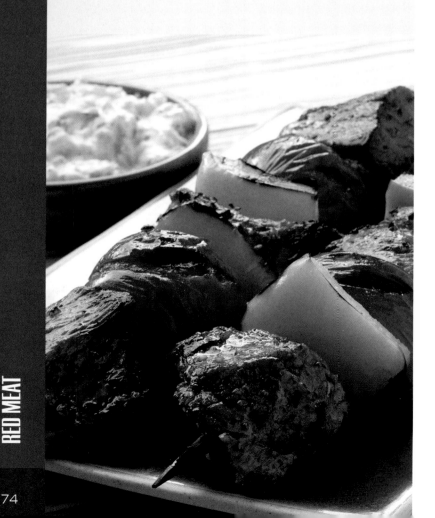

LAMB SOUVLAKI
WITH CUCUMBER-YOGURT SAUCE

SERVES: 4
PREP TIME: 20 MINUTES
MARINATING TIME: 3 TO 4 HOURS

WAY TO GRILL: DIRECT HIGH HEAT (450° TO 550°F)
GRILLING TIME: 6 TO 7 MINUTES
SPECIAL EQUIPMENT: BAMBOO SKEWERS,
    SOAKED IN WATER FOR AT LEAST 30 MINUTES

MARINADE
  ½ cup extra-virgin olive oil
  1 tablespoon finely chopped garlic
  1 tablespoon minced fresh oregano leaves or 1 teaspoon crumbled dried oregano
  1 teaspoon kosher salt
  ¼ teaspoon freshly ground black pepper

  1 boneless leg of lamb, about 1½ pounds, trimmed of excess fat, cut into 1½-inch chunks
  2 medium red or green bell peppers, cut into 1-inch squares
  24 large cherry tomatoes

SAUCE
  ½ English cucumber, coarsely grated
  1 cup plain Greek-style yogurt
  2 tablespoons minced red onion
  1 teaspoon finely grated lemon zest
  1 tablespoon fresh lemon juice
  ½ teaspoon minced garlic
    Kosher salt
    Freshly ground black pepper

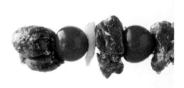

1. In a small bowl whisk the marinade ingredients. Thread the lamb chunks, pepper squares, and tomatoes alternately onto skewers. Place in a shallow dish, pour the marinade over the skewers, and turn to coat them evenly. Cover and refrigerate for 3 to 4 hours, turning occasionally. Allow to stand at room temperature for 20 to 30 minutes before grilling.

2. Squeeze the grated cucumber to remove as much liquid as possible. Transfer the cucumber to a small bowl and stir in the yogurt, onion, lemon zest, lemon juice, and garlic. Season to taste with salt and pepper. Cover and refrigerate until serving.

3. Prepare the grill for direct cooking over high heat. Brush the cooking grates clean. Remove the skewers from the dish and discard the marinade. Grill the skewers over **direct high heat**, with the lid closed as much as possible, until the meat is cooked to your desired doneness, 6 to 7 minutes for medium rare, turning occasionally. Serve the skewers warm with the sauce.

PORCINI-RUBBED VEAL CHOPS WITH HERBED MASCARPONE

SERVES: 4
PREP TIME: 15 MINUTES

WAY TO GRILL: DIRECT MEDIUM HEAT (350° TO 450°F)
GRILLING TIME: ABOUT 6 MINUTES
SPECIAL EQUIPMENT: SPICE MILL

MASCARPONE
⅓ cup mascarpone cheese
1 teaspoon minced fresh sage
¼ teaspoon kosher salt
¼ teaspoon freshly ground black pepper

¼ cup dried porcini mushrooms
2 teaspoons kosher salt
1 teaspoon freshly ground black pepper

4 veal rib chops, each about 8 ounces and 1 inch thick
Extra-virgin olive oil

1. In a small bowl mix the mascarpone ingredients. Cover and let stand at room temperature for 1 hour.

2. Using a spice mill, grind the mushrooms into a powder (this should yield 2 tablespoons). Put the powder into a small bowl and mix with the salt and pepper. Pour some oil onto a sheet pan and then sprinkle the seasoning over the oil. Dredge the chops through the oil mixture to coat them evenly. Cover and let stand at room temperature for 20 to 30 minutes before grilling. Prepare the grill for direct cooking over medium heat.

3. Brush the cooking grates clean. Grill the chops over **direct medium heat**, with the lid closed as much as possible, until cooked to your desired doneness, about 6 minutes for medium rare, turning once. Remove from the grill and let rest for 3 to 5 minutes. Serve the chops hot with the herbed mascarpone.

If your impression of veal comes mostly from over-breaded and overcooked cutlets, you owe it to yourself to try this chop. Quickly grilling a lean, bone-in veal chop over a fragrant fire, Tuscan style, results in a succulent, tender taste experience.

WAY TO PREP VEAL CHOPS

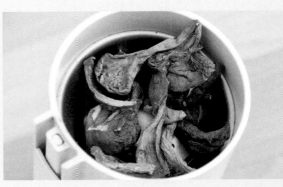

1. Dried porcini mushrooms star in this veal chop recipe. Pulverize them first in a spice mill or coffee grinder.

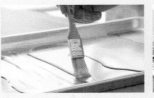 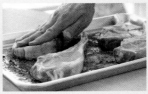

2. Pour some good olive oil onto a sheet pan and sprinkle the pulverized mushrooms along with salt and pepper, over the oil.

3. Press the veal chops into the oil and seasonings.

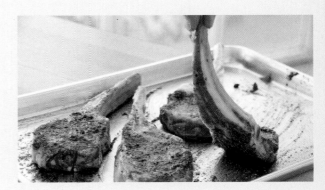

4. Drag each chop back and forth on both sides to get an even coating.

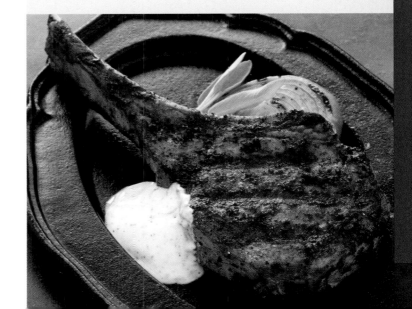

WAY TO FRENCH A RACK OF LAMB

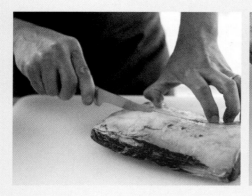

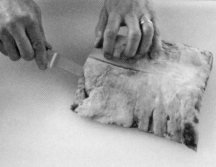

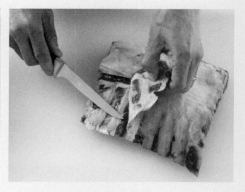

1. Frenching means removing the fat on the bones extending from a rack (or chop) and cleaning them thoroughly for a nice presentation.

2. Each rack of lamb has a "fat cap" that runs on top of the rib bones and meat. Make a cut through the fat at the base of the bones.

3. Use the knife to help lift off the fat cap.

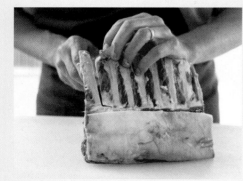

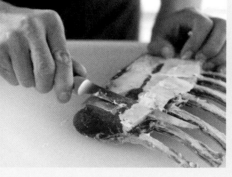

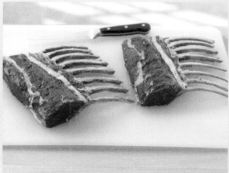

4. Use your knife to cut out the rib meat between the bones and to scrape the bones clean.

5. Then trim off the fat clinging to the loin meat, to prevent flare-ups.

6. Ideally the meat will be pinkish red, not purple. A dark color indicates an older animal.

WAY TO GRILL RACK OF LAMB

Lamb chops are a buttery-soft luxury. You can certainly grill them individually, but they are likely to be juicier and more succulent if you grill whole racks first and then cut them into chops.

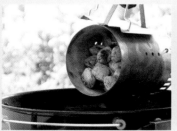

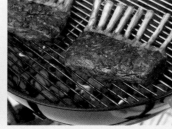

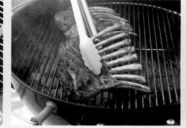

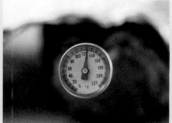

1. Prepare your grill by spreading the coals over one-half to three-quarters of the charcoal grate.

2. Grill the lamb as much as possible over direct heat.

3. If flare-ups occur, move the racks to the other side of the grill, over indirect heat.

4. Once the internal temperature reaches 125°F, remove the racks from the grill, loosely tent them with foil, and let them rest for about 5 minutes before cutting them into chops.

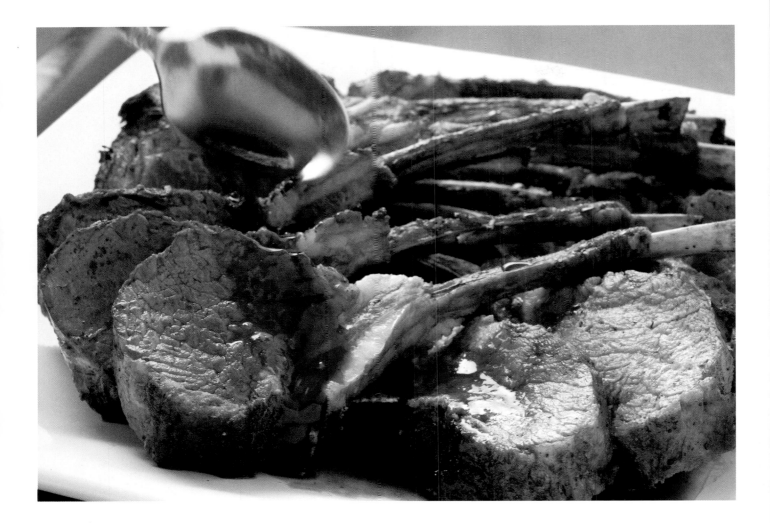

RACK OF LAMB WITH ORANGE-POMEGRANATE SYRUP

SERVES: 4 TO 6
PREP TIME: 40 MINUTES

WAY TO GRILL: DIRECT MEDIUM HEAT (350° TO 450°F)
GRILLING TIME: 15 TO 20 MINUTES

  2 lamb racks, 1 to 1½ pounds each

PASTE
  2 tablespoons extra-virgin olive oil
  1 tablespoon minced garlic
  1 tablespoon prepared chili powder
  2 teaspoons kosher salt
  1 teaspoon freshly ground black pepper

SYRUP
  ½ cup fresh orange juice
  ¼ cup pomegranate juice
  2 tablespoons honey
  1 tablespoon balsamic vinegar
  ½ teaspoon kosher salt

1. French the lamb racks as shown on the previous page.

2. In a small bowl mix the paste ingredients. Spread the paste over the lamb racks and allow them to stand at room temperature for 20 to 30 minutes before grilling.

3. In a small saucepan combine the orange juice, pomegranate juice, honey, and balsamic vinegar. Bring to a boil over high heat. Once boiling, reduce the heat to medium and simmer until the liquid has reduced to about ⅓ cup, 15 to 20 minutes. Season the light syrup with the salt and let cool. (You can refrigerate the syrup for up to 3 days.)

4. Prepare the grill for direct cooking over medium heat. Brush the cooking grates clean. Grill the lamb, bone sides down first, over **direct medium heat**, with the lid closed as much as possible, until cooked to your desired doneness, 15 to 20 minutes for medium rare, turning once or twice and moving the racks over indirect heat if flare-ups occur. Remove from the grill when the internal temperature reaches 125°F. Let the lamb rest for 5 minutes before carving into chops (the temperature will rise about 5 degrees during resting).

5. If necessary, warm the syrup over low heat until it reaches your desired consistency. Serve the lamb warm with the syrup drizzled on top.

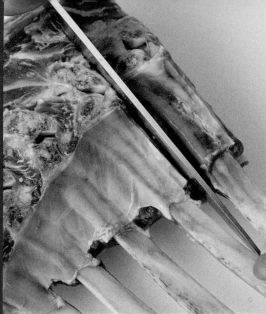

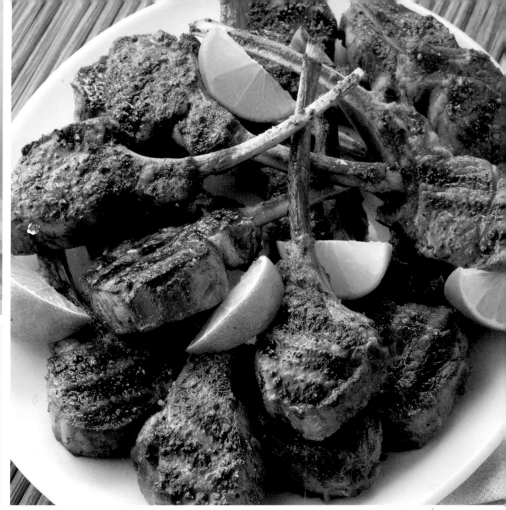

Of course you can buy pre-cut lamb rib chops, but cutting them yourself from a frenched rack of lamb will probably save you some money and assure you that each chop is the same thickness. For a clear look at where the bones are, face the meaty side of each rack down on a cutting board. Cut right between each pair of ribs.

LAMB CHOPS WITH INDIAN SPICES

SERVES: 4
PREP TIME: 10 MINUTES
MARINATING TIME: 1 TO 2 HOURS

WAY TO GRILL: DIRECT HIGH HEAT (450° TO 550°F)
GRILLING TIME: 4 TO 6 MINUTES

MARINADE
¼ cup extra-virgin olive oil
2 tablespoons fresh lime juice
1 tablespoon minced garlic
1½ teaspoons kosher salt
1 teaspoon ground coriander
1 teaspoon ground cumin
½ teaspoon ground ginger
½ teaspoon freshly ground black pepper

16 rib lamb chops, each about ¾ inch thick, trimmed of excess fat

1. In a small bowl whisk the marinade ingredients.

2. Arrange the chops on a large, rimmed plate. Spoon or brush the marinade over the chops, turning to coat them evenly. Cover with plastic wrap. Refrigerate for 1 to 2 hours.

3. Remove the chops from the refrigerator 20 to 30 minutes before grilling. Prepare the grill for direct cooking over high heat.

4. Brush the cooking grates clean. Grill the chops over **direct high heat**, with the lid closed as much as possible, until nicely marked on both sides and grilled to your desired doneness, 4 to 6 minutes for medium rare, turning once.

5. Remove the chops from the grill and let rest for 3 to 5 minutes. Serve warm.

LAMB CHOPS IN UZBEK MARINADE

SERVES: 4
PREP TIME: 10 MINUTES
MARINATING TIME: 3 TO 5 HOURS

WAY TO GRILL: DIRECT HIGH HEAT (450° TO 550°F)
GRILLING TIME: ABOUT 8 MINUTES

MARINADE/SAUCE

- 1 small yellow onion, cut into chunks
- 4 canned plum tomatoes
- ½ cup extra-virgin olive oil
- 4 large garlic cloves
- 2 tablespoons red wine vinegar
- 1 tablespoon sweet paprika
- 1 tablespoon dried thyme
- 1 tablespoon ground coriander
- 2 teaspoons ground cumin
- 2 teaspoons kosher salt
- ½ teaspoon ground cayenne pepper
- ½ teaspoon freshly ground black pepper

- 8 lamb loin chops, each about 1½ inches thick
  Extra-virgin olive oil

1. In the bowl of a food processor, process the marinade ingredients until very smooth, 1 to 2 minutes.

2. Arrange the chops side by side in a shallow dish. Pour the marinade over the chops and turn to coat them on all sides. Cover with plastic wrap and marinate in the refrigerator for 3 to 5 hours.

3. Remove the chops from the dish and wipe off most of the marinade. Discard the marinade. Lightly brush the chops with oil and let stand at room temperature for 20 to 30 minutes before grilling. Prepare the grill for direct cooking over high heat.

4. Brush the cooking grates clean. Grill the chops over **direct high heat**, with the lid closed as much as possible, until the chops are cooked to your desired doneness, about 8 minutes for medium rare, rotating and turning them once or twice for even cooking. Each time you lift the chops off the grate to rotate them or turn them over, place them down on a clean area of the grate, and brush away the bits of marinade that will cling to the grate as you go.

5. Remove the chops from the grill and let rest for 3 to 5 minutes. Serve warm.

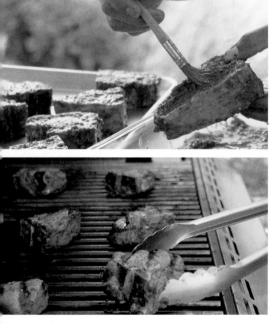

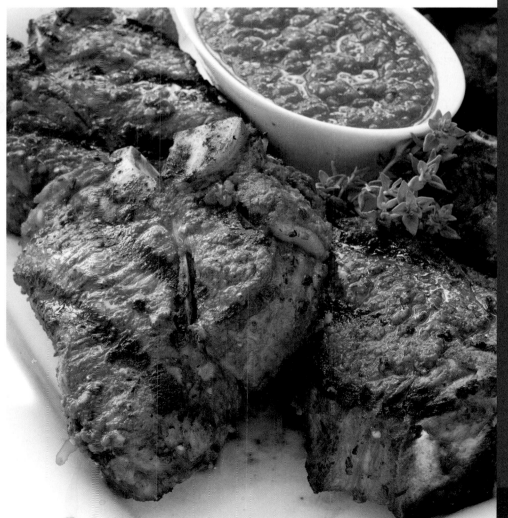

After marinating lamb chops in a thick, coarse puree, wipe off most of the marinade before putting the chops on the grill. Otherwise, the coating would prevent the chops from searing nicely and developing a good char on the outside. Don't worry; the flavors of the marinade will have imbued the meat itself.

WAY TO MAKE BASIL-GARLIC OIL

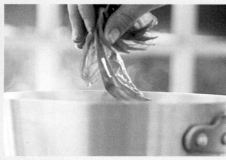

1. Bring a saucepan of salted water to a boil. Add the basil leaves and let them cook (blanch) for 10 seconds.

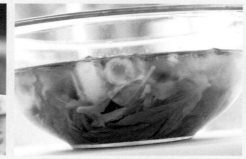

2. Immediately remove the basil with a slotted spoon and plunge the leaves into a bowl of ice water to stop the cooking and to retain the green color.

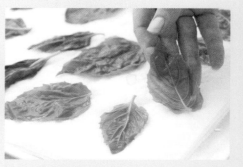

3. Lay the basil leaves on paper towels and pat them dry.

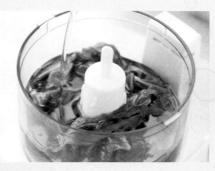

4. Combine the basil leaves, oil, and garlic in a food processor or blender.

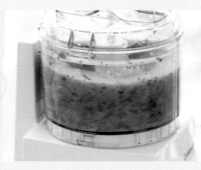

5. Process until the basil is pureed, and then season the mixture with salt and crushed red pepper flakes.

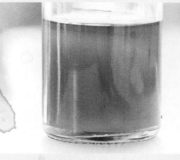

6. Drizzle the basil-garlic oil over grilled meats. Save any remaining oil by straining out the solids and storing it in the refrigerator for up to a week.

WAY TO PREP SHOULDER CHOPS

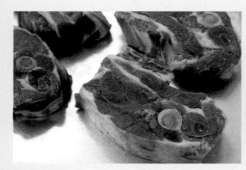

1. Lamb shoulder chops typically cost about one-third the price of loin and rib chops, and their flavor is excellent.

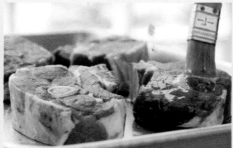

2. First brush them with good olive oil and some bold seasonings like herbes de Provence.

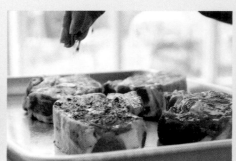

3. Their texture, though, can be a little tough, so it's best to slow-cook them over indirect heat, which renders them tender.

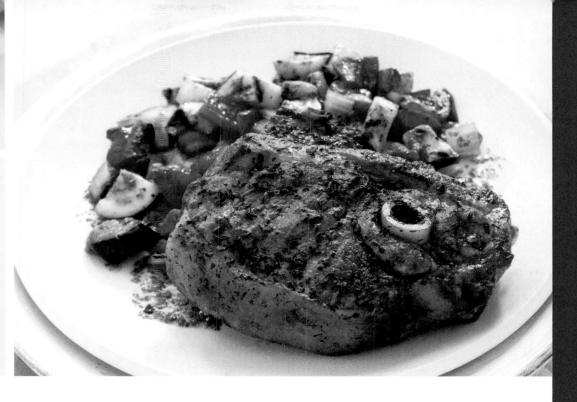

HERBES DE PROVENCE

Herbes de Provence is an aromatic blend of dried herbs frequently used in the south of France. It typically includes thyme, marjoram, parsley, tarragon, lavender, celery seed, and bay leaf.

LAMB SHOULDER CHOPS WITH RATATOUILLE SALAD AND BASIL-GARLIC OIL

SERVES: 4
PREP TIME: 25 MINUTES

WAY TO GRILL: DIRECT AND INDIRECT MEDIUM HEAT
(350° TO 450°F)
GRILLING TIME: 51 TO 58 MINUTES

OIL
1 tablespoon plus ½ teaspoon kosher salt, divided
1 cup packed fresh basil leaves
¾ cup extra-virgin olive oil
1 medium garlic clove, peeled
¼ teaspoon crushed red pepper flakes

RATATOUILLE
1 large red bell pepper
1 medium eggplant, cut into ½-inch slices
2 small zucchini, cut in half lengthwise
1 medium yellow onion, cut crosswise into 4 thick slices
Extra-virgin olive oil
4 plum tomatoes
Kosher salt
Freshly ground black pepper

2 teaspoons herbes de Provence
4 lamb shoulder chops, 10 to 12 ounces each

1. Bring a small saucepan of water, with 1 tablespoon of the salt, to a boil over high heat. Add the basil leaves and blanch them for 10 seconds. Immediately remove the basil and plunge them into a bowl of ice water. Transfer to paper towels and pat away the excess water. In a food processor or blender, process the basil, oil, and garlic until the basil is pureed. Season with the remaining ½ teaspoon salt and the red pepper flakes. Pour into a small pitcher and set aside.

2. Prepare the grill for direct and indirect cooking over medium heat.

3. Remove the stem, ribs, and seeds from the bell pepper and cut into 4 pieces. Lightly brush the eggplant, zucchini, and onion with oil. Brush the cooking grates clean. Grill all the vegetables over **direct medium heat** until the bell pepper is charred and blistered, the eggplant, zucchini, and onion are tender, and the tomato skins are seared and blistered, 6 to 8 minutes, turning occasionally. Transfer the vegetables to a platter as they are done, and season to taste with salt and pepper. Cut the vegetables into chunks and drizzle with 2 tablespoons of basil-garlic oil. Set aside.

4. In a small bowl mix 2 teaspoons kosher salt, ½ teaspoon pepper and the herbes. Lightly brush or spray the lamb with oil and season with the spices.

5. Brush the cooking grates clean. Grill the lamb over **indirect medium heat**, with the lid closed as much as possible, until the chops are fork tender, 45 to 50 minutes, turning once or twice.

6. Place equal portions of ratatouille on each of 4 dinner plates. Add a chop to each plate and garnish with another drizzle of basil-garlic oil on the plate around the lamb and vegetables.

WAY TO CUT SHORT RIBS

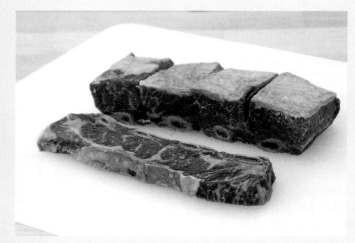

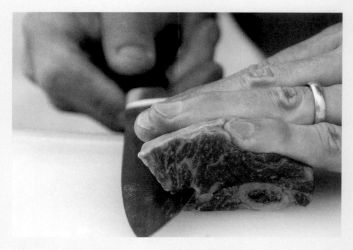

1. Short ribs are cut two different ways for Korean barbecue. You can buy "flanken-style" short ribs, like what you see toward the bottom of this picture, or you can buy "English-style" short ribs, like the thicker pieces toward the top of this picture.

2. To prepare the English-style short ribs, begin by making a horizontal cut just over the bone of each rib.

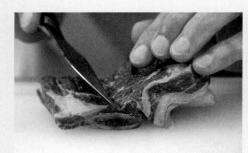

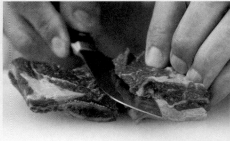

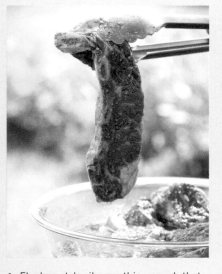

3. Stop just before you cut all the way through the meat.

4. Continue to make horizontal cuts and butterfly the meat until it is about ½ inch thick.

5. Then cut very shallow slits in the meat to tenderize it.

WAY TO GRILL FLANKEN-STYLE RIBS

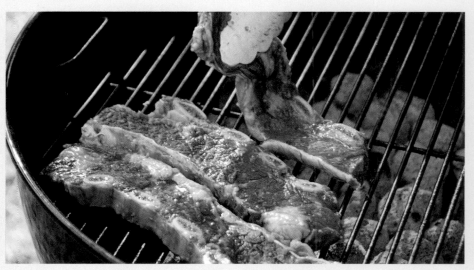

1. Flanken-style ribs are thin enough that they require no cutting. Simply marinate them for a few hours in the refrigerator. When you lift them, let the excess liquid drip back into the bowl before laying them on the grill.

2. Grill the ribs over direct hight heat, leaving the lid off so that you can keep an eye on them and turn them as they char.

KOREAN BEEF BARBECUE

SERVES: 4 TO 6
PREP TIME: 10 MINUTES
MARINATING TIME: 2 TO 4 HOURS

WAY TO GRILL: DIRECT HIGH HEAT (450° TO 550°F)
GRILLING TIME: 3 TO 5 MINUTES

MARINADE
- 1 Asian pear (baseball size), peeled, cored, and roughly chopped
- 3 scallions, trimmed and roughly chopped
- 6 large garlic cloves
- 2 cups water
- ¾ cup soy sauce
- ⅓ cup granulated sugar
- ¼ rice vinegar

- 12 flanken-style beef ribs, about 4 pounds total and ½ inch thick
- 2 tablespoons toasted sesame seed

1. In the bowl of a food processor, finely chop the pear, scallions, and garlic. Add the remaining marinade ingredients. Process until well combined.

2. Put the ribs in a large bowl and pour in the marinade. Mix well to coat the ribs evenly. Cover and refrigerate for 2 to 4 hours.

3. Prepare the grill for direct cooking over high heat.

4. Brush the cooking grates clean. One at time, lift the ribs and let the liquid and solid bits fall back into the bowl. Discard the marinade. Grill the ribs over **direct high heat**, with the lid open, until they are nicely charred on both sides and cooked to a medium or medium-rare doneness, 3 to 5 minutes, turning occasionally. Remove from the grill and sprinkle with the sesame seeds.

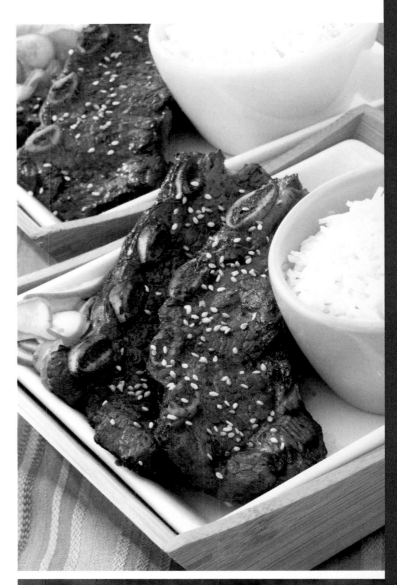

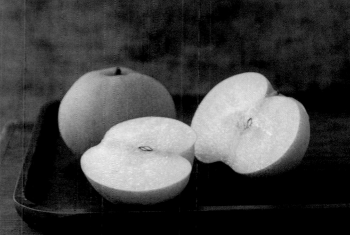

The crisp, translucent flesh of Asian pears makes a sweet juice that is excellent for marinating beef.

WAY TO BARBECUE BEEF RIBS

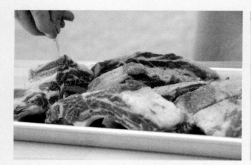

1. Look for the meatiest beef ribs you can find and season them generously.

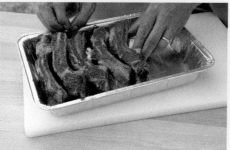

2. Line them up on their sides in a foil pan.

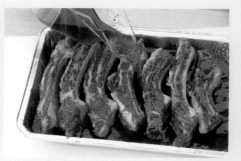

3. Add beef broth to create a moist cooking environment.

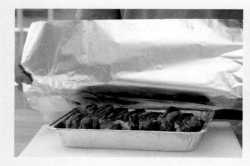

4. The foil will trap steam and help to tenderize the meat.

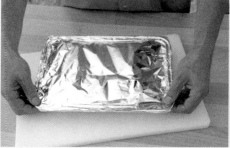

5. Seal the edges tightly so that the liquid does not evaporate.

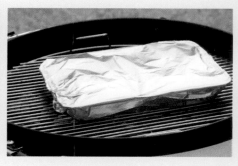

6. The ribs should cook over indirect heat, with the lid closed, for the first hour.

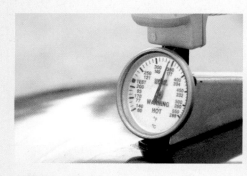

7. It's important to maintain the grill's temperature at about 350°F.

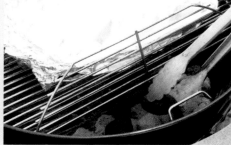

8. At the start of the second hour, add more charcoal to maintain the heat.

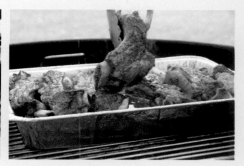

9. Turn the ribs over so they cook evenly.

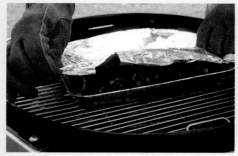

10. Seal the pan again for the second hour of cooking.

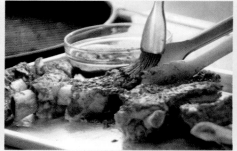

11. Remove the ribs from the pan and brush them with the sauce.

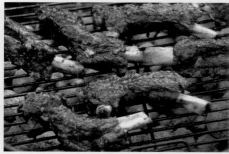

12. Finish them over direct heat for a beautifully caramelized surface.

BEEF RIBS WITH BARBACOA SAUCE

SERVES: 2 TO 4
PREP TIME: 45 MINUTES

WAY TO GRILL: INDIRECT AND DIRECT MEDIUM HEAT
   (350° TO 450°F)
GRILLING TIME: ABOUT 2¼ HOURS
SPECIAL EQUIPMENT: LARGE DISPOSABLE FOIL PAN,
   CAST-IRON SKILLET

RUB
   2   teaspoons granulated garlic
   1   teaspoon ground cinnamon
   1   teaspoon kosher salt
   1   teaspoon freshly ground black pepper

   ½   rack beef ribs (7 ribs), about 5 pounds
   2   cups beef broth

SAUCE
   3   dried ancho chile peppers
   1   cup finely chopped onion
   1   teaspoon dried oregano
   1   teaspoon ground cumin
   1   medium garlic clove, minced
   2   tablespoons cider vinegar
   1   tablespoon light brown sugar
   ¾   teaspoon kosher salt
   ½   cup ketchup

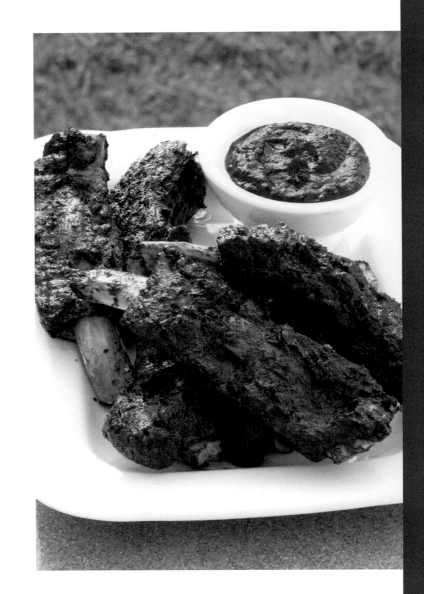

1. In a small bowl combine the rub ingredients.

2. Prepare the grill for indirect and direct cooking over medium heat.

3. Cut the rack into individual ribs and arrange them on a sheet pan. Evenly coat each rib with the rub and then place them side by side in a large disposable foil pan, layering a few ribs if necessary. Add the beef broth to the pan and tightly cover with aluminum foil.

4. Place the pan over **indirect medium heat**, close the lid, and cook for 1 hour. After the first hour, using tongs and wearing insulated barbecue mitts, carefully remove the aluminum foil cover and turn the ribs over. Put the foil cover back on the pan and continue to cook over **indirect medium heat** for another hour. If using a charcoal grill, to maintain the heat, add 5 to 8 unlit briquettes to each pile of lit charcoal about every hour.

5. While the ribs are cooking, make the sauce. Heat a cast-iron skillet over medium-high heat. Add the chiles and cook, occasionally pressing the chiles against the bottom of the skillet, until the chiles are lightly toasted, pliable, and dark brick red in spots, 3 to 5 minutes. The chiles may start to puff while in the pan. Let the toasted chiles cool until easy to handle. Split the chiles open and remove and discard the stems, seeds, and ribs. Transfer to a bowl and cover with 2½ cups hot tap water.

Let stand until the chiles soften, about 20 minutes. Strain into a small bowl, reserving the chile soaking liquid.

6. In a blender combine the soaked chiles, onion, oregano, cumin, and garlic. Add ½ cup of the reserved soaking liquid and blend to make a thick paste, adding more reserved liquid if necessary. In a medium saucepan over medium heat, add the chile paste, vinegar, brown sugar, and salt and bring to a boil, stirring often. Reduce the heat to medium-low and cook until slightly thickened, about 5 minutes. Remove from the heat and stir in the ketchup. Transfer to a bowl and allow to cool.

7. When the ribs are tender and the meat has visibly shrunk back from the bones, wearing insulated barbecue mitts, carefully remove the pan from the grill. Remove the ribs from the pan drippings and place them on a sheet pan. Discard the pan and the drippings. Liberally brush the ribs with the sauce and then grill the ribs over **direct medium heat** for 3 to 5 minutes. Brush the ribs again with more sauce, turn them over and grill for an additional 3 to 5 minutes. Transfer the ribs to a platter and let rest for 5 minutes. Serve with the remaining sauce.

LEG OF LAMB
WITH MOROCCAN SPICES

SERVES: 6 TO 8
PREP TIME: 20 MINUTES
MARINATING TIME: 1 HOUR

WAY TO GRILL: DIRECT AND INDIRECT HIGH HEAT
    (450° TO 550°F)
GRILLING TIME: 21 TO 27 MINUTES

MARINADE
  ½ cup chopped yellow onion
  1 tablespoon grated lemon zest
  ¼ cup fresh lemon juice
  3 tablespoons extra-virgin olive oil
  2 garlic cloves
1½ teaspoons crushed red pepper flakes
  1 teaspoon ground coriander
  1 teaspoon ground cumin
  1 teaspoon paprika
  1 teaspoon ground ginger
  1 teaspoon kosher salt

  1 boneless leg of lamb, about 3 pounds, butterflied
    and trimmed of any excess fat and sinew

1. In a food processor combine the marinade ingredients and pulse to make a smooth paste, scraping down the sides of the bowl as necessary. Place the lamb in a large, resealable plastic bag and pour in the marinade. Press the air out of the bag and seal tightly. Turn the bag to distribute the marinade and refrigerate for 1 hour. Allow the lamb to stand at room temperature for 20 to 30 minutes before grilling. Prepare the grill for direct and indirect cooking over high heat.

2. Remove the lamb from the bag, letting the marinade cling to the lamb. Discard the marinade in the bag. Brush the cooking grates clean. Grill the lamb over **direct high heat**, with the lid closed as much as possible, until nicely browned on both sides, about 6 minutes, turning once. Then slide the lamb over **indirect high heat** and cook, with the lid closed, to your desired doneness, 15 to 20 minutes for medium rare. Remove the lamb from the grill and let rest for about 5 minutes before carving. Cut the lamb across the grain into thin diagonal slices and serve warm.

WAY TO BUTTERFLY LEG OF LAMB

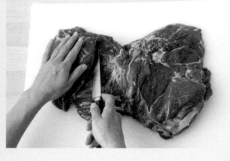

1. A boneless leg of lamb is actually several muscles held together. The different muscles have various shapes and thicknesses.

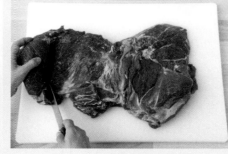

2. In order to grill the whole leg evenly, you need to make the thickest parts thinner.

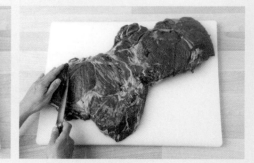

3. You do that by making angled cuts at the thickness you want and then spreading the meat open like a book.

PANIOLO TRI-TIP ROAST WITH ORANGE BARBECUE SAUCE

SERVES: 6
PREP TIME: 20 MINUTES

WAY TO GRILL: DIRECT AND INDIRECT MEDIUM HEAT
    (350° TO 450°F)
GRILLING TIME: 23 TO 30 MINUTES

PASTE

    2   tablespoons extra-virgin olive oil
    2   tablespoons minced fresh ginger
    2   tablespoons light brown sugar
    2   teaspoons coarse sea salt or *alaea* (Hawaiian sea salt)
    2   teaspoons minced garlic
    1   teaspoon chile-garlic sauce, such as Sriracha

    1   tri-tip roast, about 2 pounds and 1½ inches thick, fat and silver skin removed

SAUCE

    1   cup thawed frozen orange juice concentrate
    2   tablespoons packed light brown sugar
    2   tablespoons apple cider vinegar
    2   tablespoons soy sauce

1. In a medium bowl combine the paste ingredients. Coat the roast evenly with the paste. Let the roast stand at room temperature for 20 to 30 minutes before grilling. Prepare the grill for direct and indirect cooking over medium heat.

2. In a medium saucepan over medium heat, combine the sauce ingredients. Cook, whisking frequently, until thickened and reduced to about ¾ cup, 10 to 15 minutes. Set aside. Reheat just before serving.

3. Brush the cooking grates clean. Grill the roast over **direct medium heat** until well marked on both sides, 8 to 10 minutes, turning once. Move the tri-tip over **indirect medium heat** and cook to your desired coneness, 15 to 20 minutes for medium rare, turning every 5 minutes or so. Keep the lid closed as much as possible during grilling. Remove the roast from the grill, tent with foil, and let rest for 5 to 10 minutes. Cut the roast across the grain into thin slices. Serve warm with the sauce.

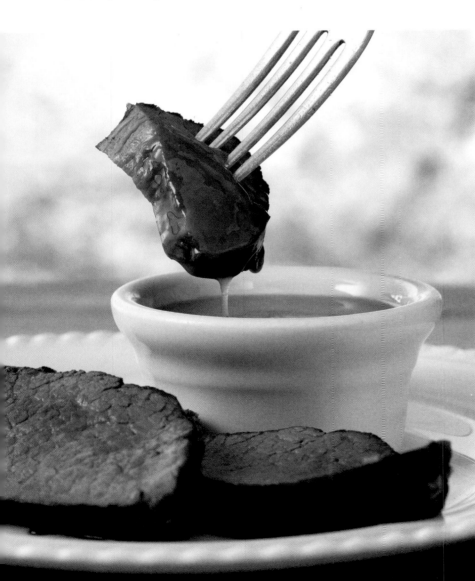

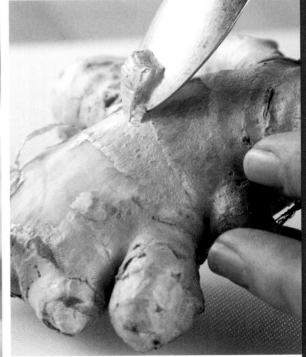

Much of what gives this Hawaiian-style tri-tip roast such great flavor is the paste, which features fresh ginger. Before mincing the ginger, scrape off the skin with the back of a spoon. Also, be careful not to overcook the tri-tip roast. It's a very lean cut of meat and it's best served medium rare.

WAY TO PREP BEEF TENDERLOIN

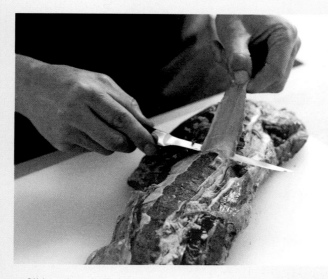

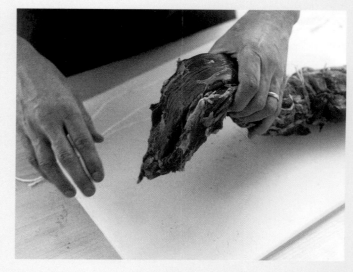

1. Slide a sharp knife just under any large clumps of fat, being careful not to cut into the meat. Also remove the strips of silver skin, which are tough and chewy.

2. Tie the "cleaned" roast every couple of inches to make it even and compact. Because the tail is thinner than the rest of the roast, fold it underneath and tie it snugly for a more even thickness end to end.

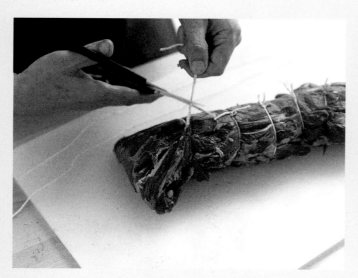

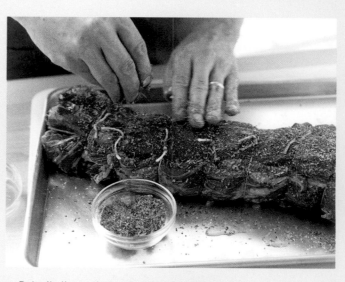

3. Cut off the loose ends of the twine.

4. Rub oil all over the roast and season it with herbs and spices.

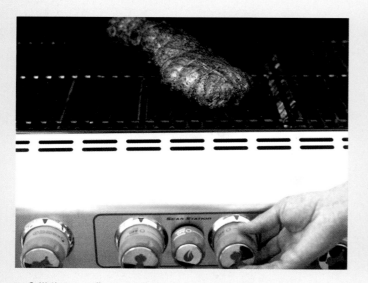

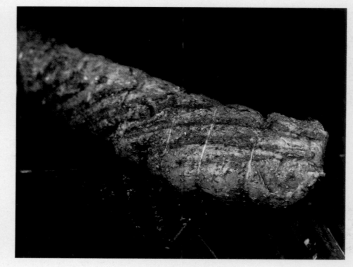

5. Grill the roast first over direct heat to brown it on all sides.

6. Finish cooking it over indirect heat so that the exterior does not burn before the interior is cooked.

HERB-CRUSTED BEEF TENDERLOIN ROAST WITH WHITE WINE CREAM SAUCE

SERVES: 10 TO 12
PREP TIME: 40 MINUTES

WAY TO GRILL: DIRECT AND INDIRECT MEDIUM HEAT
(350° TO 450°F)
GRILLING TIME: 35 TO 45 MINUTES
SPECIAL EQUIPMENT: BUTCHER'S TWINE

RUB
1½ tablespoons dried tarragon
2½ teaspoons kosher salt
2 teaspoons freshly ground black pepper
1½ teaspoons dried thyme
1 teaspoon rubbed dried sage, packed

1 whole beef tenderloin, 6 to 7 pounds, untrimmed
Extra-virgin olive oil

SAUCE
½ cup minced shallot
½ cup rice vinegar
1½ teaspoons dried tarragon
¼ teaspoon dried thyme
½ cup dry white wine
½ cup reduced-sodium chicken broth
1½ cups whipping cream
½ cup packed minced fresh Italian parsley

Kosher salt

1. In a small bowl mix the rub ingredients.

2. Trim and discard the excess fat and silver skin from the tenderloin. Part of the thin "tail" end of the tenderloin may separate as it is trimmed, but leave it connected to the main muscle as much as possible. Lay the tenderloin out flat and straight, with the smoothest side up, aligning the narrow pieces at the tail end. Neatly fold the tail end of the tenderloin under itself to form an even thickness (one end may be larger). Tie the roast snugly with butcher's twine at 2-inch intervals. Secure the folded end with two strings. Lightly coat the roast with oil. Season the roast all over with the rub.

3. Let the roast stand at room temperature for 30 minutes to 1 hour before grilling. Prepare the grill for direct and indirect cooking over medium heat.

4. In a large skillet over high heat, combine the shallot, vinegar, tarragon, and thyme, and cook until the vinegar evaporates, 3 to 4 minutes, stirring often. Add the wine and broth and boil until reduced to about ½ cup, 3 to 4 minutes. Add the cream and boil until the surface is covered with large, shiny bubbles and the sauce is reduced to about 1½ cups, 5 to 7 minutes. Remove from the heat, adjust the seasonings, and set aside. Reheat and add parsley just before serving.

5. Brush the cooking grates clean. Sear the roast over **direct medium heat** for about 15 minutes, turning a quarter turn once every 3 to 4 minutes. Then slide the roast over **indirect medium heat** and cook until it reaches your desired doneness, 20 to 30 minutes for medium rare (125° to 130°F), turning once. Keep the lid closed as much as possible during grilling. Remove from the grill, loosely tent with foil, and let rest for 10 to 15 minutes. The temperature will rise 5 to 10 degrees during this time.

6. Snip and remove all the twine from the roast. Cut the meat crosswise into ½- to 1-inch slices. Season to taste with salt. Serve warm with the sauce.

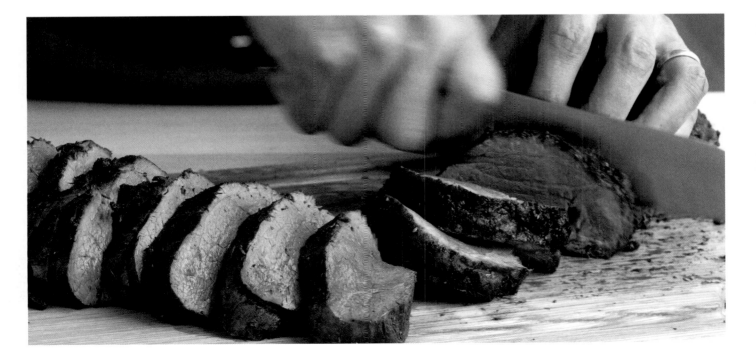

WAY TO PREP RIB ROAST

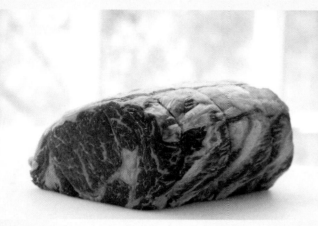

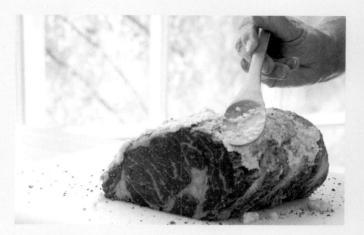

1. For a special occasion, consider buying a rib roast a few days before you plan to serve it and dry-aging it in your refrigerator (for safety reasons, never do this for more than 4 days). Patted dry and set on a rack over a sheet pan in the refrigerator, the meat will develop more concentrated flavors and a softer texture.

2. After you have seasoned the meat, let it stand at room temperature for 30 to 40 minutes so that the outer ring of the roast won't overcook before the center reaches your ideal temperature on the grill.

WAY TO SMOKE A RIB ROAST

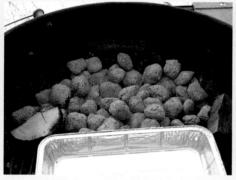

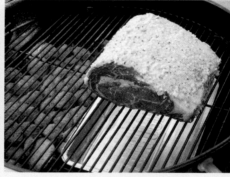

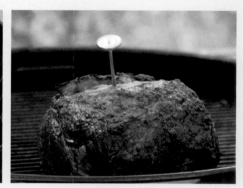

1. Spread a layer or two of lit coals on one-half of the charcoal grate. Position some wood chunks alongside the coals. On the opposite side, set up a water pan, which will absorb some heat and release it slowly.

2. Initially position the roast with the thicker end toward the coals.

3. An instant-read thermometer takes all the guesswork out of doneness. For medium rare, remove the roast when it hits the 120° to 125°F range. The internal temperature will climb another 10 degrees or so as the meat rests.

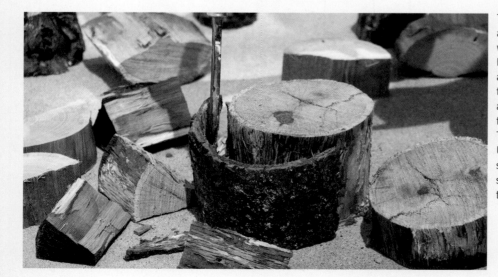

The sweet, haunting aromas of smoldering oak are a distinctive part of this recipe. Bags of wood chunks are pretty easy to find in stores, but if you happen to have dried oak logs lying around, you can make your own chunks. Saw the logs into smaller sections and use a chisel and hammer to break off most of the bark; it tends to add a bit of bitterness to the smoke. Then split the wood into fist-sized pieces. Unlike wood chips, chunks don't need to be soaked. Alongside the coals, they will burn slowly and permeate the meat with a taste of the great outdoors.

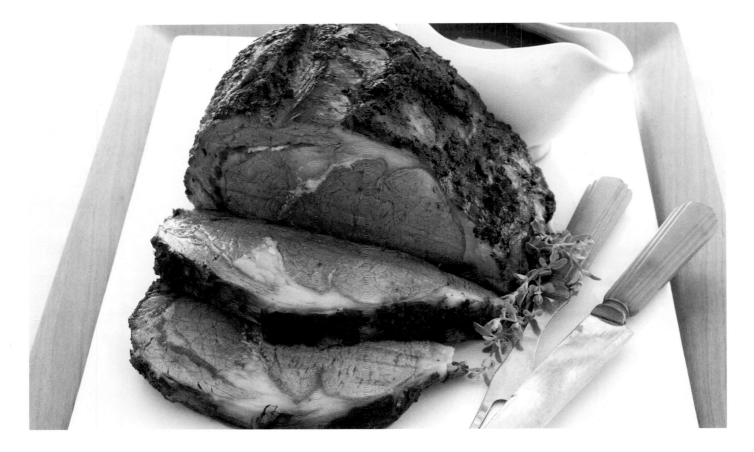

OAK-SMOKED BONELESS RIB ROAST WITH SHIRAZ SAUCE

SERVES: 10
PREP TIME: 30 MINUTES

WAY TO GRILL: INDIRECT MEDIUM HEAT (350° TO 375°F)
GRILLING TIME: ABOUT 1½ HOURS
SPECIAL EQUIPMENT: LARGE DISPOSABLE FOIL PAN,
   INSTANT-READ THERMOMETER

1	boneless rib roast, about 5½ pounds, trimmed of excess surface fat
	Kosher salt
	Freshly ground black pepper
¼	cup Dijon mustard
⅓	cup coarsely grated yellow onion
3	garlic cloves, minced
2	oak wood chunks (not soaked)

SAUCE

3	tablespoons unsalted butter, cold, divided
3	tablespoons minced shallot
1	garlic clove, minced
4	cups beef stock, preferably homemade
1½	cups Shiraz wine
1	tablespoon soy sauce
1½	teaspoons tomato paste
¼	teaspoon dried thyme
½	bay leaf

1. Season the roast with 2 teaspoons salt and 1 teaspoon pepper. In a small bowl mix the mustard, onion, and garlic. Spread over the top of the roast. Allow the roast to stand at room temperature for 30 to 40 minutes before grilling.

2. Prepare the grill for indirect cooking over medium heat (see instructions at left). Add 2 wood chunks alongside the coals. Brush the cooking grates clean. Position the roast with the thicker end facing the coals. Grill over **indirect medium heat**, with the lid closed as much as possible, until the internal temperature reaches 120° to 125°F for medium rare, about 1½ hours, rotating the roast 180 degrees halfway through the grilling time. Keep the grill's temperature between 350° and 375°F.

3. In a medium, heavy-bottomed saucepan over medium heat, melt 1 tablespoon of the butter (keep the remaining butter refrigerated). Add the shallot and cook until softened, about 2 minutes. Add the garlic and cook until fragrant, about 1 minute. Add the stock, wine, soy sauce, tomato paste, thyme, and bay leaf, and bring to a boil over high heat. Cook, uncovered, until reduced to about 2 cups, about 30 minutes. Season to taste with salt and pepper. Remove the bay leaf. Keep the sauce warm.

4. Remove the roast from the grill, loosely cover with aluminum foil, and let rest for 20 to 30 minutes. The internal temperature will rise another 10 degrees or so during this time. Carve the roast into ½-inch slices, reserving the juices. Just before serving, whisk the remaining 2 tablespoons cold butter into the sauce, and stir in the carving juices. Serve warm with the sauce.

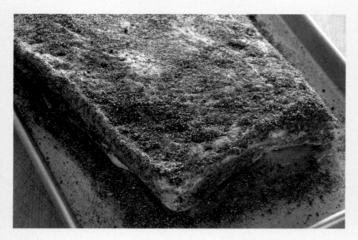

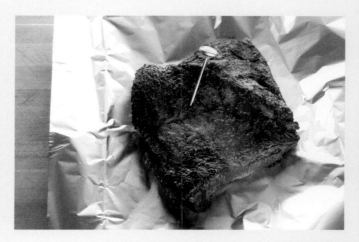

1. The first layer of flavor to apply is the sweet heat of a good spice rub and mustard. Next, cook the seasoned brisket on a smoker for 4 to 5 hours so that it absorbs a good amount of flavorful wood smoke. The brisket should be in a large disposable foil pan to catch some of the juices, and the thick layer of fat should be on top so that it bastes the meat below it.

2. When the internal temperature of the meat reaches 160°F, take it out of the foil pan and double-wrap the brisket in aluminum foil. This will trap some moisture and help to break down the tough fibers in the meat.

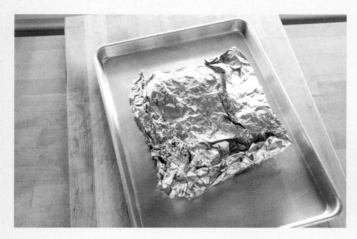

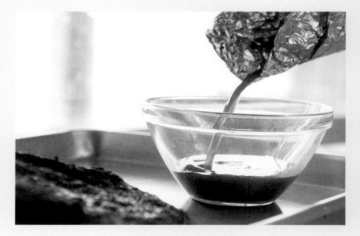

3. When the internal temperature reaches 190° to 195°F in the thickest section, remove the brisket from the smoker and let the precious meat juices collect in the foil. The brisket will stay warm and continue to cook for an hour or two.

4. Carefully unwrap the foil, set the brisket aside, and bend the foil to funnel the juices into a serving bowl.

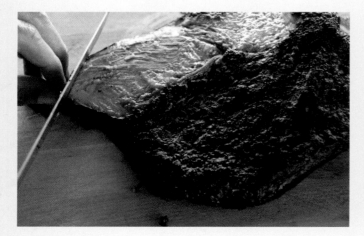

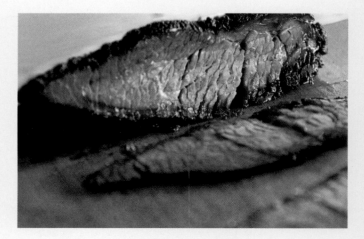

5. Slice a section of fat from the top side of the brisket so you can see which way the grain of the meat runs. For the sake of tenderness, you want to slice against the grain.

6. Slice the brisket nice and thin with a sharp knife. That beautiful pink ring is a result of the wood smoke. Now spoon those meat juices over the top and have at it.

TRULY BARBECUED BRISKET

SERVES: 6
PREP TIME: 15 MINUTES
MARINATING TIME: 6 TO 8 HOURS

WAY TO GRILL: INDIRECT LOW HEAT (225° TO 250°F)
GRILLING TIME: 6 TO 8 HOURS, PLUS 1 TO 2 HOURS
    RESTING TIME
SPECIAL EQUIPMENT: LARGE DISPOSABLE FOIL PAN,
    INSTANT-READ THERMOMETER

RUB
- 4 teaspoons kosher salt
- 2 teaspoons ancho chile powder
- 2 teaspoons light brown sugar
- 2 teaspoons granulated garlic
- 2 teaspoons paprika
- 1 teaspoon celery seed
- 1 teaspoon coarsely ground black pepper

- 1 brisket (flat cut), 5 to 6 pounds, untrimmed
- ¼ cup yellow mustard
- 6 hickory or oak wood chunks (not soaked)
- 2 cups favorite barbecue sauce

1. In a small bowl mix the rub ingredients.

2. Lay the brisket, fat side up, on a large cutting board. Trim the layer of fat to a ½-inch thickness. Turn the brisket over and trim any hard fat or thin membrane covering the meat.

3. Season the brisket evenly with the mustard and then the rub. Cover and refrigerate for 6 to 8 hours.

4. Place the brisket, fat side up, in a large disposable foil pan.

5. Prepare your smoker, following manufacturer's instructions, for indirect cooking over low heat.

6. Place the pan with the brisket on the cooking grate. Smoke the brisket, starting with 2 chunks of wood, at 225° to 250°F, until the internal temperature of the meat reaches 160° to 170°F, 4 to 5 hours. Every hour or so, add another chunk of wood to the coals and, if necessary, add more coals to maintain the temperature of the smoker at 225° to 250°F.

7. When the internal temperature of the meat has reached 160° to 170°F, the collagen in the meat will have dissolved. At that point, remove the brisket and pan from the smoker (close the lid to maintain the heat). Baste the brisket with some of the juices and fat collected in the pan. Then wrap the brisket in 2 large sheets of heavy-duty aluminum foil. Discard the pan.

8. Return the brisket to the smoker and cook until the internal temperature of the brisket reaches 190° to 195°F in the thickest section, 2 to 3 hours, without adding more wood chunks. The

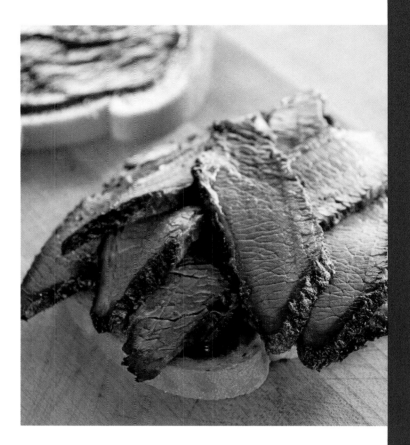

probe of the thermometer should slide in and out of the brisket with just a little resistance.

9. Remove the brisket from the smoker and let it rest inside the foil at room temperature for 1 to 2 hours. It will stay hot and continue to tenderize.

10. Carefully unwrap the brisket, being careful not to lose any of the juices inside the foil. Move the brisket to a large cutting board. Pour the juices into a small bowl.

11. If necessary, cut off a small chunk of brisket to identify the direction of the grain. Cut the brisket across the grain into ⅛-inch slices. Spoon or brush some of the juices over the slices. Serve warm with barbecue sauce on the side.

■■■

Brisket is the Mt. Everest of barbecue. Not only is it huge, but it also poses challenges all along the way. If your first couple of attempts don't work out exactly as you had hoped, persevere. The rewards of mastering your own barbecued brisket are unspeakably good. Among a cadre of outdoor cooks you will have earned long-standing respect and admiration.

■■■

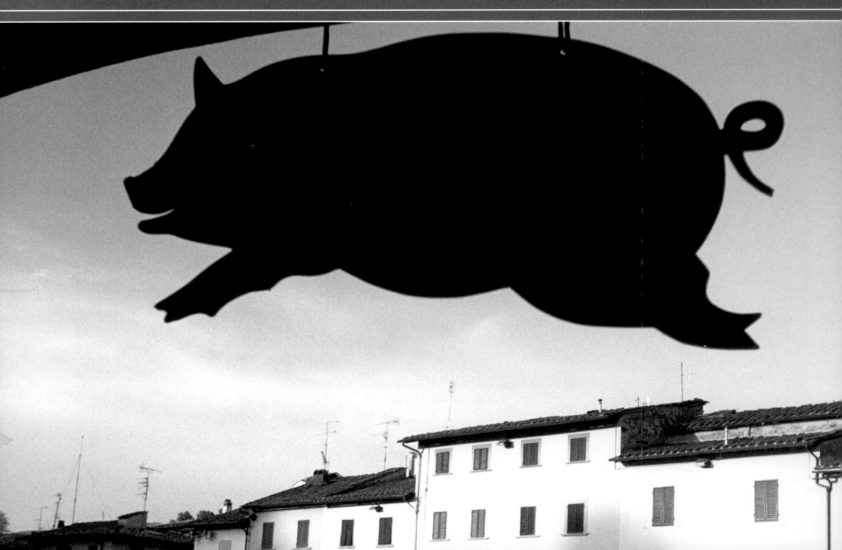

WAY TO GRILL™
PORK

TECHNIQUES

RECIPES

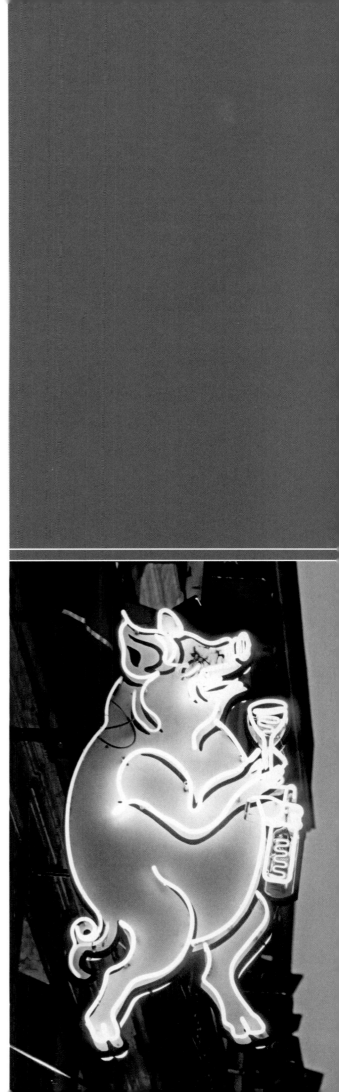

WAY TO GRILL BRATWURST

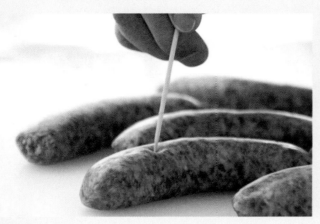

1. Before cooking, prick several small holes in each bratwurst to prevent them from bursting open.

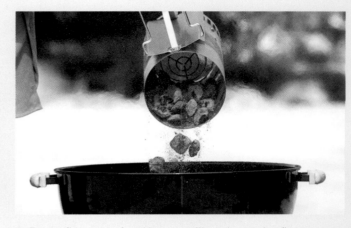

2. For the first stage of cooking, you will need a very hot fire on one side of the cooking grate.

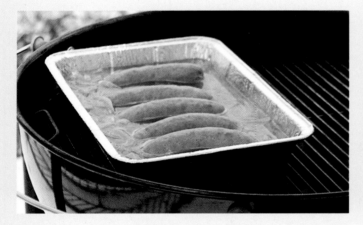

3. Arrange the bratwurst in a single layer in a foil pan with hard cider and sliced onions.

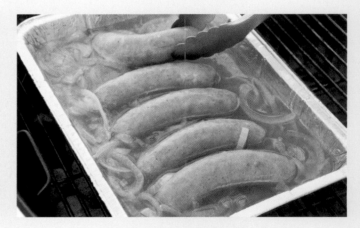

4. Simmer the bratwurst for about 20 minutes, turning them occasionally. If the liquid boils, slide the pan over indirect heat.

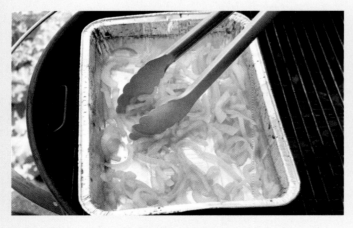

5. Strain the onions and return them to the pan to caramelize with brown sugar.

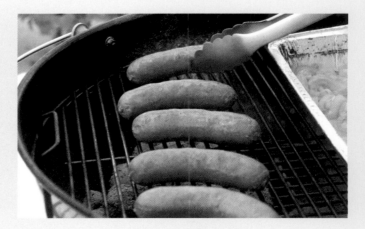

6. Finish grilling the bratwurst over direct heat to lightly char the surfaces.

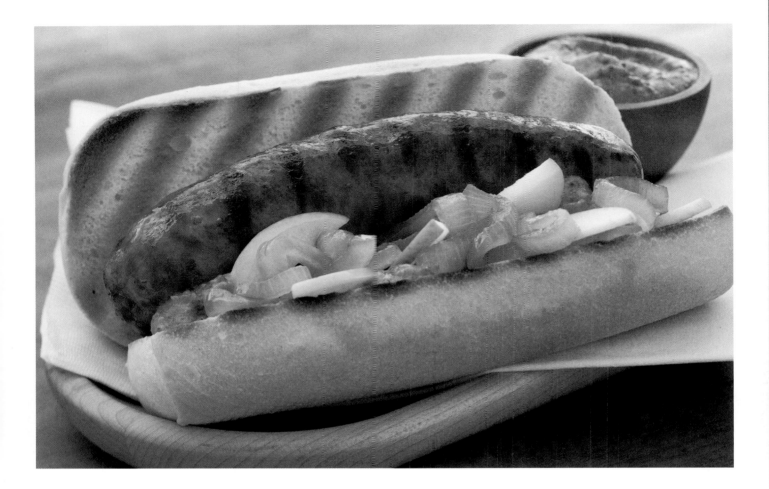

CIDER-SIMMERED BRATS WITH APPLES AND ONIONS

SERVES: 5
PREP TIME: 15 MINUTES

WAY TO GRILL: DIRECT HIGH HEAT (450° TO 550°F) AND
DIRECT MEDIUM HEAT (350° TO 450°F)
GRILLING TIME: 6 TO 8 MINUTES
SPECIAL EQUIPMENT: 2 LARGE DISPOSABLE FOIL PANS

MUSTARD
    2 tablespoons apple butter
    2 tablespoons Dijon mustard
    2 tablespoons whole-grain mustard

    2 bottles (12 ounces each) hard apple cider
    2 medium yellow onions, halved and cut into ¼-inch slices
    5 fresh bratwurst, pierced several times
    1 tablespoon brown sugar
    5 submarine sandwich buns, halved lengthwise
    2 Granny Smith apples, cored and thinly sliced

1. In a small bowl mix the mustard ingredients. Cover and let
stand at room temperature until ready to serve.

2. Prepare the grill for direct and indirect cooking over high
heat. Brush the cooking grates clean. Put the hard cider,

onions, and bratwurst into a large disposable foil pan. Place
the pan over **direct high heat** and bring the liquid to a simmer.
Keep the grill lid closed as much as possible. Continue
simmering until the brats are evenly colored and have lost their
raw look, about 20 minutes, turning them occasionally. If the
liquid starts to boil, move the pan over indirect heat to prevent
the bratwurst from splitting open.

3. Lower the temperature of the grill to medium heat. Transfer
the brats to another large disposable aluminum pan. Strain the
onions in a colander over the pan with the brats (the liquid will
keep the brats warm while you cook the onions). Return the
onions to the original pan and stir in the brown sugar. Cook the
onions over **direct medium heat**, with the lid closed as much
as possible, until they are golden brown, about 15 minutes,
stirring occasionally. Move the onions over indirect heat to keep
them warm.

4. Remove the brats from the liquid and grill them over
direct medium heat until browned, 6 to 8 minutes, turning
once or twice. During the last minute, place the buns on the
grill to toast.

5. Place the brats in the buns. Spread each with the mustard,
and top with the glazed onions and a few apple slices. Serve hot.

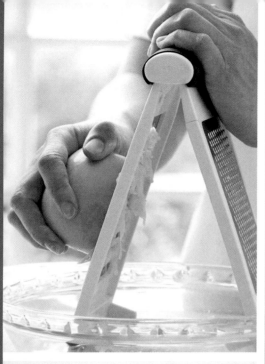

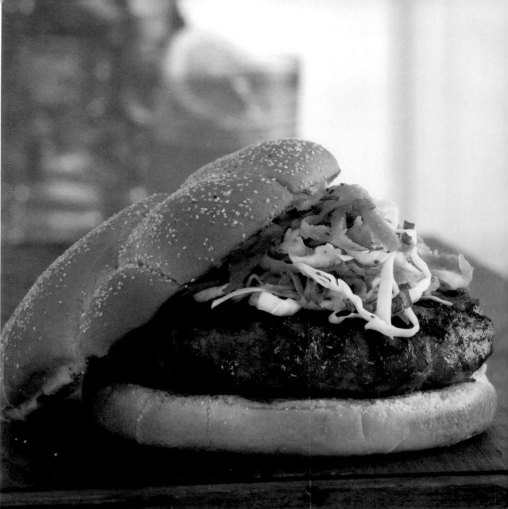

One key to the juiciness of these burgers is mixing applesauce into the ground pork. Another key is including green apples in the slaw. A box grater conveniently separates the moist flesh of a cored apple from its tough skins.

PORK BURGERS WITH APPLE-TARRAGON SLAW

SERVES: 4
PREP TIME: 20 MINUTES

WAY TO GRILL: DIRECT MEDIUM HEAT (350° TO 450°F)
GRILLING TIME: 12 TO 15 MINUTES

SLAW
- 2 cups thinly sliced green cabbage
- ½ cup coarsely grated tart green apple
- ½ cup coarsely grated carrot
- 2 tablespoons finely chopped fresh tarragon
- 2 tablespoons cider vinegar
- 1 tablespoon granulated sugar
- ½ teaspoon celery seed
- ¼ teaspoon kosher salt

PATTIES
- 1½ pounds ground pork
- ⅓ cup applesauce
- 1½ teaspoons kosher salt
- 1 teaspoon hot sauce, or to taste
- ½ teaspoon freshly ground black pepper

- 4 hamburger buns

1. In a large bowl mix the slaw ingredients. Cover and refrigerate until ready to assemble the burgers.

2. In a large bowl gently mix the patty ingredients. Gently shape into 4 patties of equal size and thickness, each about ¾ inch thick. With your thumb or the back of a spoon, make a shallow indentation about 1 inch wide in the center of each patty. Prepare the grill for direct cooking over medium heat.

3. Brush the cooking grates clean. Grill the patties over **direct medium heat**, with the lid closed as much as possible, until cooked through, 12 to 15 minutes, turning once when the patties release easily from the grate without sticking. During the last minute of grilling time, toast the buns, cut sides down, over **direct medium heat**. Place the burgers on the buns and top with the slaw. Serve warm.

BUTTERMILK BISCUITS
WITH PEPPER JELLY–GLAZED HAM

SERVES: 6
PREP TIME: 20 MINUTES

WAY TO GRILL: INDIRECT HIGH HEAT (ABOUT 400°F) AND
   DIRECT MEDIUM HEAT (350° TO 450°F)
GRILLING TIME: 16 TO 21 MINUTES

BISCUITS
  4 cups all-purpose flour
  4 teaspoons baking powder
  1 teaspoon baking soda
  1 teaspoon kosher salt
  1 cup solid vegetable shortening, cold
  1½ cups buttermilk, cold
  1 tablespoon unsalted butter, melted

  1 cup medium or hot jalapeño jelly, divided
  2 pounds ham steak, about ½ inch thick

1. Prepare the grill for indirect cooking over high heat.

2. In a large bowl combine the flour, baking powder, baking
soda, and salt. Cut in the shortening with your fingertips or
a pastry blender until the mixture resembles coarse bread
crumbs. Add the buttermilk and stir just until the mixture sticks
together. Turn the dough out onto a lightly floured surface and
knead lightly for 20 to 30 seconds. Lightly dust your hands
with flour and gently pat out the dough to a thickness of about
¾ inch. Dip a 2½-inch round biscuit cutter in flour and cut out
rounds of dough. Gather scraps of dough and pat out, using a
light touch so you don't overwork the dough; cut to make a total
of 12 biscuits. Place the biscuits close together on a greased
baking sheet. Brush the tops with melted butter.

3. Grill the sheet of biscuits over **indirect high heat** (keeping
the grill's temperature as close to 400°F as possible) until
the biscuits are lightly browned, 12 to 15 minutes, checking
occasionally and moving or rotating the sheet as needed so the
bottoms of the biscuits do not burn. Keep the grill lid closed as
much as possible. Remove the biscuits from the grill and set
aside to keep warm.

4. Prepare the grill for direct cooking over medium heat.

5. In a small saucepan over low heat, warm ⅓ cup of the
jalapeño jelly until it melts. Brush the cooking grates clean. Grill
the ham steaks over **direct medium heat**, with the lid closed
as much as possible, until the ham is nicely marked and crispy
on the edges, 4 to 6 minutes, turning once and basting with
jalapeño jelly before and after turning.

6. Cut the ham into pieces about the same size as the biscuits.
Split each biscuit horizontally. Serve the ham warm in biscuits
with the remaining jalapeño jelly on top.

WAY TO MAKE
BUTTERMILK BISCUITS

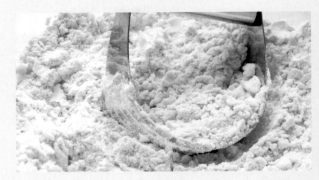

1. In a medium bowl mix the dry ingredients first. Add cold
vegetable shortening. Use a pastry blender or fork to "cut in"
the fat until the mixture resembles coarse crumbs with a few
larger clumps.

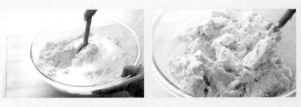

2. Add buttermilk and stir just until the mixture
comes together.

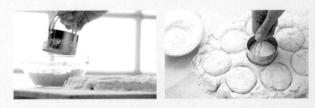

3. Pat the dough on a floured surface into a disk about ¾ inch
thick. Use a floured biscuit cutter to cut out rounds of dough.

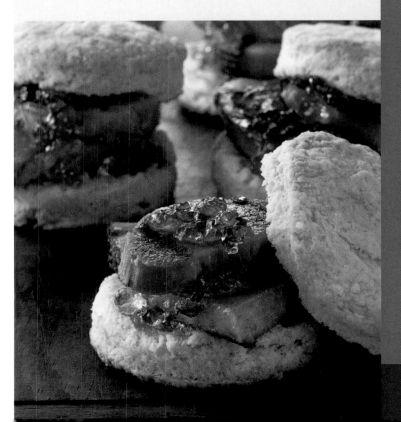

WAY TO GRILL PORK CHOPS
5 THINGS YOU NEED TO KNOW

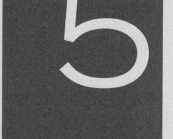

1 NOT YOUR GRANDFATHER'S PORK

Today's pigs come to market younger and smaller than the pigs of yesteryear. They have had less time to develop much collagen and connective tissue—that is, the stuff that can make pork chewy. Therefore, pork chops are definitely tender enough for grilling. That's the good news.

2 IT'S BRINE TIME

The bad news is that today's pigs are also much leaner than the pigs of yesteryear. In fact, pork chops are about as lean as chicken today, which means it doesn't take long for them to dry out on the grill. So it is always a good idea to brine pork chops first. Brining means soaking them in a flavorful salty liquid that the meat can absorb, giving them more moisture (and flavor) from the start.

3 CHOOSE YOUR CHOP WELL

Pork chops are cut from a pig's loin, which runs from the shoulder to the hip. The chops from the shoulder (blade chops and country-style ribs) are the most marbled and flavorful, but also the chewiest of the group. The chops from the hip (sirloin chops) are quite dry and tough, so I don't recommend those for grilling. The chops from the mid-section of the loin (rib chops and loin chops) can be quite tender and juicy, if you grill them right.

4 EASY DOES IT

We don't serve pork chops charred on the outside and rare or medium rare in the middle, like steaks. We serve them with a relatively even doneness from top to bottom. This means a gentler heat on the grill so that the centers of the chops can reach the right degree of doneness well before the outsides are overdone.

5 THAT TOUCH OF PINK

There is really only one correct doneness level for pork chops. You'll know it when you see it and when you taste it. As the chop cooks, the color of the meat inside will turn from reddish-pink to a very light pink. That's it. Stop there. If you cook pork chops any further than that, the meat will be gray and bland.

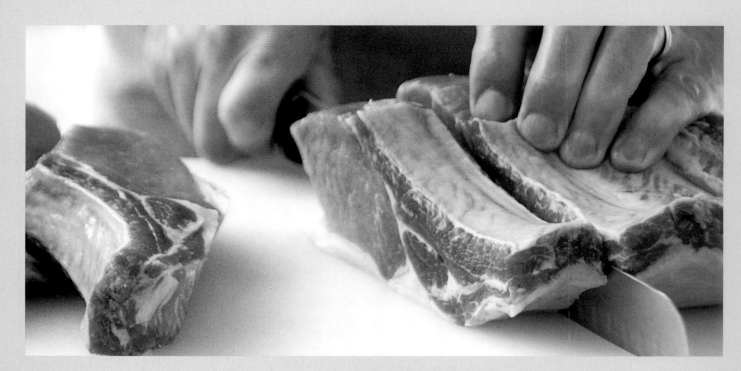

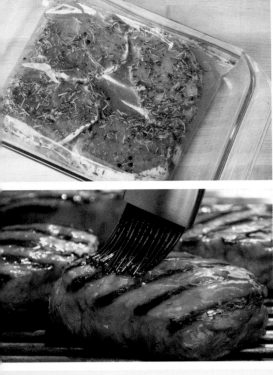

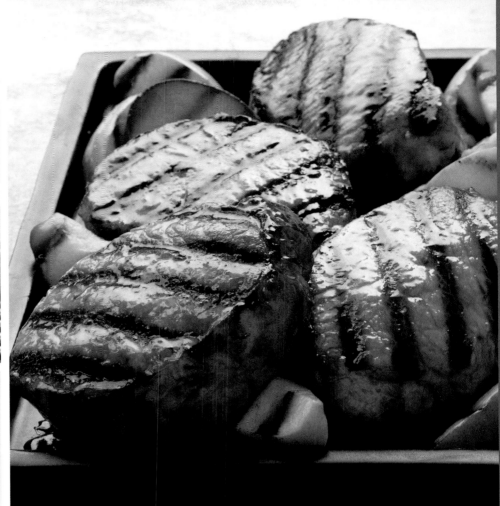

Good grilling is all about layering flavors from the inside out. In this recipe, pork chops benefit dramatically from a hard-cider brine that penetrates right to the middle of the meat, plus an apple-brandy glaze that coats the outside.

CIDER-BRINED PORK CHOPS WITH GRILLED APPLES

SERVES: 4
PREP TIME: 15 MINUTES
BRINING TIME: 1 TO 1½ HOURS

WAY TO GRILL: DIRECT MEDIUM HEAT (350° TO 450°F)
GRILLING TIME: ABOUT 12 MINUTES

BRINE
- 1½ cups hard apple cider
- ½ cup kosher salt
- 1 tablespoon dried rosemary
- 1 tablespoon dried sage
- 1½ teaspoons dried thyme
- ½ teaspoon whole black peppercorns

- 4 center-cut pork loin chops, each about 12 ounces and 1½ inches thick, trimmed of excess fat
  Extra-virgin olive oil

GLAZE
- 6 tablespoons apple jelly
- 2 tablespoons unsalted butter
- 2 tablespoons Calvados or applejack (apple brandy)

- 4 Granny Smith apples, each cut into 6 wedges and cores removed

1. In a large bowl mix the brine ingredients. Put the chops in a large, resealable plastic bag and pour in the brine. Press the air out of the bag and seal tightly. Place the bag in a bowl or a rimmed dish and refrigerate for 1 to 1½ hours, turning the bag every 30 minutes.

2. Remove the chops from the bag and discard the brine. Rinse the chops under cold water and pat dry with paper towels. Lightly brush or spray the chops with oil and let stand at room temperature for 20 to 30 minutes before grilling. Prepare the grill for direct cooking over medium heat.

3. In a small saucepan over medium-low heat, warm the jelly and butter, stirring until the jelly melts. Remove from the heat and stir in the Calvados. If the glaze cools, reheat gently until fluid. Set aside half of the glaze to serve as a sauce with the grilled pork. Brush the remaining glaze all over the apple slices and then the chops.

4. Brush the cooking grates clean. Grill the chops over **direct medium heat**, with the lid closed as much as possible, until they are slightly pink in the center, about 10 minutes, turning once. Remove the chops from the grill and let rest for 3 to 5 minutes. While they rest, grill the apples over **direct medium heat** until crisp-tender, about 2 minutes, turning once. Serve the chops and apples warm with the reserved glaze.

WAY TO PREP LEEKS

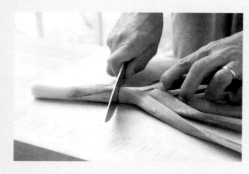 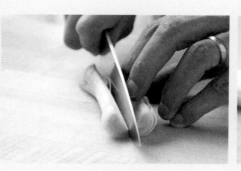 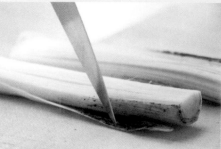

1. Remove the tough green tops from small, slender leeks and trim off just enough of the root end to get rid of the stringy parts.

2. Cut each leek in half lengthwise to expose the many layers inside, making sure to leave some root end intact so the layers remain attached.

3. Because leeks grow underground, you will often find dirt and sand trapped between the layers. Spread the layers open under running water to clean them before grilling.

WAY TO MAKE PORK PAILLARDS

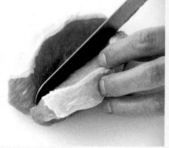 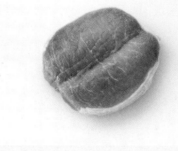 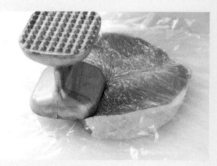

1. Begin with boneless center-cut pork chops at least 1 inch thick. Cut into the middle of the fat side to within about ½ inch of the other side, so that each chop opens up like a butterfly.

2. Flatten the meat with the palm of your hand and trim off any excess fat around the perimeter.

3. Lay each chop between 2 large sheets of plastic wrap. Use the flat side of a meat tenderizer (or the bottom of a small, heavy skillet) to flatten the meat to an even thickness of about ¼ inch.

WAY TO GRILL PORK PAILLARDS

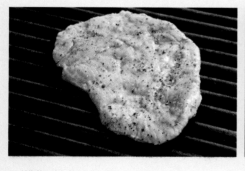 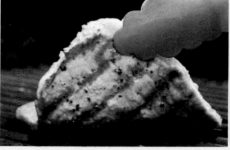 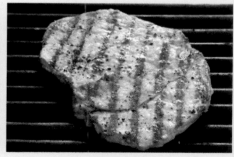

1. While thick pork chops do best over medium heat, thinly pounded paillards should be grilled quickly over very high heat.

2. Grill the first side of each paillard with the lid closed until it has nice grill marks, usually about 3 minutes.

3. The second side should need no more than 1 minute to finish cooking.

PORK PAILLARDS
WITH ROMESCO SAUCE

SERVES: 4
PREP TIME: 25 MINUTES

WAY TO GRILL: DIRECT LOW HEAT (250° TO 350°F) AND
    DIRECT HIGH HEAT (450° TO 550°F)
GRILLING TIME: 19 TO 24 MINUTES

  4 boneless center-cut pork chops, 6 to 7 ounces each
      and about 1 inch thick
      Extra-virgin olive oil
      Kosher salt
      Freshly ground black pepper
  8 small leeks, no wider than 1 inch in diameter, optional

SAUCE
  ¾ cup roughly chopped roasted red bell pepper
  ⅓ cup slivered almonds, toasted
  1 tablespoon ketchup
  1 tablespoon extra-virgin olive oil
  1 tablespoon fresh lemon juice
  1 teaspoon roughly chopped garlic
  ½ teaspoon paprika
  ⅛ teaspoon ground cayenne pepper

  1 tablespoon finely chopped fresh Italian parsley

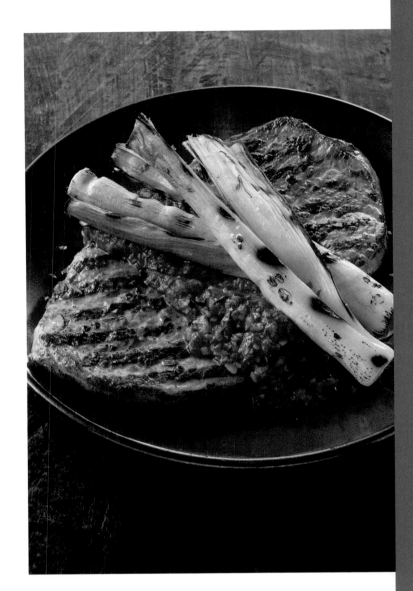

1. Butterfly each chop from the fat side and trim them of excess fat. One at a time, place each chop between 2 sheets of plastic wrap and pound to an even ¼-inch thickness. Lightly brush or spray the paillards with oil and season all sides with salt and pepper.

2. Remove the dark green tops off of each leek, cutting about 2 inches above the point where the leaves begin to darken. Trim just enough of each root end to remove the stringy parts, but leave enough of each root end so the layers remain attached. Cut each leek in half lengthwise. Remove the tough outer leaves on each leek. Rinse the leeks under water, opening up the layers to remove any dirt. Pat dry. Lightly coat the leeks with oil and season to taste with salt and pepper.

3. Prepare the grill for direct cooking over low heat.

4. Brush the cooking grates clean. Grill the leeks over **direct low heat**, with the lid closed as much as possible, until softened and slightly charred on all sides, 15 to 20 minutes, turning every couple of minutes for even cooking, and moving over indirect heat if the leeks become too dark before they are tender.

5. In a food processor combine the sauce ingredients. Pulse until you get a semi-smooth consistency. Season to taste with salt.

6. Increase the temperature of the grill to high heat. Brush the cooking grates clean. Grill the paillards over **direct high heat** for about 3 minutes on the first side, turning when the meat is nicely marked. The second side will need only a minute to finish cooking.

7. Transfer the paillards, with the first grilled side facing up, to a serving platter or individual plates. Divide the sauce evenly and spoon over the meat. Arrange two leeks on top of each paillard. Garnish with some parsley over the top.

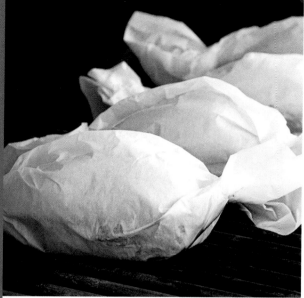

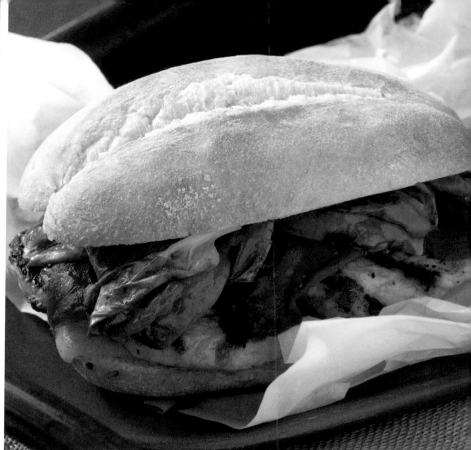

Once the sandwiches are assembled, you can reheat the meat and melt the cheese by wrapping each sandwich in parchment paper or aluminum foil and grilling them over direct medium heat, turning them occasionally.

PORK, ROASTED PEPPER, AND PEPPER JACK SANDWICHES

SERVES: 4
PREP TIME: 30 MINUTES
MARINATING TIME: 30 MINUTES

WAY TO GRILL: DIRECT HIGH HEAT (450° TO 550°F)
    AND DIRECT MEDIUM HEAT (350° TO 450°F)
GRILLING TIME: 18 TO 22 MINUTES

MARINADE
    2 tablespoons fresh lemon juice
    1 teaspoon dried oregano
    1 teaspoon finely chopped fresh rosemary
    1 teaspoon minced garlic
    1 teaspoon kosher salt
    ¼ teaspoon crushed red pepper flakes
    ⅓ cup extra-virgin olive oil

    6 boneless center-cut loin pork chops, each 2 to 4 ounces
       and about ½ inch thick, trimmed of excess fat
    2 red bell peppers
    4 crusty French rolls, split in half crosswise
    4 slices pepper jack cheese
    1 cup baby spinach, rinsed and dried

1. In a small bowl combine the lemon juice, oregano, rosemary, garlic, salt, and red pepper flakes. Whisk in the oil. Reserve 2 tablespoons of the marinade to use as a dressing.

2. Working with 1 chop at a time, place each chop between two sheets of plastic wrap. Using a flat meat tenderizer, pound the chop until it is an even ¼ inch thick. When all the chops are

pounded, place them in a large, resealable plastic bag, arrange them flat, and pour in the marinade. Press the air out of the bag and seal tightly. Turn the bag to distribute the marinade, place the bag on a plate, and let marinate at room temperature for 30 minutes. Prepare the grill for direct cooking over high heat.

3. Brush the cooking grates clean. Grill the peppers over *direct high heat*, with the lid closed as much as possible, until blackened and blistered all over, 10 to 12 minutes, turning every 3 to 5 minutes. Place the peppers in a bowl and cover with plastic wrap. Let stand for 10 to 15 minutes. Remove the peppers from the bowl and peel away and discard the charred skins. Cut off the tops and remove the seeds. Cut lengthwise into ½-inch-wide strips.

4. Remove the chops from the bag and discard the marinade. Sear the chops over *direct high heat*, with the lid closed as much as possible, about 4 minutes, turning once. During the last minute of grilling, toast the cut sides of the rolls over direct heat.

5. In a medium bowl toss the spinach with the 2 tablespoons of reserved marinade. Build the sandwiches with a slice of cheese, 1 to 1½ pork chops, cut to fit the roll, strips of roasted pepper, and spinach.

6. Lower the temperature of the grill to medium heat. Completely wrap each sandwich in a 12x12-inch sheet of parchment paper, twisting the ends in opposite directions to enclose the sandwiches. Grill over *direct medium heat* until the cheese melts and the sandwiches are hot, 4 to 6 minutes. Serve warm.

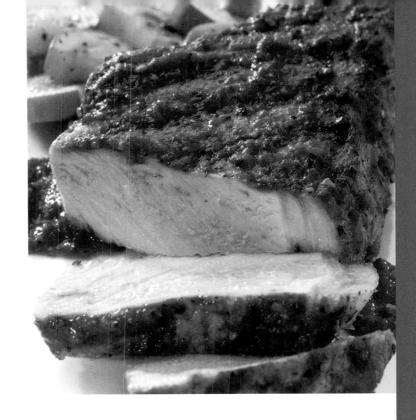

PORK LOIN CHOPS
WITH SOFRITO BARBECUE SAUCE

SERVES: 4
PREP TIME: 30 MINUTES

WAY TO GRILL: DIRECT MEDIUM HEAT (350° TO 450°F)
GRILLING TIME: 7 TO 9 MINUTES

SAUCE
1½ cups ¼-inch-diced yellow onion
  3 tablespoons extra-virgin olive oil
  1 small bay leaf
  1 tablespoon finely chopped garlic
  1 tablespoon sherry vinegar
  ½ cup apple juice
  1 can (14 ounces) fire-roasted tomatoes
  1 teaspoon paprika
  ½ teaspoon dried oregano
  ¼ teaspoon crushed red pepper flakes
  ¼ teaspoon kosher salt
  ¼ teaspoon freshly ground black pepper

RUB
  1 teaspoon kosher salt
  ½ teaspoon paprika
  ½ teaspoon dried oregano
  ½ teaspoon freshly ground black pepper

  4 bone-in pork loin rib chops, each ¾ to 1 inch thick
      Extra-virgin olive oil

1. In a medium skillet over medium heat, combine the onion, oil, and bay leaf. When the onion starts to sizzle, adjust the heat to medium-low and cook until the onions are evenly browned, about 30 minutes, stirring frequently, adding the garlic to the skillet after 15 minutes. Add the vinegar to the caramelized onion and garlic, and cook until it has almost evaporated. Then add the apple juice. Simmer until the liquid in the pan has reduced by half. Add the rest of the sauce ingredients and continue to simmer for about 5 minutes.

2. Remove the bay leaf. Transfer the sauce to a food processor or blender and puree until smooth. Reserve ½ cup of the sauce for basting and the rest to serve with the chops.

3. In a small bowl combine the rub ingredients. Lightly coat the chops with oil and season with the rub. Let the chops stand at room temperature for 20 to 30 minutes before grilling. Prepare the grill for direct cooking over high heat.

4. Brush the cooking grates clean. Grill the chops over **direct medium heat**, with the lid closed as much as possible, until they are nicely marked on each side, 4 to 5 minutes, turning once. Then brush both sides with the reserved sauce and continue grilling until the sauce cooks into the meat a bit and the centers are barely pink, 3 to 4 minutes, turning once or twice. Remove the chops from the grill and let rest for 2 to 3 minutes. Serve warm with the reserved sauce.

WAY TO GRILL PORK CHOPS WITH SOFRITO BARBECUE SAUCE

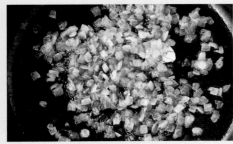

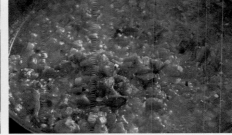

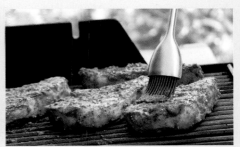

1. In Spain and throughout much of Latin America, it is common to begin sauces with a *sofrito*, that is, slowly browned onions and garlic followed by tomatoes.

2. Combined with apple juice and spices, this *sofrito* becomes a barbecue sauce. Use it for brushing onto the chops and as a dipping sauce.

3. Mark the pork chops well on both sides before brushing on the sauce. Then let the sauce flavors cook into the meat.

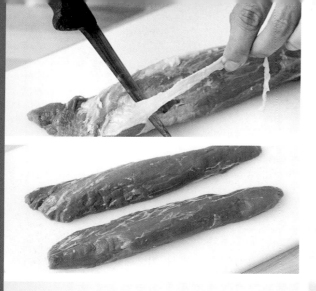

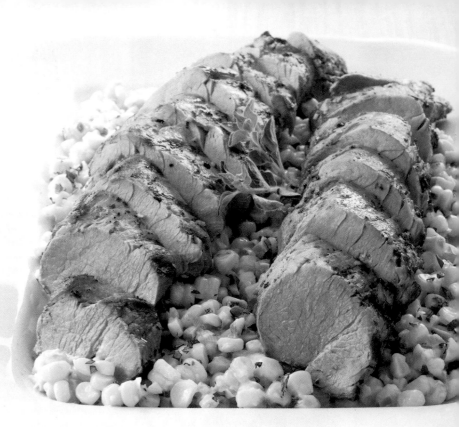

To remove the tough silver skin from the surface, slip the tip of a narrow, sharp knife under a piece of silver skin. Then grab the loosened end and stretch it taut. Slide the knife just over the pinkish meat below, angling it upward to avoid cutting into the meat. The goal is to "clean" the tenderloins without losing any more meat than necessary.

PORK TENDERLOINS WITH CREAMY CORN

SERVES: 4 TO 6
PREP TIME: 25 MINUTES
MARINATING TIME: 1 TO 3 HOURS

WAY TO GRILL: DIRECT MEDIUM HEAT (350° TO 450°F)
GRILLING TIME: 25 TO 30 MINUTES

PASTE
- 3 large garlic cloves
- ¼ cup fresh oregano leaves and tender stems
- 1 teaspoon kosher salt
- ¼ cup extra-virgin olive oil
- 2 tablespoons cider vinegar
- ½ teaspoon freshly ground black pepper

- 2 pork tenderloins, about 1 pound each

- 5 ears fresh corn, husked
  Extra-virgin olive oil
- ½ cup finely chopped red onion
- 3 scallions, thinly sliced crosswise
- 1 cup heavy cream
- ¼ teaspoon kosher salt
- ⅛ teaspoon freshly ground black pepper
- 1 tablespoon finely chopped fresh oregano
  Hot sauce, optional

1. Roughly chop the garlic, then sprinkle the oregano and salt over the garlic. Continue to chop until the garlic and oregano are minced. Periodically use the side of your knife blade to press the garlic on the cutting board and create a paste. Transfer the garlic paste to a bowl and mix in the oil, vinegar, and pepper.

2. Trim the pork tenderloins of surface fat and silver skin. Brush the paste all over the surface of the meat. Cover and refrigerate for 1 to 3 hours. Allow the meat to stand at room temperature for 20 to 30 minutes before grilling. Prepare the grill for direct cooking over medium heat.

3. Lightly brush the ears of corn with oil. Brush the cooking grates clean. Grill the corn over **direct medium heat**, with the lid closed as much as possible, until browned in spots and barely tender, about 10 minutes, turning occasionally. Using a sharp knife, cut the corn kernels off the cobs.

4. In a medium skillet over medium heat, warm 2 tablespoons of olive oil. Add the onion and scallions; cook for 3 to 4 minutes, stirring occasionally. Add the corn kernels, cream, salt, and pepper. Mix well. Reduce the heat to low, and simmer until about half of the cream has evaporated, 5 to 7 minutes. Add the oregano and a couple dashes of hot sauce, if desired. Set aside.

5. Grill the pork over **direct medium heat**, with the lid closed as much as possible, until the outsides are evenly seared and the centers are barely pink, 15 to 20 minutes, turning about every 5 minutes. The internal temperature of the tenderloins should be 150°F when fully cooked.

6. Remove the pork from the grill and let rest for 3 to 5 minutes before slicing. Meanwhile, warm the corn mixture over medium heat. Cut each tenderloin crosswise into slices about ½ inch thick. Arrange the slices on a platter or individual plates. Serve warm with the creamy corn.

PORK TENDERLOINS
WITH SMOKED PAPRIKA ROUILLE

SERVES: 6
PREP TIME: 15 MINUTES

WAY TO GRILL: DIRECT MEDIUM HEAT (350° TO 450°F)
GRILLING TIME: 27 TO 35 MINUTES

ROUILLE
+ 2 medium red bell peppers
+ 2–3 small garlic cloves
+ ¾ teaspoon kosher salt
+ 1 cup plain bread crumbs
+ 3 tablespoons fresh lemon juice
+ ¾ teaspoon smoked paprika
+ ⅔ cup extra-virgin olive oil

+ 2 pork tenderloins, about 1 pound each
   Extra-virgin olive oil
+ ½ teaspoon kosher salt
+ ¼ teaspoon freshly ground black pepper

1. Prepare the grill for direct cooking over medium heat. Brush the cooking grates clean. Grill the peppers over **direct medium heat**, with the lid closed as much as possible, until blackened and blistered all over, 12 to 15 minutes, turning every 3 to 5 minutes. Place the peppers in a bowl and cover with plastic wrap. Let stand for 10 to 15 minutes. Remove the peppers from the bowl and peel away and discard the charred skins, tops, and seeds.

2. In a blender or food processor, mince the garlic first, and then add the roasted peppers, salt, and bread crumbs. Add the lemon juice and paprika and, with the motor running, slowly add the oil. Blend until very smooth and orangey-red in color. If the rouille is too thick, add about 1 tablespoon of water. Season to taste with more salt, if needed.

3. Trim the tenderloins of any surface fat and silver skin. Lightly brush with oil and season evenly with the salt and pepper. Allow the meat to stand at room temperature for 20 to 30 minutes before grilling.

4. Grill the tenderloins over **direct medium heat**, with the lid closed as much as possible, until the outsides are evenly seared and the centers are barely pink, 15 to 20 minutes, turning about every 5 minutes. The internal temperature of the tenderloins should be 150°F when fully cooked.

5. Remove the pork from the grill and let rest for 3 to 5 minutes. Cut each tenderloin crosswise into thin slices. Serve warm or at room temperature with the rouille.

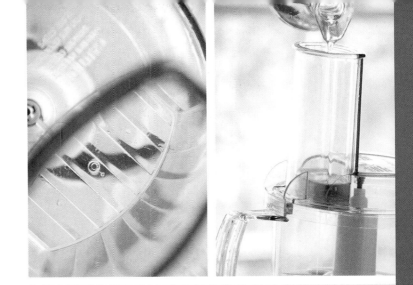

A *rouille* is a rust-colored garlicky paste that it is traditionally added to bouillabaisse (fish stew), but if you thin out a *rouille* with a bit more extra-virgin olive oil, it also makes a very nice sauce. The key to a smooth texture is adding the oil very slowly while the paste whirs in a food processor or blender. Some food processors have a handy little hole in the feed tube that prevents too much oil from pouring into the emulsion all at once.

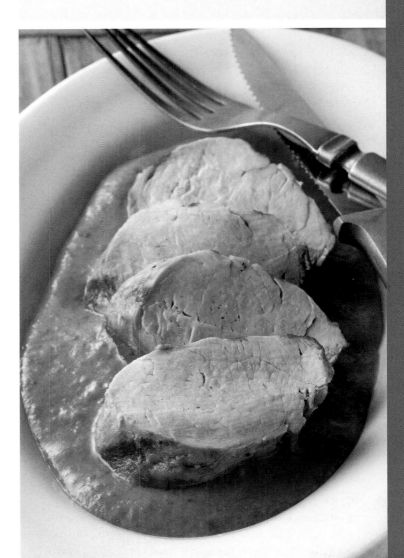

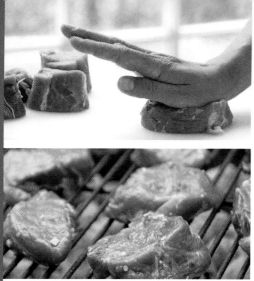

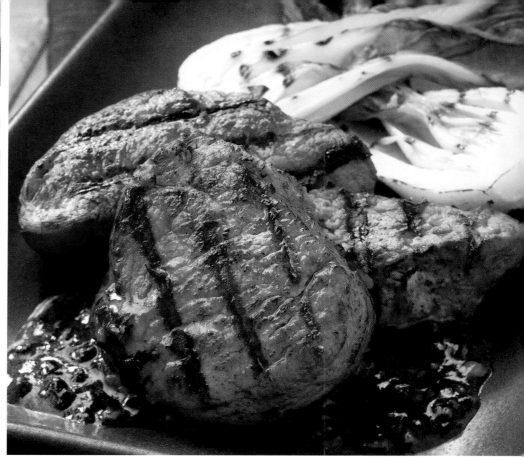

Cut each pork tenderloin crosswise into pieces about 1½ inches thick. Use the heel of your hand to flatten each piece into a medallion about 1 inch thick. For juicy results, marinate the medallions for at least 1 hour, and then grill them gently over medium heat until barely pink in the center.

PORK MEDALLIONS WITH ASIAN BLACK BEAN SAUCE

SERVES: 4
PREP TIME: 25 MINUTES
MARINATING TIME: 1 HOUR

WAY TO GRILL: DIRECT MEDIUM HEAT (350° TO 450°F)
GRILLING TIME: 4 TO 5 MINUTES

MARINADE
- ½ teaspoon grated orange zest
- ¼ cup fresh orange juice
- ¼ cup Chinese rice wine or dry sherry
- 2 tablespoons soy sauce
- 1 tablespoon hoisin sauce
- 1 tablespoon minced fresh ginger
- 1 tablespoon toasted sesame oil
- ¼ teaspoon crushed red pepper flakes

- 2 pork tenderloins, about 1 pound each, trimmed of silver skin

SAUCE
- 2 tablespoons Chinese fermented black beans
- ½ cup low-sodium chicken broth
- 2 tablespoons Chinese rice wine or dry sherry
- 1 tablespoon soy sauce
- 1 teaspoon granulated sugar
- 1½ teaspoons cornstarch
- 1 tablespoon peanut or vegetable oil
- 2 teaspoons peeled and minced fresh ginger
- 1 garlic clove, minced
- 2 tablespoons fresh orange juice

1. In a medium bowl whisk the marinade ingredients.

2. Cut off the thin, tapered end from each tenderloin and reserve for another use, or marinate and grill along with the medallions. Cut each tenderloin crosswise into 6 equal pieces, each about 1½ inches thick. One at a time, stand the pork rounds on a work surface and, using the heel of your hand, slightly flatten into a round medallion about 1 inch thick. Place the medallions in a large, resealable plastic bag and pour in the marinade. Press the air out of the bag and seal tightly. Turn the bag several times to distribute the marinade and refrigerate for at least 1 hour, turning the bag occasionally.

3. In a small bowl filled with warm water, soak the fermented black beans for 10 to 20 minutes. Drain well. Coarsely chop the beans and set aside. In a medium bowl whisk the broth, rice wine, soy sauce, and sugar until the sugar dissolves. Sprinkle in the cornstarch and stir to dissolve. Set aside.

4. In a small saucepan over medium-high heat, warm the oil. Add the ginger and garlic, and stir until softened, about 20 seconds. Stir in the beans, then the broth mixture, and bring to a full boil, stirring constantly, until the sauce is slightly thickened. Remove from the heat and stir in the orange juice.

5. Prepare the grill for direct cooking over medium heat. Brush the cooking grates clean. Remove the pork from the bag and discard the marinade. Grill the medallions over **direct medium heat**, with the lid closed as much as possible, until the outsides are evenly seared and the centers are barely pink, 4 to 5 minutes, turning once. Remove from the grill and let rest for 2 to 3 minutes. Serve hot with the black bean sauce.

SODA-BRINED PORK LOIN WITH CHERRY-CHIPOTLE GLAZE

SERVES: 4 TO 6
PREP TIME: 25 MINUTES
BRINING TIME: 1 TO 2 HOURS

WAY TO GRILL: DIRECT AND INDIRECT HIGH HEAT
 (450° TO 550°F)
GRILLING TIME: 33 TO 42 MINUTES
SPECIAL EQUIPMENT: LARGE DISPOSABLE FOIL PAN

 4 cups Dr. Pepper® (do not use diet soda)
 ½ cup kosher salt
 1 boneless center-cut pork loin, 3 to 4 pounds

GLAZE
 1 jar (9 ounces) tart cherry preserves
 ½ cup Dr. Pepper®
 ½ cup water
 1–2 tablespoons minced canned chipotle in adobo
 4 teaspoons Dijon mustard

 Vegetable oil

1. Pour the soda into a large bowl and slowly add the salt (the mixture will foam up quite a bit so be sure to use a bowl large enough to prevent overflowing). Stir until the salt dissolves completely, 1 to 2 minutes. Place a large, disposable plastic bag inside a large bowl, and carefully pour the brine into the bag.

2. Trim excess fat and silver skin from the pork. Submerge the pork in the brine, seal the bag, and refrigerate for 1 to 2 hours.

3. In a small bowl combine the glaze ingredients.

4. Remove the pork from the bag and discard the brine. Pat dry with paper towels. Lightly coat the pork with oil and let stand at room temperature for 20 to 30 minutes before grilling. Prepare the grill for direct and indirect cooking over high heat.

5. Brush the cooking grates clean. Sear the pork over **direct high heat**, with the lid closed as much as possible, until the surface is well marked but not burned, 8 to 12 minutes, turning once.

6. Place a large disposable foil pan over **indirect high heat** and pour the glaze into the pan. Transfer the pork to the pan and turn to coat with the glaze. Grill the pork over **indirect high heat**, with the lid closed as much as possible, until barely pink in the center and the internal temperature reaches 145° to 150°F, 25 to 30 minutes, turning in the glaze every 8 to 10 minutes. If the glaze gets too thick or starts to scorch, add a little water or more soda to the pan. Transfer the pork to a cutting board and let rest for about 5 minutes. Cut the pork crosswise into ½-inch-thick slices and serve with the remaining pan sauce on the side.

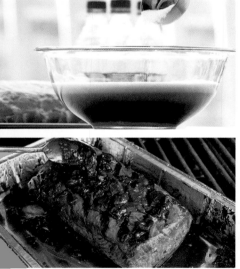

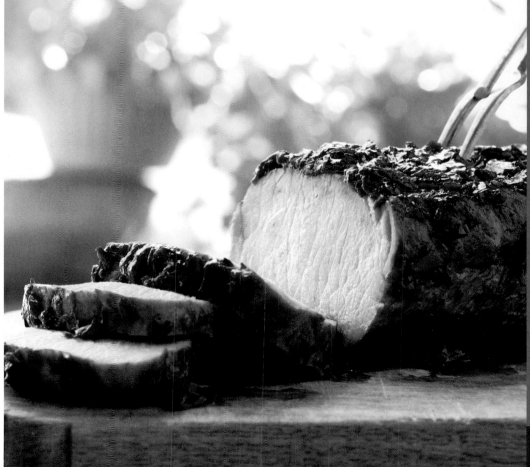

If it's not treated right, pork loin can dry out all too quickly on the grill. The surest way to prevent this is to brine it first in a sweet and savory solution, swelling the meat with moisture and flavor. Then brown the roast over direct heat and finish cooking it over indirect heat, glazing it periodically.

WAY TO MAKE ROTISSERIE PORK LOIN

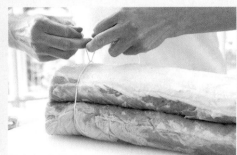

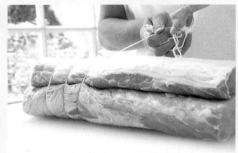

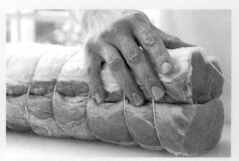

1. Large, thick pieces of meat will almost always be juicier after cooking than small narrow ones will, so improve your chances of wonderfully moist results by tying two sections of pork loin together.

2. Place one roast on top of the other, with the fat sides on the outside, and tie them together crosswise with individual lengths of butcher's twine separated by an inch or so.

3. Cut 2 very long pieces of twine, each about 4 feet. Tie one end of each piece to a crosswise piece at one end of the roast. Weave the long pieces of twine lengthwise in and out of the crosswise pieces and all the way around the length of the roast.

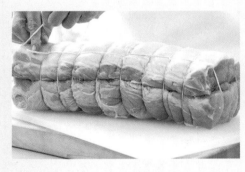

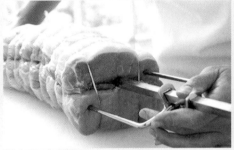

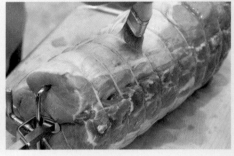

4. Tie off each lengthwise piece of twine at the knot where it began, on the first crosswise piece. The twine will hold the meat in place as it shrinks a little on the rotisserie.

5. Slide the center rod (spit) of the rotisserie between the sections of pork loin, making sure to imbed the fork prongs well inside the meat.

6. Let the meat rest at room temperature for 1 hour before cooking. Then brush it with oil and season it evenly with salt and pepper.

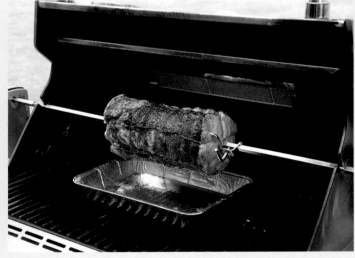

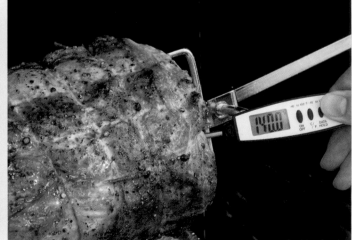

7. Natural juices baste the meat inside and out as the roast turns slowly on the rotisserie. Place a foil pan underneath to prevent grease from falling into the grill.

8. Check the internal temperature of the meat at the center of the roast. When it reaches 145° to 150°F, turn off the rotisserie and, wearing insulated barbecue mitts, remove it from the grill. While the meat rests at room temperature, it will continue to cook an additional 5° to 10°F.

PORK

ROTISSERIE PORK LOIN AGRO DOLCE

SERVES: 12 TO 14
PREP TIME: 45 MINUTES

WAY TO GRILL: INDIRECT HEAT (ABOUT 400°F)
GRILLING TIME: 1 TO 1¼ HOURS
SPECIAL EQUIPMENT: BUTCHER'S TWINE, ROTISSERIE,
    LARGE DISPOSABLE FOIL PAN

SAUCE
   2 tablespoons extra-virgin olive oil
2½ cups finely diced yellow onions
 ½ teaspoon kosher salt
  3 cups red wine
  1 cup finely diced pitted prunes
  1 cup raisins
  1 tablespoon finely grated orange zest
 ¾ cup fresh orange juice
 ⅛ teaspoon ground cloves
     Kosher salt
     Freshly ground black pepper

  2 boneless pork loin roasts, 3 to 3½ pounds each
  2 tablespoons extra-virgin olive oil
1½ teaspoons kosher salt
  1 teaspoon freshly ground black pepper

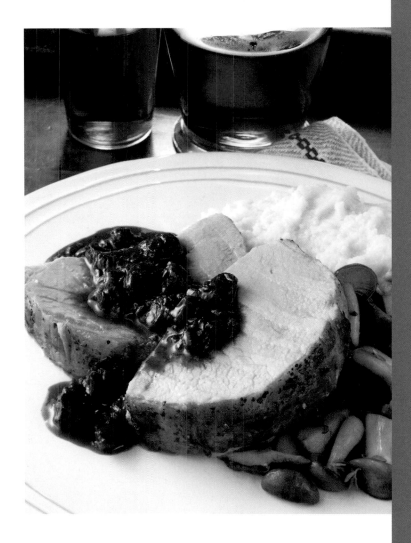

1. In a medium saucepan over medium heat, warm the oil. Add the onions and salt, and cook until the onions are quite soft, about 15 minutes, stirring often. Increase the heat to high, add the wine, and boil until reduced by half, about 8 minutes. Stir in the prunes, raisins, and orange zest, reduce the heat to medium, and cook until the fruit is tender, 5 to 10 minutes, stirring occasionally. Add the orange juice and cloves, and season to taste with salt and pepper. Keep warm.

2. Trim the pork loins to match in size and then place one roast on top of the other, making sure the sides of the roast with the layers of fat are facing outward. This fatty layer will help protect the meat while it cooks. Tie the two roasts together to make one large cylindrical roast. Allow the roast to stand at room temperature for 1 hour before grilling. Brush the roast with the oil and season with the salt and pepper.

3. Prepare the grill for rotisserie cooking over indirect heat. If your gas grill has one, turn on the infrared burner to **low** and set the outer burner control knobs to **low heat**. The temperature of the grill should be around 400°F (you may need to adjust the outer burners to medium heat).

4. Carefully slide one pronged fork onto the spit, with the tines facing inward, about 10 inches from the end of the spit. Secure the fork but do not tighten at this time. Slide the spit through the center of the roast and gently push the roast onto the fork tines so that they are deep inside the roast. Add the other pronged fork to the spit with the tines facing inward and slide down until they are firmly imbedded into the roast. Secure the fork, but do not completely tighten at this time. Wearing barbecue mitts, place the pointed end of the spit into the rotisserie motor. If necessary, adjust the roast so that it is centered on the spit and tighten the forks into place. Place the foil pan under the roast to catch any grease. Turn on the motor to begin the rotisserie.

5. Grill the roast until the internal temperature reaches 145° to 150°F, 1 to 1¼ hours. To check the temperature, turn off the rotisserie motor and insert a thermometer down the center of one of the roasts. Wearing barbecue mitts, carefully remove the spit from the grill. Gently loosen the forks and slide the roast off of the spit. Transfer the pork to a carving board, tent with foil, and let rest for 15 to 30 minutes (the roast will continue to cook an additional 5° to 10°F during this time).

6. Slice the roast and serve with the sauce.

WAY TO GRILL BONE-IN PORK LOIN

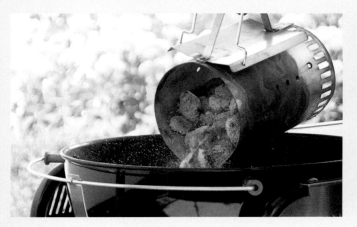

1. A moderately hot fire of about 350°F is just right for roasting a bone-in pork loin. Begin with a chimney starter filled about two-thirds full with charcoal briquettes. Let the coals burn down until they are completely covered with ash, and then dump them onto the charcoal grate.

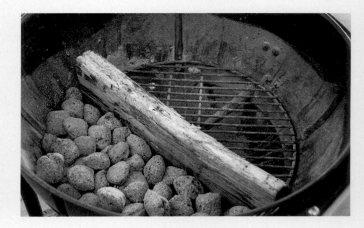

2. Spread the briquettes in a single layer over one side of the charcoal grate and lay an oak log beside them. It will smolder and smoke, filling the pork with haunting outdoorsy aromas.

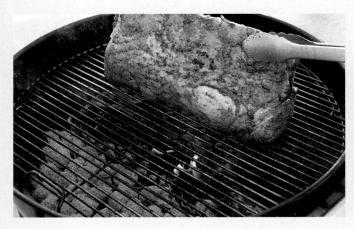

3. Cook the roast on the cooler side of the grill opposite the bed of charcoal, with the bone side facing down and the thick meaty side facing the coals. If the log catches fire, use a spray bottle filled with water to douse the flames.

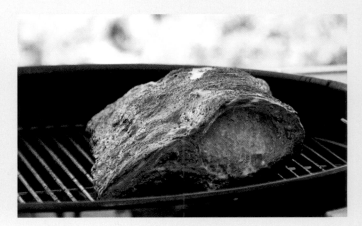

4. After cooking with the lid on for 45 minutes, rotate the roast 180 degrees so the tips of the bones are facing the coals. As the meat finishes cooking, the grill temperature should fall to about 300°F.

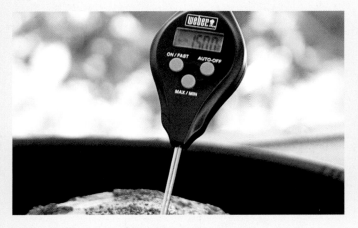

5. Remove the roast from the grill when the internal temperature reaches the range of 145° to 150°F. Loosely cover the roast with foil and let it rest for 15 minutes, which allows the juices to stay in the meat when you slice it.

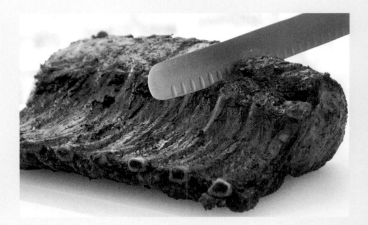

6. The easiest way to carve the roast is to turn it over so the bone side is facing up. Then you can see exactly where the bones are and slice right between them.

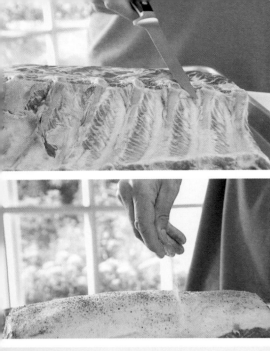

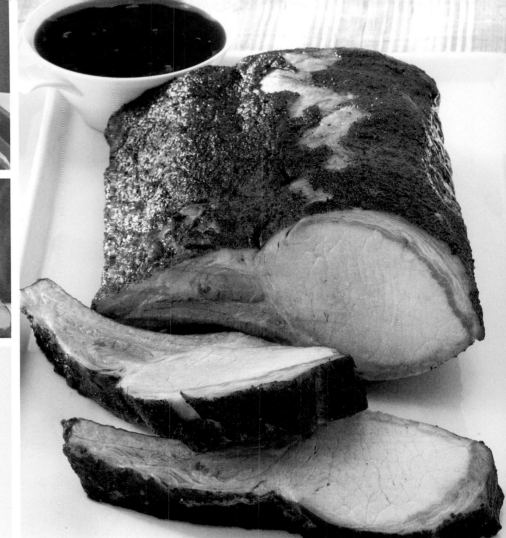

When you buy a bone-in pork loin, make sure the butcher has removed the chine bone (backbone), which runs along the top of all the rib bones. Otherwise it will be nearly impossible to slice between the ribs and serve individual chops. Also, don't be afraid to season the meat generously before cooking. It is a thick roast that can handle plenty of salt and pepper.

SMOKE-ROASTED PORK LOIN WITH RED CURRANT SAUCE

SERVES: 8
PREP TIME: 20 MINUTES

WAY TO GRILL: INDIRECT MEDIUM HEAT (300° TO 350°F)
GRILLING TIME: 1½ TO 2 HOURS

- 1 bone-in pork loin roast, 7 to 8 pounds
- 3 tablespoons extra-virgin olive oil
- 2 teaspoons kosher salt
- 1 teaspoon freshly ground black pepper

- 1 oak log, about 18 inches long and 4 inches in diameter

SAUCE
- ¾ cup red currant preserves
- ½ cup ketchup
- ½ cup apple juice
- 2 tablespoons cider vinegar
- 1 tablespoon soy sauce
- 1 tablespoon whiskey
- ½ teaspoon crushed red pepper flakes

1. Lightly coat the pork with the oil and season with the salt and pepper. Allow the pork to stand at room temperature for 30 minutes while you prepare the grill.

2. Starting with about two-thirds of a chimney of lit coals, arrange them on one-third of the charcoal grate. Place the log alongside the outer edge of the coals; do not place it directly on top of the coals. The log should slowly start to smolder but should not catch on fire. If it does catch on fire, use a spray bottle filled with water to douse the flames. Put the cooking grate in place and set the pork roast, bone side down and with the meaty section facing the fire, over *indirect medium heat* (about 350°F), with the lid closed, and cook for 45 minutes.

3. After 45 minutes, to maintain the heat, add 8 to 10 lit briquettes to the coals and rotate the meat 180 degrees so the bone section is facing the heat. Continue to cook over *indirect medium heat*, with the lid closed, until the internal temperature reaches 145° to 150°F, 45 minutes to 1¼ hours. The fire should slowly lose heat and finish cooking the roast at about 300°F.

4. In a medium saucepan over medium heat, combine the sauce ingredients. Let the sauce come to a simmer and cook until the preserves have melted and the sauce is well combined, stirring occasionally. Remove from the heat.

5. Transfer the roast to a cutting board, loosely cover with foil, and let rest 15 to 30 minutes. Slice between each bone. Serve warm with the sauce.

WAY TO BARBECUE PORK SHOULDER

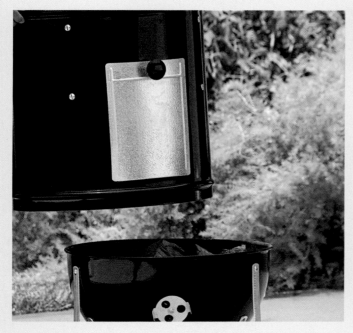

1. A water smoker can maintain temperatures between 225° and 250°F for several hours, which is just what you need to break down the connective tissue in pork shoulder roasts.

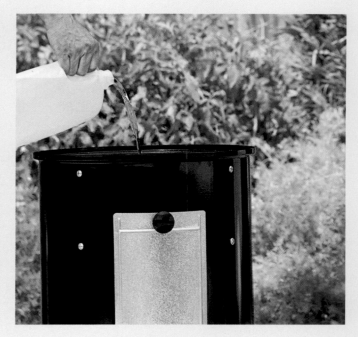

2. Fill the water pan in the middle section of the smoker. It will absorb some of the charcoal's heat and release it slowly with some humidity.

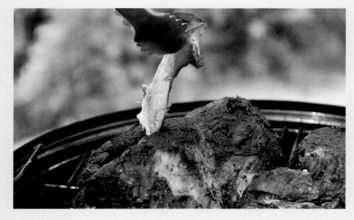

3. After 8 to 10 hours of barbecuing, the meat will be so tender that you can slide the bone out cleanly.

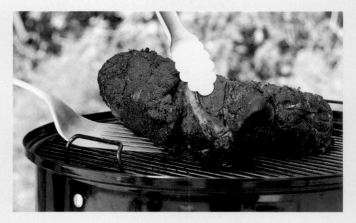

4. Ideally you will need both a spatula and a pair of tongs to remove the shoulders without the meat falling apart.

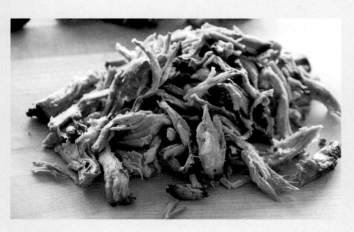

5. Shred the meat with your fingers or two forks. Discard any clumps of fat, but hold onto the crispy bits of "bark" that have developed on the outside of the meat.

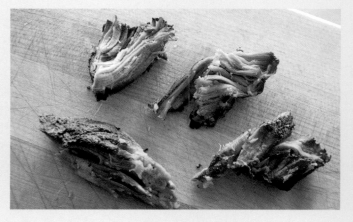

6. The pinkish color of the meat is a good sign that smoke has penetrated the surface and filled the pork with authentic barbecue flavor.

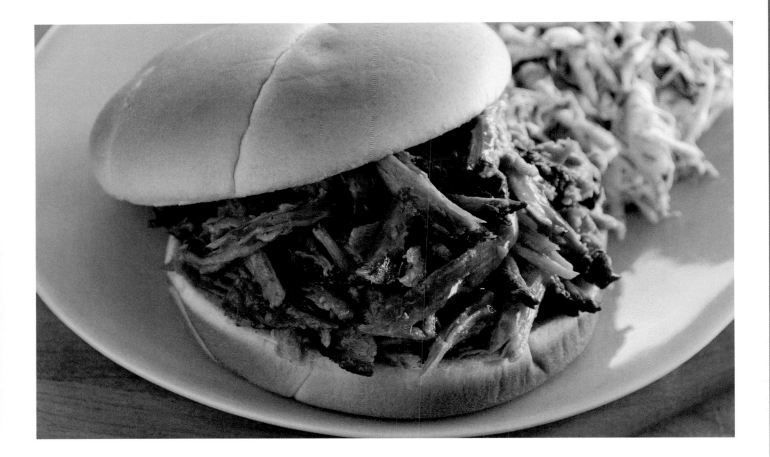

PULLED PORK SANDWICHES

SERVES: 10 TO 12
PREP TIME: 25 MINUTES

WAY TO GRILL: INDIRECT LOW HEAT (225° TO 250°F)
GRILLING TIME: 8 TO 10 HOURS

RUB
  2 tablespoons pure chile powder
  2 tablespoons kosher salt
  4 teaspoons granulated garlic
  2 teaspoons freshly ground black pepper
  1 teaspoon dry mustard

  2 bone-in pork shoulder roasts, 5 to 6 pounds each
  3 large handfuls hickory wood chips, soaked in water for at
     least 30 minutes

SAUCE
  1 cup ketchup
  ¾ cup apple cider vinegar
  ¼ cup lightly packed light brown sugar
  1½ teaspoons Worcestershire sauce
  1 teaspoon hot sauce, or to taste
  1 teaspoon kosher salt
  ½ teaspoon dry mustard
  ¼ teaspoon freshly ground black pepper

  12 hamburger buns

1. Prepare your smoker, following manufacturer's instructions, for indirect cooking over low heat.

2. In a small bowl mix the rub ingredients. Season the pork shoulders all over with the rub and press the spices into the meat.

3. Smoke the pork over *indirect low heat*, with the lid closed, adding a handful of drained wood chips to the coals every hour for the first 3 hours, until the internal temperature of the meat reaches 190°F. At this point the bone should easily slip out of the meat, and the meat should be falling apart in some areas. The total cooking time will be 8 to 10 hours. Maintain the heat of the smoker between 225° to 250°F.

4. In a large, heavy-bottomed saucepan whisk the sauce ingredients. Bring to a simmer over medium heat and cook for about 5 minutes, stirring occasionally. Taste and adjust the seasonings, if necessary. It should be spicy and tangy.

5. Transfer the pork roasts to a sheet pan and tightly cover them with aluminum foil. Let the pork rest for 30 minutes.

6. Pull the warm meat apart with your fingers or use two forks to shred the meat. Discard any large pieces of fat or sinew. In a large bowl moisten the pork with as much sauce as you like (you may not need all of the sauce). Pile the pork on hamburger buns. Serve warm with coleslaw, if desired.

WAY TO MAKE PORCHETTA

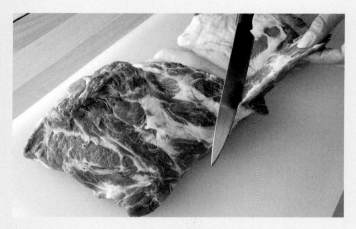

1. Trim off the relatively thin pieces of meat on the ends of the pork shoulder roast. Also trim the thick sections of the roast to create a fairly even thickness from end to end.

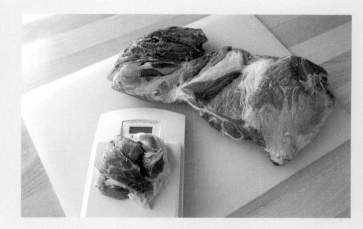

2. Ideally you will have 8 to 10 ounces of trimmed meat and fat to mix with delicious herbs, spices, garlic, and olive oil. This will be the porchetta filling.

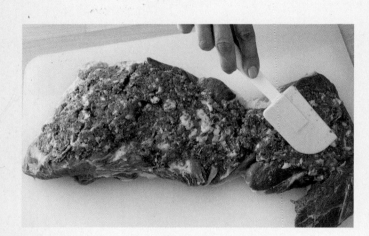

3. Pulse the ingredients in a food processor 20 to 25 times until they have the look and texture of ground sausage. Then spread the filling over the interior of the roast.

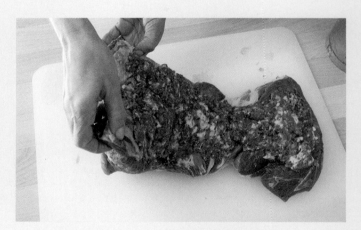

4. Leave a border along the edges of the pork roast so the filling does not spill out when you roll the meat. Press the filling into any grooves in the meat.

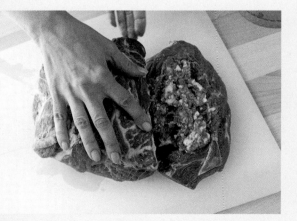

5. Now roll up the meat from one short end to the other, creating an evenly shaped and compact cylinder.

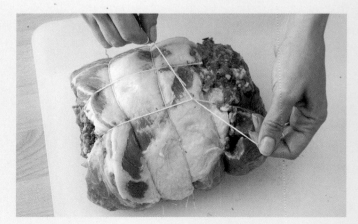

6. Use several long pieces of butcher's twine to tie the roast both crosswise and lengthwise. Let the roast stand at room temperature for 20 to 30 minutes before cooking.

PORCHETTA-STYLE PORK SHOULDER

SERVES: 6 TO 8
PREP TIME: 30 MINUTES

WAY TO GRILL: INDIRECT MEDIUM HEAT (350° TO 400°F)
GRILLING TIME: 2 TO 2½ HOURS
SPECIAL EQUIPMENT: BUTCHER'S TWINE

FILLING
- ½ cup extra-virgin olive oil
- ⅓ cup rosemary leaves, about 3 sprigs
- ¼ cup loosely packed sage leaves, about 16 large leaves
- 1 tablespoon finely grated lemon zest
- 1 tablespoon chopped garlic
- 1 teaspoon kosher salt
- ½ teaspoon whole fennel seed
- ½ teaspoon crushed red pepper flakes

- 1 boneless pork shoulder roast, about 5 pounds, butterflied, ends trimmed to produce 8 to 10 ounces meat and fat
- 1 tablespoon extra-virgin olive oil
- ½ teaspoon kosher salt
- ½ teaspoon freshly ground black pepper

1. In a food processor combine the filling ingredients and process until they form a smooth puree. Add the trimmed meat and fat, and pulse until it resembles ground sausage, 20 to 25 pulses.

2. Place the roast, skin side down, on a work surface. Evenly distribute the filling over the pork, leaving a border around the edges of the roast. Roll up the meat and tie with butcher's twine in 5 or 6 places. Rub the outside of the roast with the oil, salt, and pepper. Let the roast stand at room temperature for 20 to 30 minutes before grilling. Prepare the grill for indirect cooking over medium heat.

3. Brush the cooking grates clean. Grill the roast over *indirect medium heat*, with the lid closed, until the internal temperature reaches 180° to 185°F, 2 to 2½ hours.

4. Transfer the roast to a cutting board, loosely cover with foil, and let rest for 20 to 30 minutes. Remove the twine and carve the meat into thin slices. Serve warm.

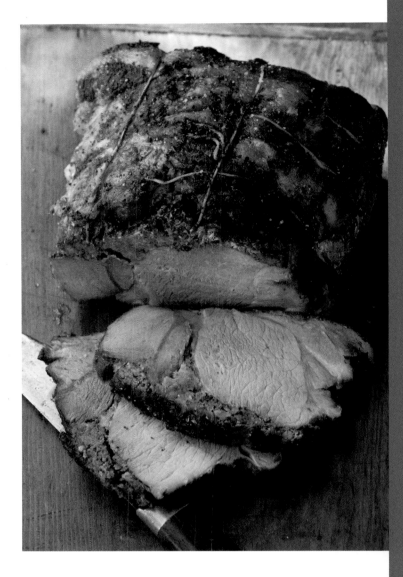

In and around Rome, Italy, porchetta is a bacchanalian dish that involves stuffing a whole pig with wild fennel, garlic, and spices, and then cooking it on a rotisserie spit. Assuming that you may not be inclined to tackle such a huge project, here's a simpler version that calls for a pork shoulder filled with the authentic flavors.

WAY TO SEASON PORK ROAST

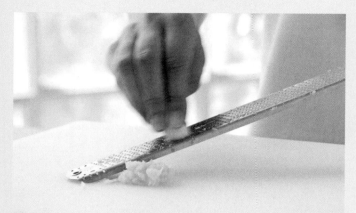

1. Grate the garlic with a microplane.

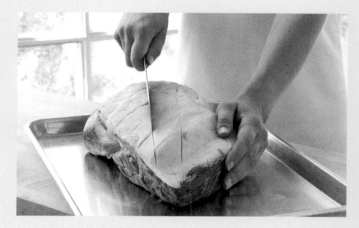

2. Make shallow crosshatch slashes about 2 inches apart through the fat but not into the flesh.

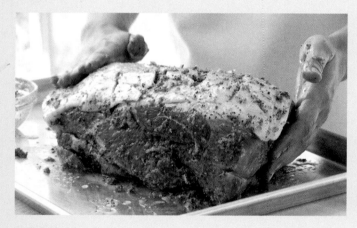

3. Smear the garlic-and-herb paste all over the roast, pressing it into the slashes and crevices.

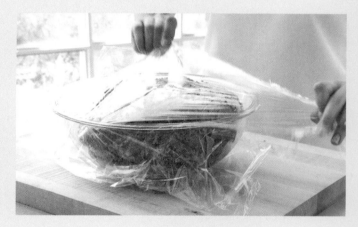

4. Cover the roast and refrigerate for 12 to 24 hours.

WAY TO GRILL PORK ROAST

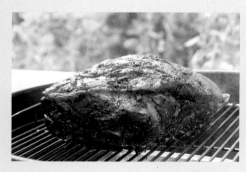

1. Cook a bone-in pork shoulder over indirect low heat (about 300°F) so that its collagen and fat will melt and make the meat succulent before the outside burns. This requires starting the fire with a charcoal chimney starter filled about halfway and adding 8 to 10 briquettes every hour or so.

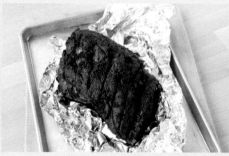

2. When the meat's internal temperature reaches 185° to 190°F, remove the roast from the grill, wrap it in foil, and let the meat rest and juices redistribute for a full hour.

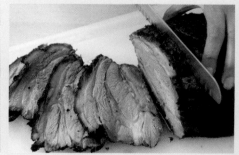

3. Cut the roast into ½-inch slices or tear the meat into bite-sized chucks. Serve with a bold garlic-citrus sauce called mojo (pronounced "mo-ho").

LATINO PORK ROAST

SERVES: 6 TO 8
PREP TIME: 30 MINUTES
MARINATING TIME: 12 TO 24 HOURS

WAY TO GRILL: INDIRECT LOW HEAT (ABOUT 250°F)
GRILLING TIME: 5 TO 7 HOURS, PLUS 1 HOUR
  RESTING TIME

PASTE
- 5 large garlic cloves
- 3 tablespoons extra-virgin olive oil
- 3 tablespoons cider vinegar
- 2 tablespoons dried oregano
- 1 tablespoon plus 2 teaspoons kosher salt
- 1 tablespoon freshly ground black pepper

- 1 bone-in pork shoulder roast (Boston butt), with an outer layer of fat, 6 to 7 pounds
- 4 handfuls oak or hickory wood chips, soaked in water for at least 30 minutes

MOJO
- Finely grated zest of 1 orange
- 1 cup fresh orange juice
- ½ cup fresh grapefruit juice
- ⅓ cup finely chopped white onion
- 2 tablespoons distilled white vinegar
- 1 small serrano chile, minced
- 1 garlic clove, finely chopped
- 1 teaspoon granulated sugar
- Kosher salt

- 3 tablespoons finely chopped fresh cilantro

1. Grate the garlic with a microplane. Transfer to a small bowl and combine with the rest of the paste ingredients.

2. Score the fat on the roast in a crosshatch pattern, about 2 inches apart, cutting through the fat just to the flesh. Rub the paste all over the roast, place the roast in a bowl, cover, and refrigerate for 12 to 24 hours. Let the roast stand at room temperature for 1 hour before grilling.

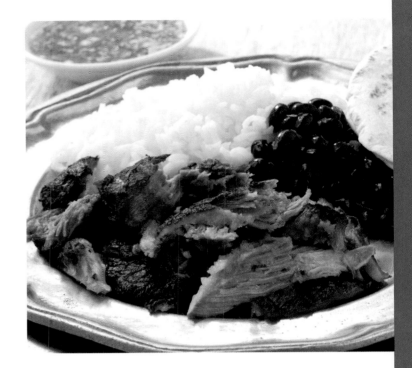

3. Prepare the grill for indirect cooking over low heat. Brush the cooking grates clean. Drain 1 handful of the wood chips and scatter them over the coals or in the smoker box of a gas grill, following the manufacturer's instructions. Grill the pork, fat side down, over **indirect low heat**, with the lid closed as much as possible, until the meat is so tender that it gives no resistance when pierced with a meat fork and the internal temperature registers 185° to 190°F, 5 to 7 hours, turning once after about 3 hours and adding 1 handful of drained wood chips each hour until they are gone. Transfer the roast to a platter and loosely cover with aluminum foil. Let rest for about 1 hour.

4. In a small serving bowl combine the mojo ingredients, including salt to taste, stirring to dissolve the sugar and salt. Cover, and set aside. Just before serving, stir in the cilantro.

5. Cut the roast into ½-inch slices (it may fall apart into chunks and not carve neatly, but that's okay). Serve warm with the mojo.

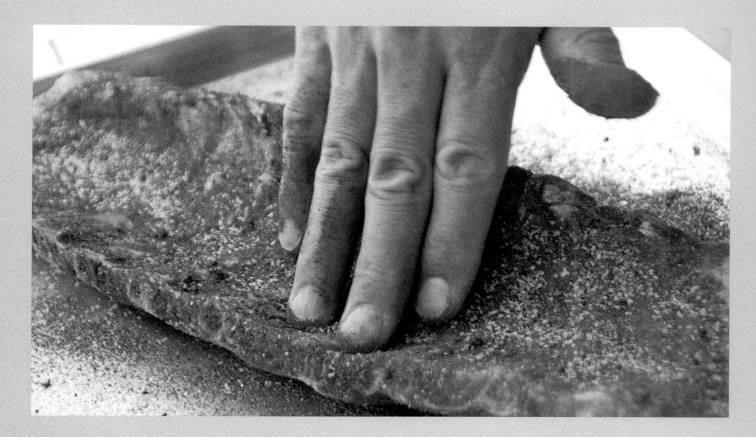

WAY TO BARBECUE PORK RIBS
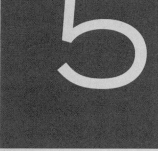 THINGS YOU NEED TO KNOW

1 STRIKE THE BALANCE

A perfectly barbecued rack of ribs achieves a seamless harmony of effects. The slightly crisp texture of a handsome, glossy surface gives way to morsels of luscious meat with a fragrant wood-smoke flavor. At each step of cooking your goal is to balance the spices, sauce, and smoke with the inherently beautiful flavor of slow-roasted pork, never letting one effect outdo the others.

2 USE WHAT YOU HAVE

You can make satisfying barbecued ribs on a gas grill, charcoal grill, or smoker. Each one is capable of slowly tenderizing the rib meat and scenting it with wood smoke, although with a gas grill, you will need a smoker box attachment.

3 WATCH THAT HEAT

The key to tender ribs is maintaining a low temperature for several hours. Spikes and valleys of heat will tighten and dry out the meat, but consistently low temperatures will produce soft and succulent meat.

4 ALL IN GOOD TIME

It's one thing to wait the required 3 to 4 hours for baby back ribs or 5 to 6 hours for spareribs, but that's not the only timing issue. You must not sauce any ribs too early, especially if you are using a sweet sauce, as the sugars will burn and threaten your precious ribs. Sauce them during the final 30 minutes of cooking, or just before you wrap them in foil.

5 WRAP 'EM UP

Wrapping ribs in foil during the final stages of cooking holds in some moisture and helps to tenderize the meat. This is a little trick that some barbecue professionals dismiss as "the Texas crutch," but you know what? It works.

WAY TO PREP BABY BACK RIBS

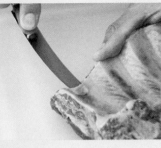 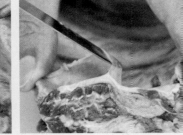 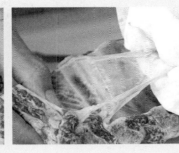 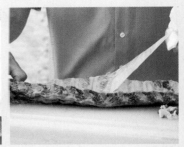

1. At one end of the rack, slide a dinner knife under the membrane and over a bone.

2. Lift and loosen the membrane until it tears.

3. Grab the edge of the membrane with a paper towel and pull it off.

4. The membrane may come off in one whole piece, or you may need to remove it in smaller pieces.

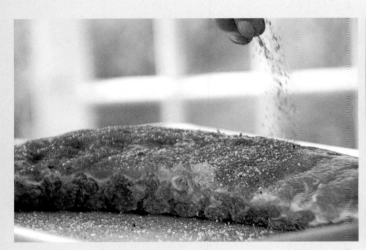 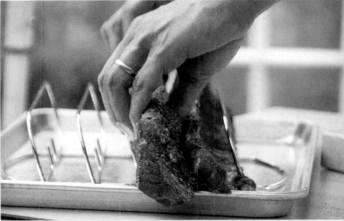

5. Season the ribs mostly on the meaty side, and press the spices into the meat so they don't fall off.

6. Stand the ribs in a rib rack to double the number of ribs you can cook in a limited grill space.

WAY TO SET UP A CHARCOAL GRILL FOR SMOKING

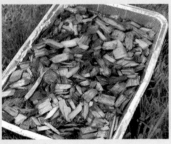 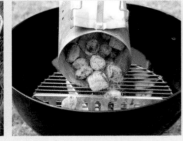 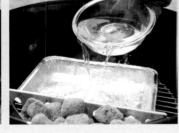 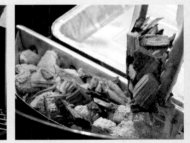

1. If you are using wood chips, soak them first in water for at least 30 minutes so that they smolder and smoke slowly rather than flame up.

2. Dump the charcoal on one side of the charcoal grate. A charcoal basket holds the coals together in a compact bunch and slows down the burning. Tap the edge of the basket with tongs every hour or so to knock the ashes through the basket holes.

3. Place a foil pan on the other side of the charcoal grate and fill it at least halfway with water to create a little steam inside the grill. The ribs will cook on the cooking grate directly above the water pan.

4. Drain some wood chips and lay them right on the coals. Replenish them after the first hour of cooking, ideally when you replenish the coals, too.

WAY TO BARBECUE BABY BACK RIBS

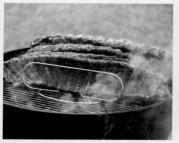
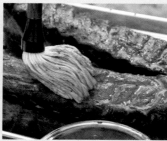
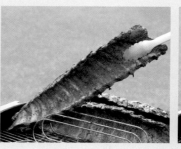
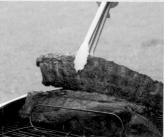

1. To protect the meat, begin with the bone side of the ribs facing the coals.

2. After the first hour of cooking, baste the ribs with a vinegar "mop."

3. Periodically swap the positions of the ribs in the rib rack for even cooking.

4. Toward the end of cooking, face the meaty sides of the ribs toward the coals to brown and crisp the surface.

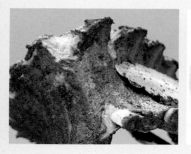
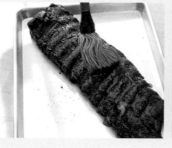
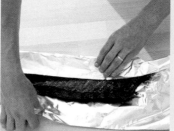
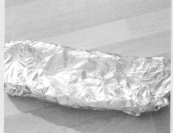

5. The meat should be tender enough that it tears when you bend a rack backwards.

6. Lightly brush each rack of ribs with sauce as it comes off the grill.

7. Wrap each rack individually in aluminum foil.

8. The ribs will stay warm and continue to cook a bit for at least 30 minutes.

SLOW GOOD BABY BACK RIBS WITH SOO-WEE SAUCE

SERVES: 4 TO 6
PREP TIME: 20 MINUTES

WAY TO GRILL: INDIRECT LOW HEAT (250° TO 300°F)
GRILLING TIME: 3 TO 4 HOURS
SPECIAL EQUIPMENT: RIB RACK

RUB
- 2 tablespoons kosher salt
- 2 tablespoons paprika
- 4 teaspoons granulated garlic
- 4 teaspoons pure chile powder
- 2 teaspoons dry mustard
- 2 teaspoons freshly ground black pepper

- 4 racks baby back ribs, 2 to 2½ pounds each

SAUCE
- 1 cup apple juice
- ½ cup ketchup
- 3 tablespoons cider vinegar
- 1 tablespoon soy sauce
- 2 teaspoons molasses
- ½ teaspoon pure chile powder
- ½ teaspoon granulated garlic
- ½ teaspoon dry mustard
- ¼ teaspoon kosher salt
- ¼ teaspoon freshly ground black pepper

MOP
- ¾ cup red wine vinegar
- ¾ cup water
- 2 tablespoons soy sauce

- 4 handfuls hickory wood chips, soaked in water for at least 30 minutes

1. Prepare a charcoal grill for indirect cooking over low heat (see page 121).

2. In a small bowl mix the rub ingredients.

3. Using a dull dinner knife, slide the tip under the membrane covering the back of each rack of ribs. Lift and loosen the membrane until it breaks, and then grab a corner of it with a paper towel and pull it off. Season the ribs all over with the rub, putting more of it on the meaty sides than the bone sides. Arrange the ribs in a rib rack, all facing the same direction. The ribs should stand at room temperature for 30 minutes to 1 hour before cooking.

4. When the fire has burned down to about 350°F, drain 2 handfuls of hickory wood chips and place them on top of the coals. The damp wood will lower the temperature a bit. Put the cooking grate in place. Place the ribs in the rack over **indirect low heat** (positioned over the foil pan) as far from the coals as possible, with the bone sides facing toward the coals. Close the lid. Close the top vent about halfway. Let the ribs cook and smoke for 1 hour. During this time, maintain the temperature between 250° and 300°F by opening and closing the top vent. Meanwhile, make the sauce and the mop.

5. In a small saucepan over medium heat, mix the sauce ingredients and let simmer for about 5 minutes. Then remove the saucepan from the heat. Taste and add more salt and pepper, if desired.

6. In a small bowl mix the mop ingredients.

7. After the first hour of cooking the ribs, add 8 to 10 unlit briquettes and the remaining 2 handfuls of wood chips (drained) to the lit coals. Move the ribs from the rack and spread them out on 2 sheet pans. Brush them generously on both sides with some of the mop. Leaving the lid off for a few minutes while you brush the ribs will help the new briquettes to light. Return the ribs to the rack, all facing the same direction, now with the bone sides facing away from the coals.

8. Close the lid and cook for another hour. During this time, maintain the temperature between 250° and 300°F by opening and closing the top vent.

9. After 2 hours of cooking, add 8 to 10 unlit briquettes to the fire. Move the ribs from the rack and spread them out on 2 sheet pans. Brush them generously on both sides with some of the mop, leaving the lid off for a few minutes while you brush the ribs to help the new briquettes to light. Return the ribs to the rack, all facing the same direction, but this time turned over so that the ends facing down before now face up. Also position any ribs that appear to be cooking faster then others toward the back of the rib rack, farther away from the coals. This time the bone sides should face the coals.

10. Close the lid and let the ribs cook for a third hour. During this time, maintain the temperature between 250° and 300°F by opening and closing the top vent.

11. After 3 hours of cooking, check to see if any rack is ready to come off the grill. They are done when the meat has shrunk back from most of the bones by ¼ inch or more. When you lift a rack by picking up one end with tongs, the rack should bend in the middle and the meat should tear easily. If the meat does not tear easily, continue to cook the ribs. The total cooking time could be anywhere between 3 to 4 hours. Not all racks will cook in the same amount of time. Lightly brush the ribs with some sauce. Transfer the racks to a clean sheet pan and brush the ribs on both sides with some sauce. Wrap each rack individually in aluminum foil and let rest for about 30 minutes. Serve warm with the remaining sauce on the side.

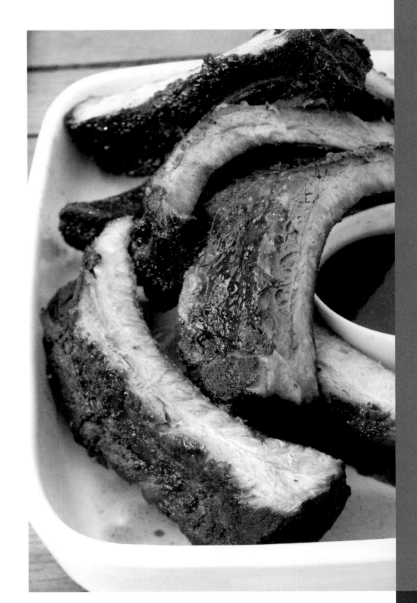

WAY TO COOK STACKED RIBS

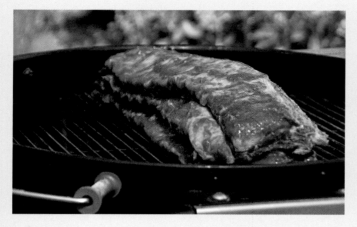

1. One space-saving solution, whether you are cooking with charcoal or gas, is to stack the racks of ribs on top of each other in the middle of the grill.

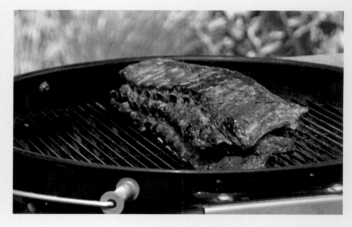

2. Cook the ribs for about 45 minutes, with the lid closed and low heat radiating from both sides of the grill.

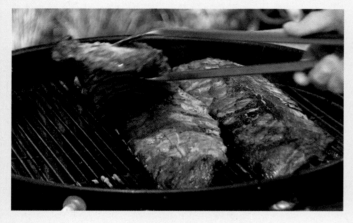

3. Then undo the stack of ribs on the cooking grate.

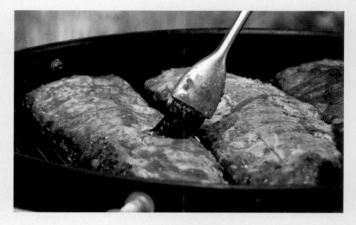

4. Baste the ribs on both sides with some reserved marinade.

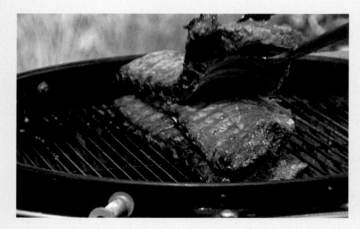

5. Stack them again, swapping the positions of the ribs by moving the top rack to the bottom, the bottom rack to the middle, and the middle rack to the top.

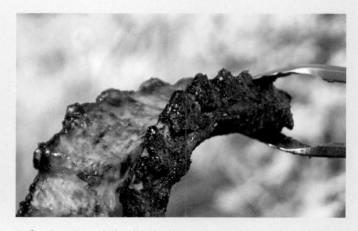

6. Continue to cook the ribs, basting and swapping positions of the racks occasionally, until the meat has shrunk back at least ¼ inch from the ends of the bones.

STACKED BABY BACK RIBS

SERVES: 6 TO 8
PREP TIME: 20 MINUTES
MARINATING TIME: 30 MINUTES

WAY TO GRILL: INDIRECT AND DIRECT LOW HEAT
(300° TO 325°F)
GRILLING TIME: 2¾ TO 3¼ HOURS

MARINADE
 1 cup sweet chili sauce
 1 cup water
    Grated zest of 3 limes
 ⅓ cup fresh lime juice
 4 large garlic cloves
 ¼ cup soy sauce
 3 tablespoons roughly chopped fresh ginger

 3 racks baby back ribs, 2 to 2½ pounds each
 1 tablespoon kosher salt

1. In a blender or food processor combine the marinade ingredients. Process for about 1 minute to puree the ingredients. Set aside 1 cup of the marinade to use as a basting sauce.

2. Remove the thin membrane from the back of each rack of ribs (see page 121). Season the ribs on the meaty sides with salt. Brush the remaining marinade over all the ribs. Let the ribs stand at room temperature for 30 minutes before cooking. Prepare the grill for indirect cooking over low heat.

3. Brush the cooking grates clean. Stack the ribs on top of each other, with the bone sides facing down, and grill over *indirect low heat*, with the lid closed, for 45 minutes.

4. Undo the stack of ribs on the grill. Brush the meaty sides with some of the reserved marinade. Stack the ribs, with the bone sides facing down, moving the top rack to the bottom, the bottom rack to the middle, and the middle rack to the top. Cook over *indirect low heat*, with the lid closed, for another 45 minutes.

5. Undo the stack of ribs on the grill again. Brush the meaty sides with some of the reserved marinade. Stack the ribs, with the bone sides facing down, moving the top rack to the bottom, the bottom rack to the middle, and the middle rack to the top. Cook over *indirect low heat*, with the lid closed, for 1 to 1½ hours. During this third round of cooking, move the relative positions of the ribs occasionally so that the racks that are browning a little faster cook in the middle of the stack and the racks that are not as brown cook at the top of the stack. As you move the ribs, brush the meaty sides with the reserved marinade.

6. Undo the stack of ribs and place them side by side, with the bone sides facing down, over *direct low heat*. Brush with a little more of the reserved marinade and continue cooking until the meat is very tender and has shrunk back from the ends of the bones, 10 to 15 minutes, turning occasionally to prevent burning.

7. Transfer the racks to a sheet pan, cover with foil, and let rest for 15 minutes before cutting into individual ribs. Serve warm.

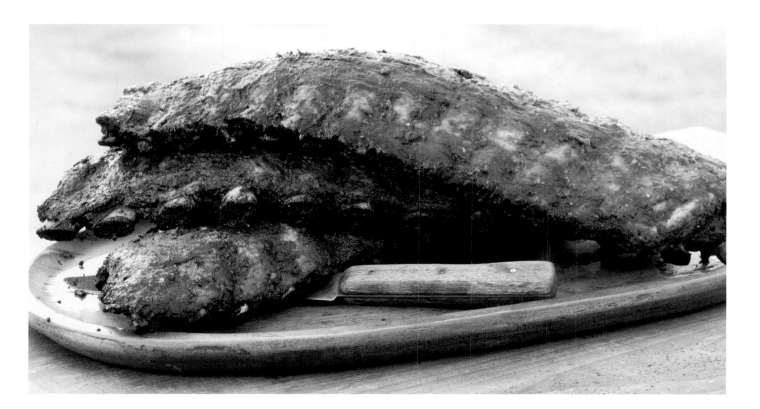

WAY TO PREP ST. LOUIS–STYLE RIBS

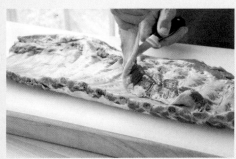

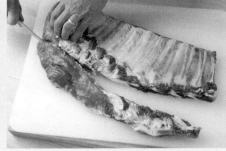

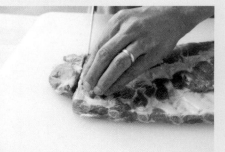

1. There is a tough flap of meat, called the skirt, hanging from the bone side of a full rack of spareribs. The first step for converting "regular" spareribs to the St. Louis-style cut is to remove that flap.

2. The next step is to cut off the long strip of cartilaginous meat, called the brisket, which runs along the bottom of the rack.

3. Then trim off any meat dangling from either end of each rack. The goal is to make a handsome rectangular rack of ribs.

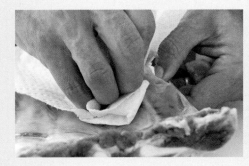

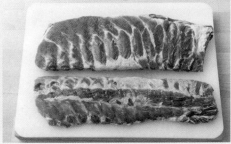

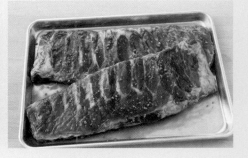

4. Use a dinner knife or some other dull instrument to get under the membrane and lift it so that you can grab an edge with paper towels. Then peel off the membrane.

5. The rack on top is a St. Louis-style cut. It is about the same length as the rack of baby back ribs, shown on the bottom, but the St. Louis-style cut is obviously wide and meatier. It's also tougher, so it requires longer cooking.

6. You can bump up the flavor and give the ribs a crispy surface by marinating them in a sweet and savory marinade for a few hours before cooking.

WAY TO USE "THE TEXAS CRUTCH"

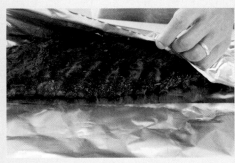

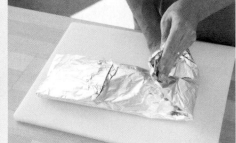

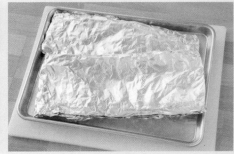

1. In the world of competition barbecue, "the Texas crutch" refers to the technique of wrapping ribs in foil during the final stages of cooking, often with some liquid trapped inside.

2. The theory is that the humidity inside the foil moistens and tenderizes the meat. Some purists shun this approach—hence the mocking sobriquet. It's unclear why the technique is associated with Texas.

3. Many barbecue teams and home cooks use the technique with great success, either finishing their ribs in foil on their smoker or just letting their ribs "rest" in foil after they have been removed from the smoker.

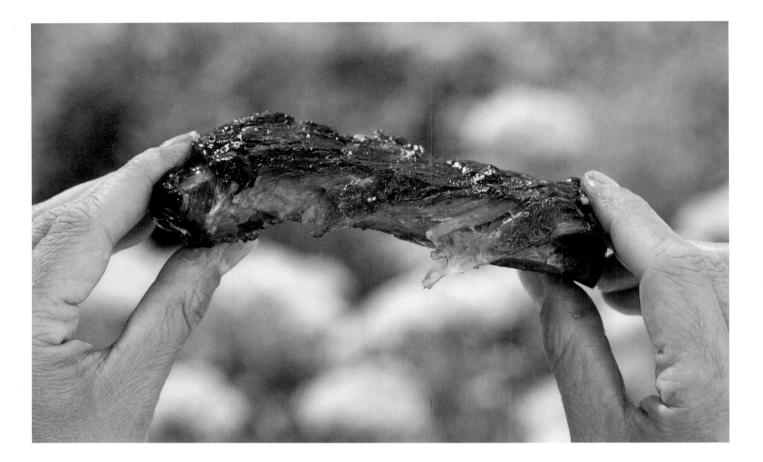

SWEET GINGER AND SOY-GLAZED SPARERIBS

SERVES: 6
PREP TIME: 30 MINUTES
MARINATING TIME: 3 HOURS

WAY TO GRILL: INDIRECT LOW HEAT (ABOUT 300°F)
GRILLING TIME: 4 TO 5 HOURS

MARINADE
- ½ cup brown sugar
- ½ cup soy sauce
- ½ cup ketchup
- ½ cup dry sherry
- 2 tablespoons minced fresh ginger
- 1½ teaspoons minced garlic

- 2 racks pork spareribs, about 4 pounds each

1. In a large bowl combine the marinade ingredients.

2. Prepare the racks of spareribs as detailed at left. Put the spareribs, meaty side up, on a cutting board. Follow the line of fat that separates the meaty ribs from the much tougher tips at the base of each rack, and cut off the tips. Turn each rack over.

Cut off the flap of meat attached in the center of each rack. Also cut off the flap of meat that hangs below the shorter end of the ribs. (The flaps and tips may be grilled separately, but they will not be as tender as the ribs.) Remove the thin membrane from the back of each rack of ribs.

3. Place the ribs in one layer on a large sheet pan. Pour the marinade over the ribs and turn to coat them evenly. Cover and refrigerate for 3 hours, turning occasionally. Remove the ribs from the pan and reserve the marinade. Allow the ribs to stand at room temperature for 30 minutes before grilling. Prepare the grill for indirect cooking over low heat.

4. Brush the cooking grates clean. Grill the ribs over **indirect low heat**, with the lid closed, for 2 hours. Remove the ribs from the grill, brush them on both sides with the reserved marinade, wrap them in aluminum foil, and continue cooking the ribs until the meat has shrunk back about ½ inch from the ends of the rib bones and the meat is tender enough to tear with your fingers, 2 to 3 hours.

5. Transfer the ribs (keep them wrapped in foil) to a large sheet pan and let rest for 30 minutes. Serve warm.

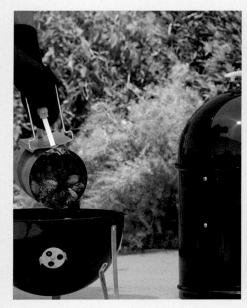
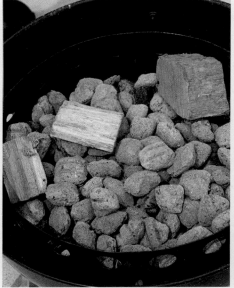
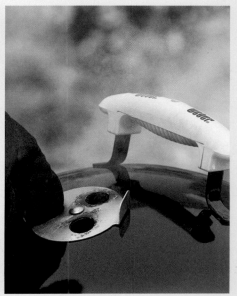

1. Fill the ring in the bottom section of the smoker with fully lit charcoal. Briquettes will burn much longer than lump charcoal, so they are a good choice for meats like pork spareribs, which require long, slow smoking.

2. Toss a few chunks of hardwood on the coals right at the start. Don't bother soaking the chunks first. They won't absorb much water, and they are large enough that they will smoke for quite a while. Put the middle section in place and immediately fill the water pan three-fourths of the way with water. The water pan gets hot fast, so don't wait to fill the pan or water will splatter all over!

3. The vent on the lid should be open right from the start. It allows much of the smoke to escape. Otherwise, the meat would be overpowered. Also, the vent keeps the air flowing so the coals stay lit.

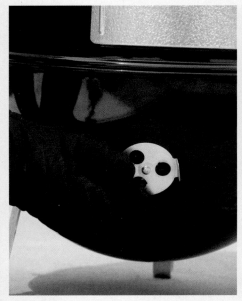
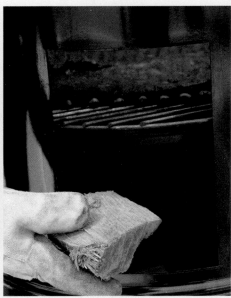
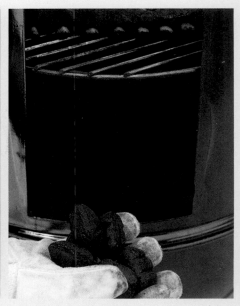

4. Regulate the temperature in the smoker by adjusting the bottom vents. If the temperature begins to fall, open the bottom vents a bit more to allow more airflow. If the temperature begins to rise, close the bottom vents to restrict airflow.

5. After the first few chunks of hardwood have burned out, open the side door and drop one or two more on the burning coals. Work quickly when the door is open so you don't allow too much air into the smoker and create havoc with the cooking temperatures.

6. If necessary, for really long cooking times, add a few more handfuls of briquettes to the coals.

SLOW-SMOKED SPARERIBS WITH SWEET-AND-SOUR BARBECUE SAUCE

SERVES: 8
PREP TIME: 30 MINUTES

WAY TO GRILL: INDIRECT LOW HEAT (225° TO 250°F)
GRILLING TIME: 5 TO 6 HOURS

RUB

- 3 tablespoons kosher salt
- 2 tablespoons pure chile powder
- 2 tablespoons light brown sugar
- 2 tablespoons granulated garlic
- 2 tablespoons paprika
- 4 teaspoons dried thyme
- 4 teaspoons ground cumin
- 4 teaspoons celery seed
- 2 teaspoons freshly ground black pepper

4 racks St. Louis-style spareribs (see page 126)

MOP

- 1 cup apple juice
- ½ cup apple cider vinegar
- 2 tablespoons Worcestershire sauce

5 fist-sized chunks hickory or apple wood (not soaked)

SAUCE

- 2 cups ketchup
- 1 cup apple juice
- ⅔ cup apple cider vinegar
- 2 tablespoons Worcestershire sauce
- 2 tablespoons honey
- 2 tablespoons reserved rub

1. Prepare your smoker, following manufacturer's instructions, for indirect cooking over low heat.

2. In a medium bowl mix the rub ingredients. Set aside 2 tablespoons for the sauce.

3. See the top of page 126, steps 1 to 4, for the way to prep St. Louis-style ribs.

4. In a small bowl mix the mop ingredients.

5. Smoke the spareribs, adding 2 wood chunks at the start of cooking and 1 chunk each hour after that, until the chunks are gone. Cook until the meat has shrunk back from the bones at least ½ inch in several places and the meat tears easily when you lift each rack, basting the ribs on both sides with the mop every 2 hours. The total cooking time could be anywhere between 5 to 6 hours. Not all racks will cook in same amount of time. Maintain the temperature of the smoker between 225° to 250°F by opening and closing the vents.

6. In a medium saucepan over medium heat, mix the sauce ingredients and cook for about 5 minutes. Remove the saucepan from the heat.

7. When the meat has shrunk back at least ½ inch in several places, lightly brush the ribs on both sides with sauce.

8. Cook the ribs for 30 to 60 minutes more. Remove them from the smoker and, if desired, lightly brush the ribs on both sides with sauce again. Then cut the racks into individual ribs. Serve warm with the remaining sauce on the side.

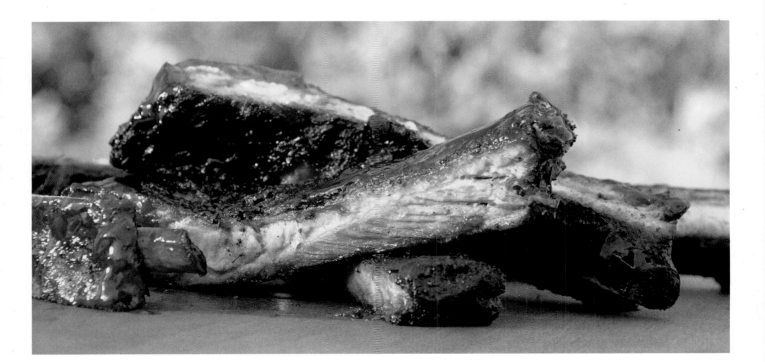

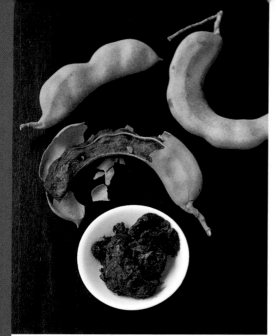

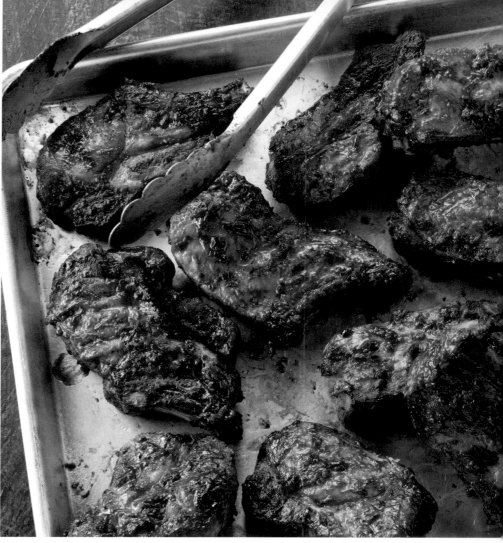

Tamarind pods (top) provide a pulp that is responsible for an addictive sour flavor in many Southeast Asian dishes. Finding the pods in the United States is a challenge, but many Asian markets here carry tamarind paste (bottom). It needs to be diluted in a liquid to use in a marinade or glaze.

TAMARIND-GLAZED COUNTRY-STYLE RIBS

SERVES: 6
PREP TIME: 10 MINUTES
MARINATING TIME: 20 TO 30 MINUTES

WAY TO GRILL: INDIRECT MEDIUM HEAT (350° TO 400°F)
GRILLING TIME: 45 TO 50 MINUTES

MARINADE
   5 ounces tamarind paste
  ⅓ cup soy sauce
  ⅓ cup light brown sugar
  ¼ cup water
  ½ teaspoon freshly ground black pepper
  ½ teaspoon granulated garlic
  ¼ teaspoon ground cayenne pepper

  12 country-style pork ribs, 3 to 3½ pounds total

1. In a medium bowl whisk the marinade ingredients. Set aside ¼ cup for brushing on the ribs during grilling.

2. Liberally brush the ribs with the marinade. Let the ribs marinate at room temperature for 20 to 30 minutes before grilling. Prepare the grill for indirect cooking over medium heat.

3. Brush the cooking grates clean. Grill the ribs over **indirect medium heat**, with the lid closed, for 20 minutes. Turn the ribs over, brush with the reserved marinade, and continue to cook for another 25 to 30 minutes.

4. Remove the ribs from the grill, tightly wrap with foil, and let rest for 30 minutes. Serve warm.

CHILE VERDE COUNTRY-STYLE RIBS

SERVES: 6 TO 8
PREP TIME: 30 MINUTES

WAY TO GRILL: DIRECT MEDIUM HEAT (350° TO 450°F)
GRILLING TIME: 30 MINUTES
SPECIAL EQUIPMENT: LARGE DISPOSABLE FOIL PAN

- 3 pounds boneless country-style pork ribs, ¾ to 1 inch thick, trimmed of fat
- 1 medium white onion, cut into ½-inch slices
- 2 jalapeño chile peppers
  Vegetable oil

RUB

- 1 tablespoon ground cumin
- 1 tablespoon packed brown sugar
- 2 teaspoons kosher salt
- 1 teaspoon pasilla or pure chile powder
- 1 teaspoon ground coriander
- 1 teaspoon dried oregano

SAUCE

- 2 cans (7 ounces each) diced green chiles with juice
- 1 can (14 ounces) fire-roasted diced tomatoes with juice
- 1 can (14 ounces) reduced-sodium chicken broth
- 1 tablespoon finely chopped garlic
- 1 teaspoon ground cumin
- 1 teaspoon dried oregano

- 12 corn or flour tortillas (7 to 8 inches)
- 1 cup sour cream
- 1 ripe medium Haas avocado, peeled and diced
- 1 cup shredded cheddar cheese
- ⅓ cup finely chopped fresh cilantro
- 2 limes, cut into wedges

1. Lightly brush the ribs, onion slices, and chiles with oil.

2. In a small bowl mix the rub ingredients. Generously coat the ribs on both sides with the rub. Allow the ribs to stand at room temperature for 20 to 30 minutes before grilling. Prepare the grill for direct cooking over medium heat.

3. Brush the cooking grates clean. Grill the ribs, onion slices, and chiles over **direct medium heat**, with the lid closed as much as possible, until the meat is well browned but still a little pink and the onions and chiles are lightly charred and softened, 10 to 12 minutes, turning once.

4. Remove the meat and vegetables from the grill and allow them to cool for a few minutes. Cut the pork into ¾-inch cubes. Coarsely chop the onions. Remove and discard the skins, seeds, and stems from the chiles and then finely chop them.

5. In a large disposable foil pan combine the sauce ingredients. Place the pan over **direct medium heat** and bring the sauce to a simmer. Add the meat and vegetables to the sauce. Keep the sauce at a simmer and cook, with the lid closed, until the pork is tender when tested with a fork, 15 to 20 minutes (if the liquid is cooking too fast, move the pan to *indirect medium heat*). Carefully slide the foil pan onto a sheet pan and remove from the grill.

6. Grill the tortillas in a single layer over **direct medium heat** just long enough to warm and soften them, about 1 minute, turning once. Stack the tortillas and wrap them in a thick kitchen towel.

7. Spoon the pork and a generous amount of sauce into warm bowls. Top with sour cream, avocado, cheese, and cilantro. Serve with warm tortillas and lime wedges.

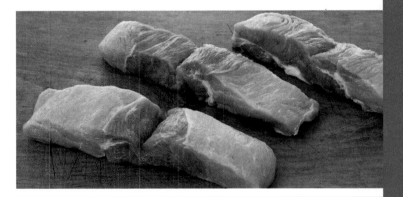

Looking more like pork chops than ribs, country-style ribs are cut from the upper shoulder. You can buy them with or without bones. Either way, the meat is a little tough, but simmering it in a spicy chile verde sauce makes it tender.

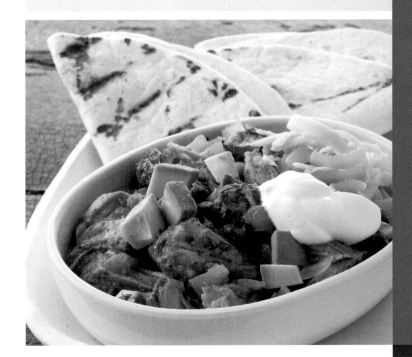

POULTRY

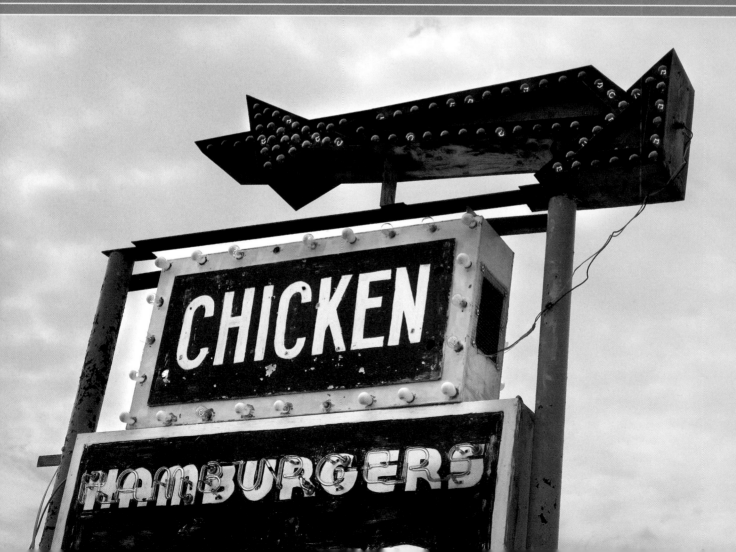

TECHNIQUES

RECIPES

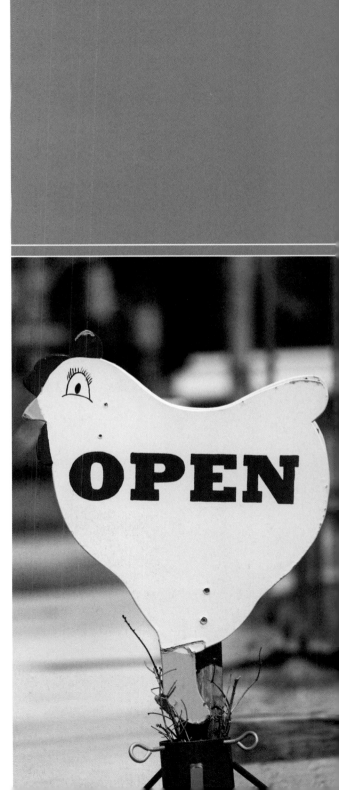

WAY TO GRILL CHICKEN INVOLTINI

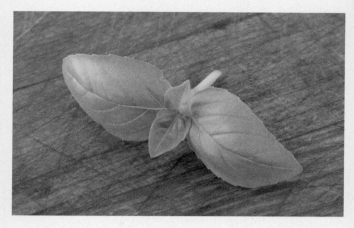

1. The brilliance of *involtini*, an Italian dish of stuffed and rolled meat, is that it allows you to fill fairly bland pieces of meat like chicken breasts with gorgeous flavors like fresh basil, prosciutto, and provolone cheese.

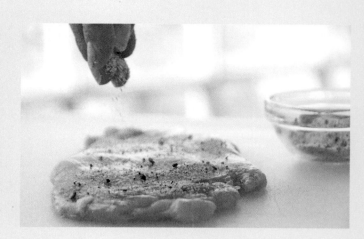

2. First flatten the chicken breasts, smooth side down, between layers of plastic wrap. Then season each one with kosher salt, granulated garlic, and freshly ground black pepper.

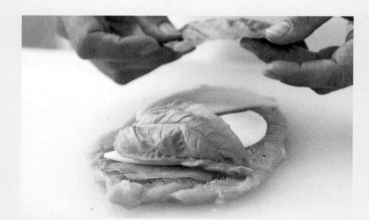

3. Lay a slice of prosciutto on each piece of chicken. Then lay down a couple pieces of cheese and a couple basil leaves.

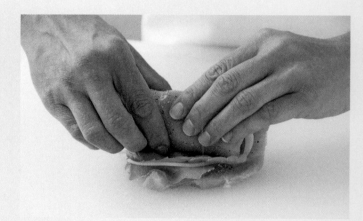

4. Roll up the chicken lengthwise, keeping it as compact as you can.

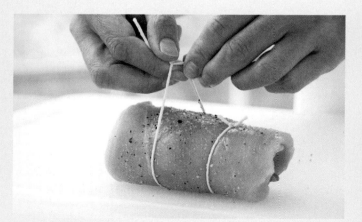

5. Tie each piece of chicken with 2 pieces of butcher's twine. Then lightly brush the surface with olive oil.

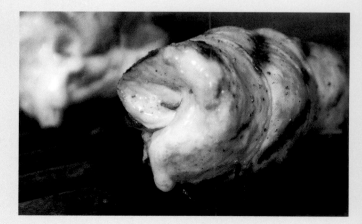

6. Grill over direct medium heat until the chicken is fully cooked and the cheese has begun to melt, about 12 minutes, turning every few minutes.

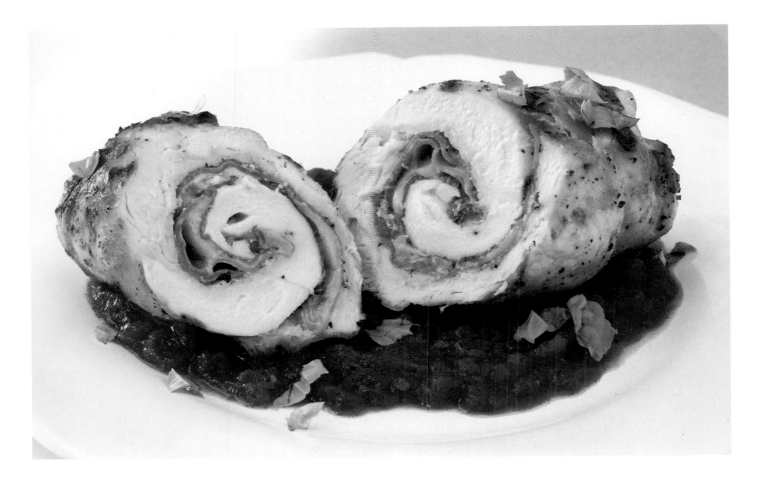

CHICKEN INVOLTINI WITH PROSCIUTTO AND BASIL

SERVES: 4
PREP TIME: 20 MINUTES

WAY TO GRILL: DIRECT MEDIUM HEAT (350° TO 450°F)
GRILLING TIME: ABOUT 12 MINUTES
SPECIAL EQUIPMENT: BUTCHER'S TWINE

- 4 boneless, skinless chicken breast halves, about 8 ounces each, tenders removed
- 1 teaspoon kosher salt
- 1 teaspoon granulated garlic
- ½ teaspoon freshly ground black pepper
- 4 very thin slices prosciutto
- 4 thin slices provolone cheese, halved
- 8 large basil leaves, plus more for garnish
  Extra-virgin olive oil
- 2 cups good-quality tomato sauce

1. Prepare the grill for direct cooking over medium heat.

2. For each piece of chicken, use about 12 inches of plastic wrap. Place the chicken, smooth side down, to one side of the plastic, about 2 inches from the edge. Fold the remaining plastic over the chicken leaving an inch or so from the folded edge. This will allow the chicken to spread out as it gets thinner. Starting from the thick side, gently pound the chicken with the flat side of a tenderizer or the bottom of a small, heavy skillet, moving to different areas with every stroke until it is about ¼ inch thick and just about doubles in size. Do not pound too hard or the chicken might break apart.

3. Season each piece of chicken on both sides with the salt, granulated garlic, and pepper. Arrange the chicken with the smooth side down on a work surface.

4. Lay a slice of prosciutto on each piece of chicken. Then lay down 2 halves of the provolone and then 2 basil leaves. Carefully roll up the chicken, keeping it snug as you work. Tie 2 pieces of butcher's twine around each piece to keep it together. Trim the loose ends of twine. Lightly brush each rolled piece of chicken with oil.

5. Brush the cooking grates clean. Grill the chicken over **direct medium heat**, with the lid closed as much as possible, until golden on all sides, about 12 minutes, turning a quarter turn every 3 minutes. Remove from the grill and let rest for 3 to 5 minutes. Meanwhile, in a small saucepan over medium-high heat, warm the tomato sauce.

6. Remove the twine from the chicken pieces, cut into slices, and serve warm on a pool of sauce. Garnish with torn pieces of basil.

WAY TO GRILL CHICKEN PAILLARDS

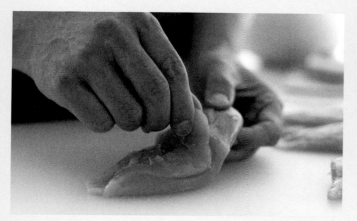

1. On the underside of some store-bought chicken breast halves is a thin strip of meat called the tender (or tenderloin). To pound the chicken breasts thinly for this recipe, remove each tender first and save it for another use.

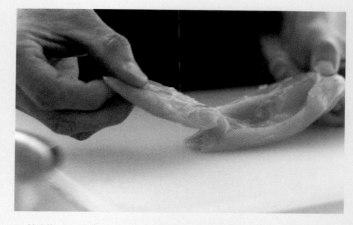

2. Holding each breast steady with one hand, use your other hand to grab the tender near the thick end of each breast and pull it off.

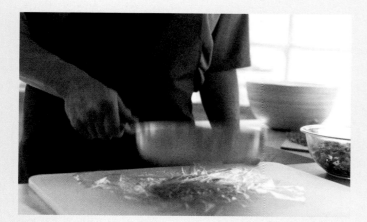

3. Place each chicken breast, smooth side down, between 2 sheets of plastic wrap and pound it to a thickness of about ¼ inch.

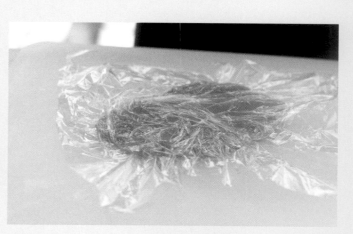

4. For an even thickness, aim the back of a small, heavy skillet at the center of each breast and push the skillet toward the thinner edges as you make contact.

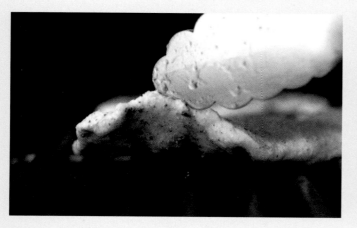

5. Using high heat, grill each chicken breast mostly on the first side. When the perimeter of the second side is turning opaque, it's time to turn the breast.

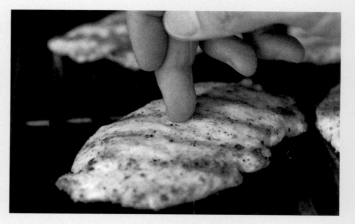

6. Check the doneness by firmness. The chicken should yield just a little to pressure. It should not be soft or hard.

CHICKEN PAILLARDS WITH TOMATO AND OLIVE RELISH

SERVES: 4
PREP TIME: 30 MINUTES

WAY TO GRILL: DIRECT HIGH HEAT (450° TO 550°F)
GRILLING TIME: 4 TO 5 MINUTES

RUB
   1   tablespoon ground fennel seed
1½ teaspoons kosher salt
  ½ teaspoon granulated garlic
  ½ teaspoon freshly ground black pepper

   4 boneless, skinless chicken breast halves, about
      6 ounces each
      Extra-virgin olive oil

RELISH
 ¾ cup ¼-inch-diced tomato
 ⅔ cup ¼-inch-diced celery heart with light green leaves
 ½ cup kalamata olives, rinsed, pitted, and cut into
      ¼-inch dice
 ½ cup green olives, rinsed, pitted, and cut into ¼-inch dice
  2 tablespoons extra-virgin olive oil
  2 teaspoons minced fresh thyme or ½ teaspoon dried
      thyme leaves
      Kosher salt

  1 lemon

1. In a small bowl combine the rub ingredients.

2. Remove the tenders from the underside of each breast (save for another use). One at a time, place each breast, smooth side down, between 2 sheets of plastic wrap and pound to an even ¼-inch thickness. Lightly brush the chicken with oil and season both sides with the rub.

3. Prepare the grill for direct cooking over high heat.

4. In a large bowl combine the relish ingredients, including salt to taste.

5. Brush the cooking grates clean. Grill the chicken, smooth side down, over **direct high heat**, with the lid closed as much as possible, until no longer pink, 3 to 4 minutes. Turn over and grill just to sear the surface, about 1 minute. Transfer the chicken, with the first grilled sides facing up, to a serving platter or individual plates. Spoon the relish over each piece and squeeze fresh lemon juice on top just before serving.

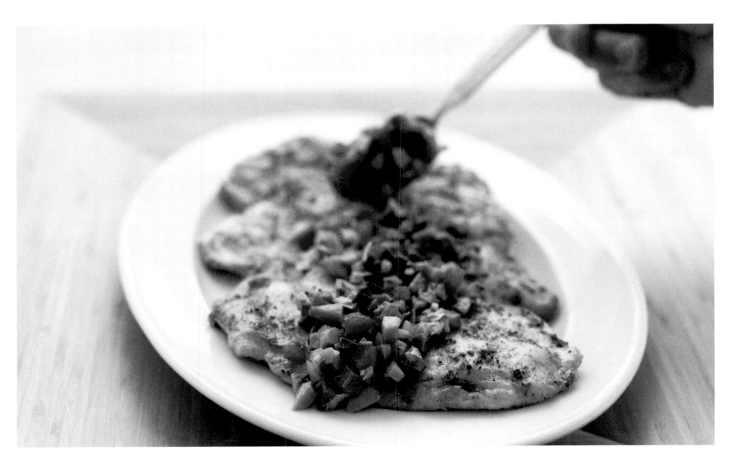

LEMON-OREGANO CHICKEN BREASTS

SERVES: 6
PREP TIME: 15 MINUTES
MARINATING TIME: 1 TO 2 HOURS

WAY TO GRILL: DIRECT MEDIUM HEAT (350° TO 450°F)
GRILLING TIME: 8 TO 12 MINUTES

MARINADE
- ¼ cup extra-virgin olive oil
- Finely grated zest and juice of 2 lemons
- 1 tablespoon dried oregano
- 1 tablespoon minced garlic
- 2 teaspoons paprika
- 1½ teaspoons kosher salt
- ½ teaspoon freshly ground black pepper

- 6 boneless, skinless chicken breast halves, about 6 ounces each

1. In a medium bowl whisk the marinade ingredients.

2. Place the breasts on a large, rimmed plate. Spoon or brush the marinade over the breasts, turning to coat them evenly. Cover with plastic wrap and refrigerate for 1 to 2 hours.

3. Prepare the grill for direct cooking over medium heat.

4. Brush the cooking grates clean. Grill the chicken, smooth side down, over **direct medium heat**, with the lid closed as much as possible, until the meat is firm to the touch and opaque all the way to the center, 8 to 12 minutes, turning once or twice. Serve warm.

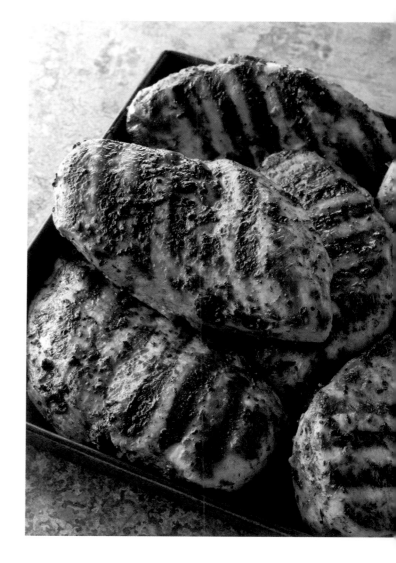

WAY TO ZEST LEMON

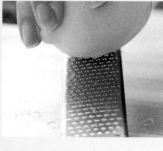
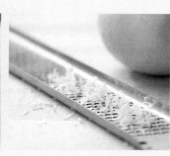

1. A microplane grater can quickly remove the outermost skin of a lemon.

2. The oil-rich zest holds a wealth of flavor, but avoid the bitter, white pith.

WAY TO JUICE LEMON

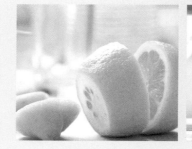
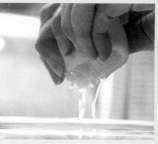

1. Cut off each end of the lemon to expose a small amount of fruit. Then cut the lemon in half.

2. This makes the lemon much easier to juice.

TANDOORI CHICKEN BREASTS WITH MANGO-MINT CHUTNEY

SERVES: 4
PREP TIME: 20 MINUTES
MARINATING TIME: 2 HOURS

WAY TO GRILL: DIRECT MEDIUM HEAT (350° TO 450°F)
GRILLING TIME: 10 TO 14 MINUTES

MARINADE
- 1 cup whole milk yogurt
- 3 tablespoons fresh lemon juice
- 1 tablespoon chopped garlic
- 1 tablespoon chopped fresh ginger
- 2 teaspoons garam masala
- 2 teaspoons kosher salt
- 1 teaspoon sweet paprika

- 4 boneless, skinless chicken breast halves, about 6 ounces each

CHUTNEY
- 2 firm ripe mangoes, sides cut from pit
- ½ tablespoon vegetable oil
- 2 tablespoons finely chopped fresh mint
- 2 tablespoons cider vinegar
- ½ teaspoon granulated sugar
- ¼ teaspoon kosher salt
- ¼ teaspoon freshly ground black pepper

Vegetable oil

1. In a food processor blend the marinade ingredients until uniform in consistency, adding 1 or 2 tablespoons of water, if needed. Place the chicken in a large, resealable plastic bag and pour in the marinade. Press the air out of the bag and seal it tightly. Turn the bag several times to distribute the marinade and refrigerate for 2 hours, turning occasionally.

2. Prepare the grill for direct cooking over medium heat.

3. Lightly brush the mango slices with the oil. Brush the cooking grates clean. Grill over **direct medium heat**, flat sides down, with the lid closed as much as possible, until they brown, about 2 minutes, without turning. Remove the mango from the grill, crosshatch the flesh in the skin, and scoop out the little pieces. In a small bowl combine the mango with the remaining chutney ingredients.

4. Remove the chicken from the bag and discard the marinade. Wipe off most of the marinade clinging to the chicken and then brush the chicken with oil. Grill over **direct medium heat**, with the lid closed as much as possible, until the meat is firm to the touch and no longer pink in the center, 8 to 12 minutes, turning once. Serve warm with the chutney.

WAY TO CUT A MANGO

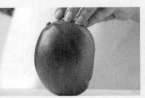

1. Inside each mango is a flat pit that runs from side to side.

2. To cut around the pit, rotate the mango so that the pit runs parallel to the blade of your knife.

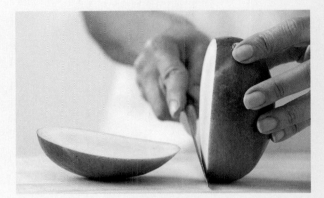

3. Cut each mango lengthwise along each side of the pit.

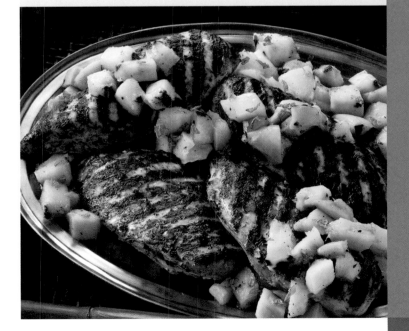

WAY TO MAKE PLUM SAUCE

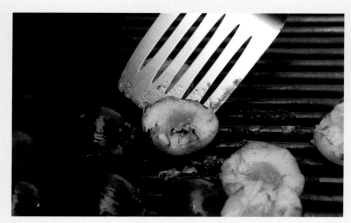

1. For the sauce, grill halved red plums until they are soft and sweet.

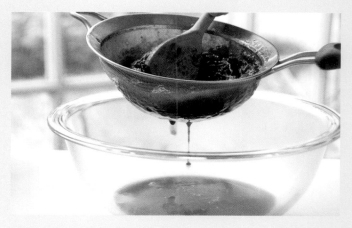

2. Then simmer the grilled plums with port, sugar, and shallots. Strain the sauce through a sieve, pressing the solids to extract as much flavor as possible.

WAY TO PREP DUCK BREASTS

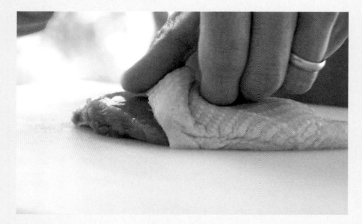

1. The skin of a duck breast is very fatty. To avoid flare-ups on the grill, one good option is to remove the skin first.

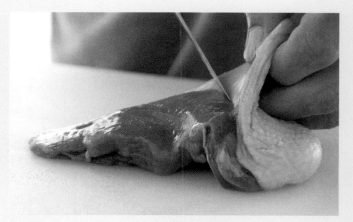

2. Lift the edge of the skin and use the sharp tip of a paring knife to separate the skin from the flesh as you pull back the skin.

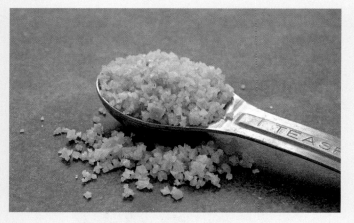

3. The secret ingredient used in both the rub and the sauce is smoked sea salt. Look for it in specialty food shops.

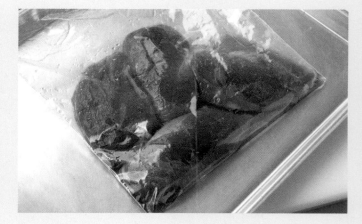

4. The salt in the rub not only adds flavor, it also breaks down some muscle fibers, making the duck more tender.

DUCK BREASTS WITH PORT WINE-PLUM SAUCE

SERVES: 4
PREP TIME: 30 MINUTES

WAY TO GRILL: DIRECT MEDIUM HEAT (350° TO 450°F)
GRILLING TIME: ABOUT 12 MINUTES

SAUCE
- 1 pound red plums, halved and pitted
- 1 tablespoon extra-virgin olive oil
- ½ cup port wine
- 3 tablespoons granulated sugar
- 1 shallot, thinly sliced
- Smoked sea salt
- Freshly ground black pepper

RUB
- 1 tablespoon smoked sea salt
- 1 tablespoon kosher salt
- 1 tablespoon brown sugar

- 4 duck breast halves, 4 to 5 ounces each, skin removed
- 1 tablespoon extra-virgin olive oil

1. Prepare the grill for direct cooking over medium heat. Brush the cooking grates clean.

2. Lightly brush the plums with the oil. Grill the plums over **direct medium heat**, with the lid closed as much as possible, until they have light grill marks and are starting to soften, about 4 minutes, turning once. Remove from the grill and place them in a medium saucepan with the port, sugar, and shallot. Bring the mixture to a boil; reduce the heat to medium, cover, and simmer for about 10 minutes, stirring occasionally. After the sauce has cooked, use a wooden spoon to gently crush the plums into the sauce. Strain the sauce through a coarse sieve into a bowl, pushing as much plum pulp as possible through the sieve. Discard the remaining plum skin and pulp. Season to taste with smoked salt and pepper. Warm the sauce just before serving.

3. In a small bowl combine the rub ingredients. Place the duck in a large, resealable plastic bag and add the rub. Seal the bag and toss to coat the duck thoroughly with the rub. Let stand at room temperature for 10 minutes. Remove the duck from the bag, pat dry with paper towels, and lightly brush with the oil.

4. Brush the cooking grates clean. Grill the duck over **direct medium heat**, with the lid closed as much as possible, until cooked to your desired doneness, about 8 minutes for medium rare, turning once. Let the duck rest for 5 minutes before serving. Slice the duck crosswise into ¼-inch slices and serve warm with the sauce.

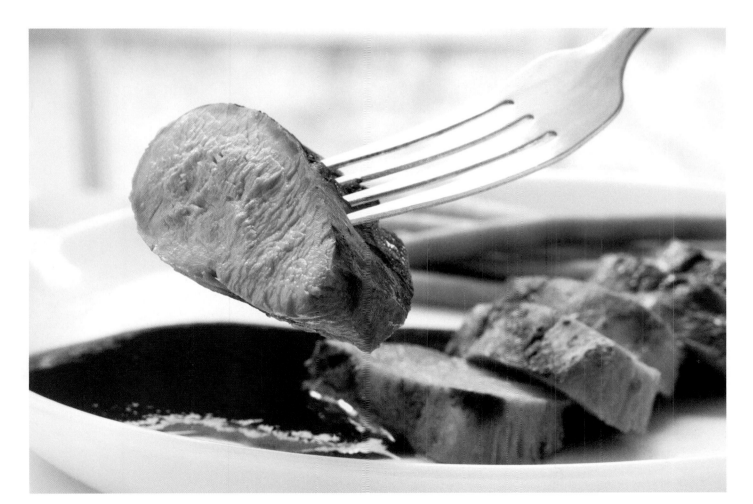

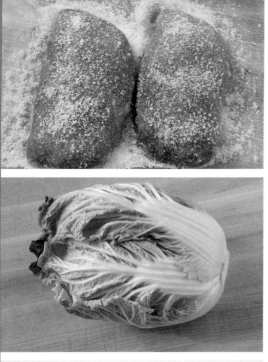

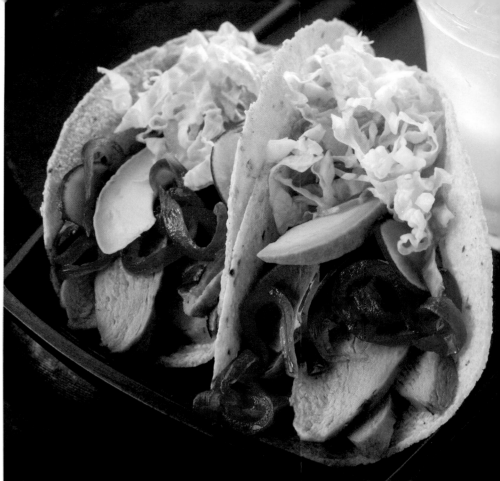

For unforeseen tacos, try salt-cured duck breasts with thinly sliced napa cabbage and cooked red onions.

DUCK BREAST TACOS WITH SOUR ORANGE-ONION SALSA

SERVES: 4 TO 6
PREP TIME: 30 MINUTES

WAY TO GRILL: DIRECT MEDIUM HEAT (350° TO 450°F)
GRILLING TIME: ABOUT 9 MINUTES

- 4 boneless duck breast halves, 4 to 6 ounces each
- 2 tablespoons kosher salt
- 2 tablespoons granulated sugar

SALSA
- 2 cups thinly sliced red onion
- ½ cup fresh orange juice
- ¼ cup fresh lime juice
- ¼ cup finely chopped poblano chile pepper
- 1 tablespoon granulated sugar
- ¼ teaspoon kosher salt
- ¼ cup chopped fresh cilantro

  Extra-virgin olive oil

- 16 corn tortillas (7 inches)
- 1 ripe Haas avocado, peeled and sliced
- ½ cup thinly sliced red radish
- 1½ cups finely sliced napa cabbage (Chinese cabbage)

1. Using a small, sharp knife, remove and discard the thick layer of fat and skin from the duck breasts (see page 140).

2. In a large bowl mix the salt and sugar, and then add the breasts and turn to coat them. Let the breasts stand at room temperature for 20 to 30 minutes before grilling, turning the breasts over once or twice.

3. In a large skillet over medium-high heat, combine the onion, orange and lime juices, chile, sugar, and salt. Cook until most of the liquid evaporates, 15 to 18 minutes, stirring occasionally to avoid any burning. Remove from the heat and stir in the cilantro.

4. Prepare the grill for direct cooking over medium heat.

5. Pat the breasts dry and generously coat them on both sides with oil.

6. Brush the cooking grates clean. Grill the breasts over **direct medium heat**, with the lid closed as much as possible, until lightly browned on each side and still rosy pink in the center, about 8 minutes, turning once. Transfer to a cutting board and, while the duck rests, grill the tortillas.

7. Brush the cooking grates clean. Grill the tortillas over **direct medium heat** for about 10 seconds on each side. Stack the grilled, hot tortillas and wrap them in a thick kitchen towel (or put them in an insulated tortilla server).

8. Thinly slice the duck and serve with the warm tortillas, salsa, avocado, radish, and cabbage.

JERK CHICKEN SKEWERS WITH HONEY-LIME CREAM

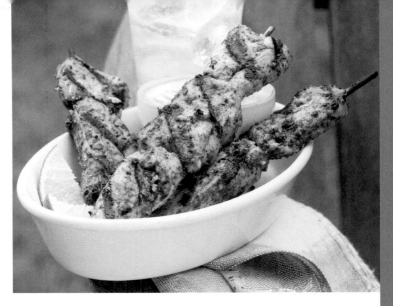

SERVES: 4 TO 6
PREP TIME: 30 MINUTES
MARINATING TIME: 2 TO 3 HOURS

WAY TO GRILL: DIRECT HIGH HEAT (450° TO 550°F)
GRILLING TIME: 6 TO 8 MINUTES
SPECIAL EQUIPMENT: RUBBER OR PLASTIC GLOVES;
   8 TO 12 BAMBOO SKEWERS, SOAKED IN WATER FOR
   AT LEAST 30 MINUTES

PASTE

- 1 habanero or Scotch bonnet chile pepper
- 1 cup lightly packed fresh cilantro leaves and tender stems
- ½ cup extra-virgin olive oil
- 4 scallions, white and light green parts, roughly chopped
- 6 medium garlic cloves
- 2 tablespoons finely chopped fresh ginger
- 2 tablespoons granulated sugar
- 1 tablespoon fresh lime juice
- 1 tablespoon ground allspice
- 2 teaspoons kosher salt
- 1 teaspoon freshly ground black pepper

- 6 boneless, skinless chicken breast halves,
  6 to 8 ounces each

SAUCE

- ½ cup sour cream
- ½ teaspoon finely grated lime zest
- 1 tablespoon fresh lime juice
- 1 tablespoon extra-virgin olive oil
- 2 teaspoons honey
- ¼ teaspoon kosher salt
- ⅛ teaspoon freshly ground black pepper

1. To avoid burning your skin, wear rubber or plastic gloves when you handle the chile. After handling the chile, do not touch your face or any other part of your body, as that might cause a burning sensation. Remove and discard the stem of the chile, then cut away and discard the hot whitish veins and seeds. Put the rest of the chile in the bowl of a food processor. Add the remaining paste ingredients and process until smooth.

2. Trim the chicken of any fat and remove the tenders. Cut the chicken lengthwise into even strips, ½ to ¾ inch thick.

3. Place the chicken strips and tenders into a large, resealable plastic bag and spoon in the paste. Work the paste into the chicken, press out the air in the bag, and seal tightly. Place in the refrigerator and let marinate for 2 to 3 hours.

4. In a small bowl whisk the sauce ingredients. Cover with plastic wrap and refrigerate. Let the sauce stand at room temperature for about 30 minutes before serving. Prepare the grill for direct cooking over high heat.

5. Wearing rubber or plastic gloves, thread the chicken strips onto the skewers, being sure to keep each skewer well within the flesh of the chicken. If you don't have rubber gloves, be sure to wash your hands thoroughly after this step.

6. Brush the cooking grates clean. Grill the skewers over **direct high heat**, with the lid closed as much as possible, until the meat is firm and the juices run clear, 6 to 8 minutes, turning once or twice. Serve warm with the sauce.

WAY TO MAKE CHICKEN SKEWERS

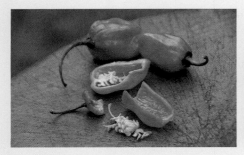

1. Wearing rubber or plastic gloves, remove and discard the incredibly spicy seeds and whitish veins in habanero chile peppers.

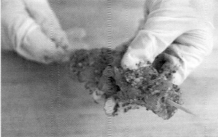

2. Marinate the chicken pieces in the pureed chile paste and thread them onto skewers. Make sure that the skewers run through the center of the chicken pieces.

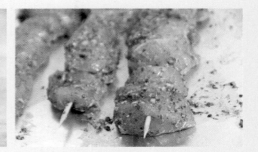

3. When you are done, you should see wood only at the tip and base of each skewer.

WAY TO PREP CHICKEN BREASTS

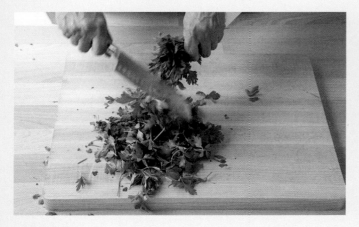

1. For a sauce of pureed parsley with olive oil, nuts, and garlic, you can use all but the tough stems of parsley. Hold the tough stems in one hand and use the other to shave off the leaves and tender stems.

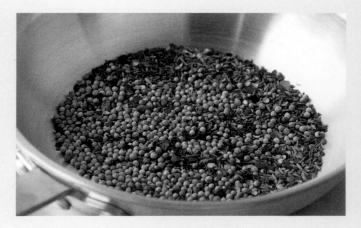

2. This Tunisian-inspired spice paste will be particularly aromatic if you cook the spices first in a dry skillet over medium heat.

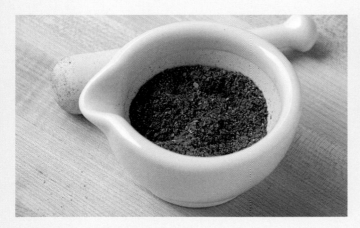

3. Crush the toasted spices with a mortar and pestle, or use a clean coffee mill or spice mill to grind them to a powder.

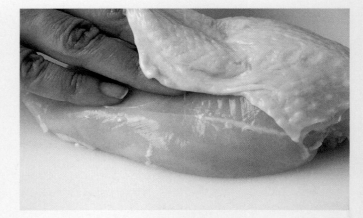

4. To get the spices right onto the meat, very gently work your fingertips under the skin at the thin end and lift the skin, but leave it attached at the other end.

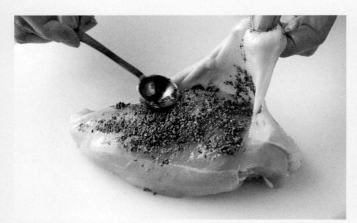

5. Spread the spice paste all over the exposed meat.

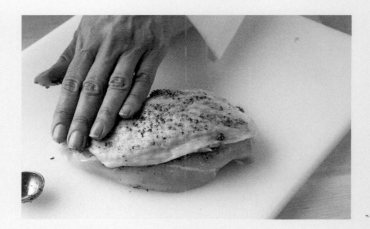

6. Lay the skin back in place and spread a bit more of the spice paste on top.

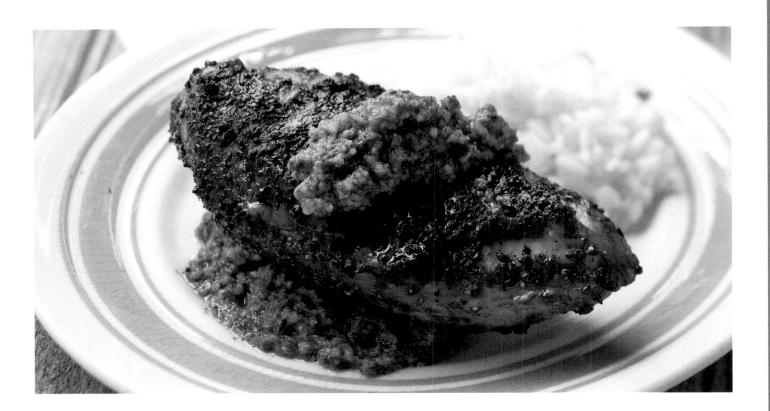

TUNISIAN CHICKEN WITH PARSLEY SAUCE

SERVES: 4

PREP TIME: 20 MINUTES

WAY TO GRILL: DIRECT AND INDIRECT MEDIUM HEAT
(350° TO 450°F)

GRILLING TIME: 23 TO 35 MINUTES

SPECIAL EQUIPMENT: MORTAR AND PESTLE OR
SPICE MILL

SAUCE
- 1½ cups lightly packed fresh Italian parsley leaves and tender stems
- ¼ cup whole unsalted almonds
- 1 medium garlic clove
- ½ cup extra-virgin olive oil
- 2 teaspoons Dijon mustard
- 1 teaspoon honey
- ¼ teaspoon kosher salt

PASTE
- 4 teaspoons coriander seed
- 2 teaspoons caraway seed
- 2 teaspoons cumin seed
- 2 teaspoons crushed red pepper flakes
- 2 tablespoons extra-virgin olive oil
- 1 teaspoon kosher salt

- 4 chicken breast halves (with bone and skin), 10 to 12 ounces each

1. In the bowl of a food processor pulse the parsley, almonds, and garlic until finely chopped. With the motor running, slowing add the oil to create an emulsion. Then mix in the mustard, honey, and salt. Emulsify the sauce again just before serving.

2. In a medium skillet over medium heat, toast the seeds and red pepper flakes until fragrant, 2 to 3 minutes. Put into a mortar and pestle or spice mill and grind to a powder. Transfer to a bowl and add the oil and salt. Stir to make a paste.

3. Using your fingertips, carefully lift the skin from the chicken breasts, leaving the skin closest to the breastbone attached. Rub 1 teaspoon of the paste under the skin of each chicken breast, then lay the skin back in place and rub the remaining paste evenly over all the pieces of chicken. Place the chicken on a plate and cover with plastic wrap. Let the chicken stand at room temperature for 20 to 30 minutes before grilling. Prepare the grill for direct and indirect cooking over medium heat.

4. Brush the cooking grates clean. Grill the chicken, skin side down, over **direct medium heat** until the skin is browned, 3 to 5 minutes. Turn over the chicken and continue to cook over **indirect medium heat**, with the lid closed, until the meat is opaque all the way to the bone, 20 to 30 minutes. Transfer to a platter and let rest for 5 to 10 minutes. Serve the chicken warm with the sauce.

WAY TO GRILL CHICKEN WINGS

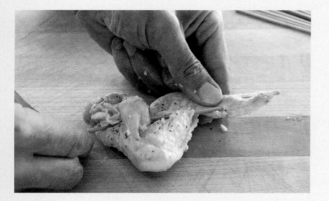

1. You don't have to use skewers to grill chicken wings. You'll get great results without them, but skewers are helpful for spreading the wings flat, as if they were "in flight."

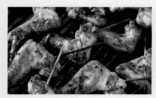 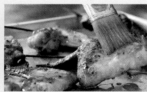

2. The flatter the wings, the more contact they have with the cooking grate. That means crispier skins and more flavors.

3. Brushing them with a honey-garlic glaze just before serving helps, too.

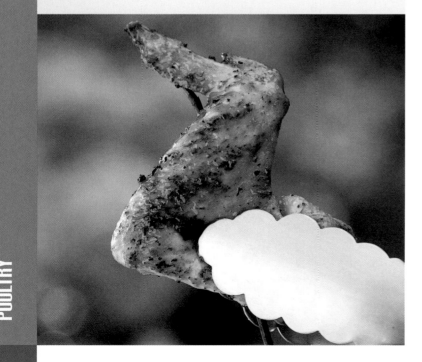

HONEY-GARLIC CHICKEN WINGS

SERVES: 4 TO 6 AS AN APPETIZER
PREP TIME: 20 MINUTES
MARINATING TIME: UP TO 4 HOURS

WAY TO GRILL: DIRECT AND INDIRECT MEDIUM HEAT (350° TO 450°F)
GRILLING TIME: 19 TO 25 MINUTES
SPECIAL EQUIPMENT: 12 BAMBOO SKEWERS, SOAKED IN WATER FOR AT LEAST 30 MINUTES

MARINADE
  6 tablespoons fresh lemon juice, divided
  1 tablespoon finely chopped garlic
  1 teaspoon kosher salt
  ½ teaspoon freshly ground black pepper

  2 pounds chicken wings
  ½ cup honey
  1 tablespoon hot sauce, or to taste

1. In a large bowl combine 3 tablespoons of the lemon juice, the garlic, salt, and pepper. Add the wings and toss to coat them evenly. Cover and refrigerate for up to 4 hours.

2. In a small bowl combine the remaining 3 tablespoons of lemon juice, the honey, and hot sauce.

3. Prepare the grill for direct and indirect cooking over medium heat.

4. Thread each wing on a bamboo skewer, being sure to skewer each portion of the wing all the way up into the cartilage in the wing tip and then spreading it out as if it were "in flight."

5. Brush the cooking grates clean. Brown the wings over **direct medium heat** for 4 to 5 minutes, turning once. Then move the wings over **indirect medium heat** and cook until the meat is no longer pink at the bone, 15 to 20 minutes, basting with the honey mixture once or twice during the last 10 minutes of grilling time. Keep the lid closed as much as possible during grilling. Remove the wings from the grill, brush once more with the glaze, and serve warm.

HICKORY DRUMETTES
WITH BOURBON-MOLASSES GLAZE

SERVES: 6 TO 8 AS AN APPETIZER
PREP TIME: 20 MINUTES

WAY TO GRILL: INDIRECT MEDIUM HEAT (350° TO 450°F)
GRILLING TIME: 20 TO 30 MINUTES

RUB
- 1   tablespoon smoked paprika
- 2   teaspoons dry mustard
- 1   teaspoon kosher salt
- ½   teaspoon granulated garlic
- ½   teaspoon granulated onion
- ¼   teaspoon ground chipotle chile

- 20 chicken wing drumettes, about 3 pounds

GLAZE
- 2   tablespoons soy sauce
- 2   tablespoons bourbon
- 1   tablespoon unsulphured (light) molasses
- 1   tablespoon unsalted butter

- 2   handfuls hickory wood chips, soaked in water for at least 30 minutes

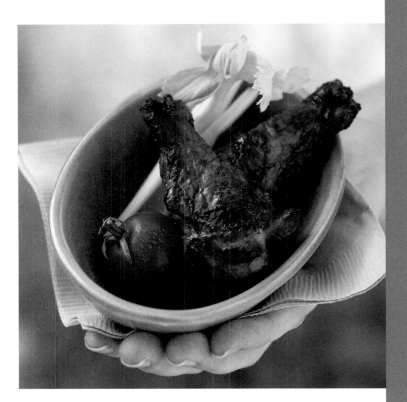

1. In a large bowl mix the rub ingredients. Add the drumettes and toss to coat them evenly.

2. Prepare the grill for indirect cooking over medium heat.

3. In a small, heavy-bottomed saucepan, bring the glaze ingredients to a boil over high heat and cook just until the butter melts. Transfer to a small bowl and let cool.

4. Drain and scatter the wood chips over lit charcoal or put them in the smoker box of a gas grill, following manufacturer's instructions. Brush the cooking grates clean. Grill the wings over **_indirect medium heat_**, with the lid closed as much as possible, until the meat is no longer pink at the bone, 20 to 30 minutes, turning and basting with the glaze once or twice during the last 20 minutes of cooking. Serve warm.

WAY TO GRILL CHICKEN DRUMETTES

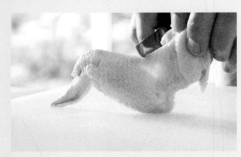

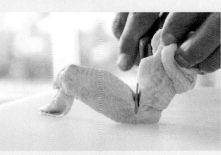

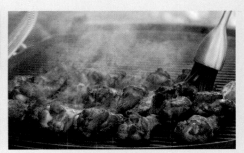

1. Each chicken wing has three parts: a wing tip (left), a two-bone middle section (middle), and an upper wing (right).

2. The upper wing is called the "drumette" because it looks like a little drumstick.

3. Grill drumettes over indirect heat to break down some of the chewy characterisic of the meat, and give them some good hickory smoke and a sweet boozy glaze.

WAY TO PREP WHOLE CHICKEN LEGS

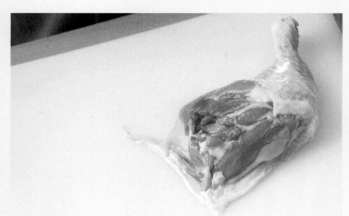

1. Turn each chicken leg skin-side down and trim off the excess skin. The fat under that skin tends to melt into the grill and pose a threat of flare-ups.

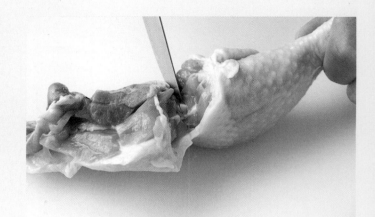

2. The meat near the joint of a chicken leg will take the longest to cook. So cut an opening between the drumstick and thigh to expose that innermost meat and speed up its cooking time.

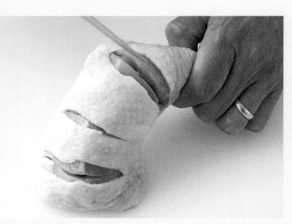

3. Making some slashes on the outside of the leg will allow the marinade to penetrate faster and deeper.

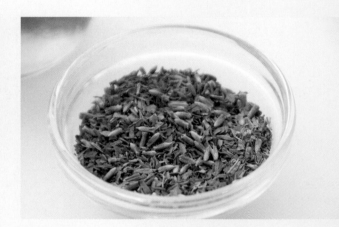

4. The Provençal flavors in this recipe come primarily from a blend of dried herbs that usually includes thyme, marjoram, parsley, tarragon, lavender, celery seed, and bay leaf. It is sold as herbes de Provence.

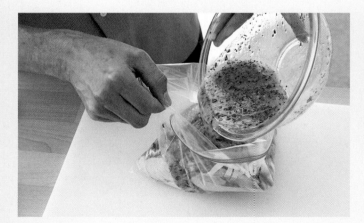

5. Pour the marinade over the chicken in a large, resealable plastic bag. Press the air out of the bag, seal it tightly, and turn it several times, making sure to coat all of the pieces evenly.

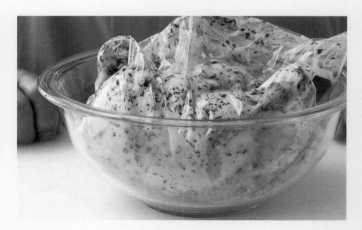

6. When you are dealing with raw chicken and a messy marinade, it's always a good idea to avoid spills by putting the bag in a bowl before refrigerating it.

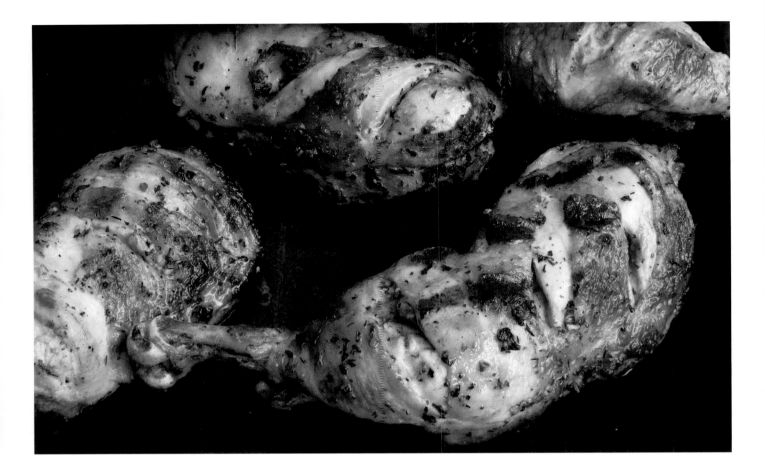

PROVENÇAL MARINATED CHICKEN LEGS

SERVES: 6
PREP TIME: 15 MINUTES
MARINATING TIME: 4 TO 8 HOURS

WAY TO GRILL: INDIRECT MEDIUM HEAT (350° TO 450°F)
GRILLING TIME: 50 MINUTES TO 1 HOUR

MARINADE
- 1 cup dry white wine
- ⅓ cup extra-virgin olive oil
- 3 tablespoons whole-grain mustard
- 3 tablespoons white wine vinegar
- 2 tablespoons herbes de Provence
- 3 garlic cloves, minced
- 2 teaspoons kosher salt
- ½ teaspoon crushed red pepper flakes

- 6 whole chicken legs, 10 to 12 ounces each

1. In a medium bowl whisk the marinade ingredients.

2. Using a sharp paring knife, cut a few deep slashes into the meaty parts of each chicken leg. Place them in a large, resealable plastic bag and pour in the marinade. Press the air out of the bag and seal tightly. Turn the bag to distribute the marinade. Refrigerate for 4 to 8 hours, turning occasionally.

3. Prepare the grill for indirect cooking over medium heat.

4. Remove the chicken from the bag, letting the herbs cling to the chicken. Discard the marinade. Brush the cooking grates clean. Grill the chicken over **indirect medium heat**, with the lid closed as much as possible, until the juices run clear and the internal temperature reaches 170°F in the thickest part of the thigh (not touching the bone), 50 minutes to 1 hour, turning once. If desired, to crisp the skin, grill the chicken over **direct medium heat** during the last 5 minutes of grilling time, turning once. Remove from the grill and cut into thighs and drumsticks.

Boneless chicken pieces do well grilled quickly over direct heat, but bone-in pieces take longer and direct heat alone would burn them, so use indirect heat (or both direct and indirect) for bone-in pieces.

WAY TO ROAST DUCK LEGS

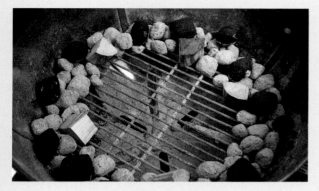

1. Duck legs have so much fat under their skins that they are prone to flare-ups if you try grilling them over direct heat, but the "ring of fire" gives you ample room in the center of the cooking grate to smoke-roast them safely over indirect heat.

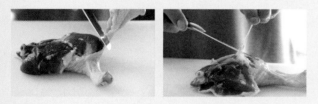

2. While the charcoal burns down to the right temperature and the wood chunks begin smoking, trim any fat hanging from the edges of the duck legs.

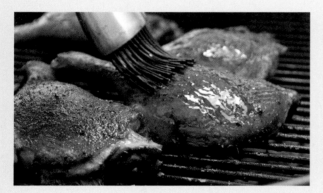

3. Cook the duck legs, skin side up, until dark brown and crispy. Brush on the orange-hoisin glaze near the end of the cooking time so that it does not burn.

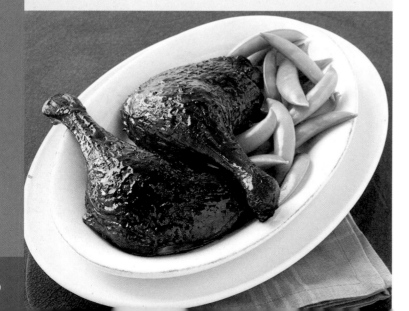

SLOW-ROASTED DUCK LEGS WITH HOISIN-ORANGE GLAZE

SERVES: 4
PREP TIME: 10 MINUTES

WAY TO GRILL: INDIRECT MEDIUM HEAT (ABOUT 325°F)
GRILLING TIME: ABOUT 1 HOUR

GLAZE
- ¼ cup orange marmalade
- ¼ cup fresh orange juice
- ¼ cup mirin (rice wine)
- 2 tablespoons hoisin sauce
- ½ teaspoon crushed red pepper flakes

RUB
- 2 teaspoons kosher salt
- ¾ teaspoon freshly ground black pepper
- ¾ teaspoon Chinese five-spice powder

- 8 whole duck legs, 6 to 8 ounces each, trimmed of excess fat
- 5 apple wood chunks (not soaked)

1. Prepare the grill for indirect cooking over medium heat using the ring-of-fire configuration (see photo above).

2. In a small saucepan over medium-high heat, combine the glaze ingredients. Bring to a simmer to melt the marmalade and then remove from the heat.

3. In a small bowl combine the rub ingredients and then season the duck evenly with the rub.

4. Add the wood chunks directly onto burning coals. As soon as the wood starts to smoke, grill the duck, skin side up, over ***indirect medium heat***, with the lid closed as much as possible, until the duck is evenly browned and crispy and is fully cooked, about 1 hour. During the last 15 to 20 minutes of grilling time, turn and baste the duck with the glaze every 5 to 10 minutes. Serve warm.

WAY TO BARBECUE CHICKEN

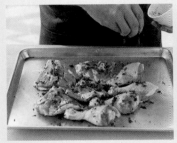

1. Season the chicken thighs and drumsticks with the spices.

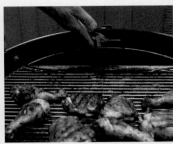

2. After browning the chicken first over direct heat, move it to indirect heat to smoke and finish cooking.

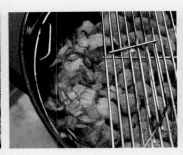

3. A couple handfuls of damp wood chips should provide smoke for 20 to 30 minutes.

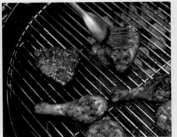

4. Spices, smoke, and finally a light coating of sauce. That's a triple play of flavor.

TRIPLE PLAY BARBECUED CHICKEN

SERVES: 4
PREP TIME: 30 MINUTES

WAY TO GRILL: DIRECT AND INDIRECT MEDIUM HEAT
(350° TO 450°F)
GRILLING TIME: 43 TO 45 MINUTES

SAUCE
2 tablespoons extra-virgin olive oil
½ cup finely chopped yellow onion
2 teaspoons minced garlic
1 cup ketchup
½ cup lemon-lime carbonated beverage (not diet)
¼ cup fresh lemon juice
¼ cup light brown sugar, packed
2 tablespoons whole-grain mustard

RUB
2 teaspoons smoked paprika
2 teaspoons kosher salt
Finely grated zest of 1 lemon
½ teaspoon granulated garlic
½ teaspoon freshly ground black pepper

4 whole chicken legs, 10 to 12 ounces each, cut into thighs and drumsticks
2 handfuls hickory wood chips, soaked in water for at least 30 minutes

1. In a medium saucepan over medium heat, cook the oil, onion, and garlic until golden, about 10 minutes, stirring often. Add the rest of the sauce ingredients and stir to combine. Bring the sauce to a simmer, reduce the heat to low, and cook until slightly thickened, 10 to 15 minutes, stirring often.

2. In a small bowl mix the rub ingredients. Sprinkle the rub evenly all over the chicken pieces. Let the chicken stand at room temperature for 20 to 30 minutes before grilling. Prepare the grill for direct and indirect cooking over medium heat.

3. Brush the cooking grates clean. Grill the chicken, skin side down, over **direct medium heat,** with the lid closed as much as possible, until golden brown, 8 to 10 minutes, turning occasionally. Move the chicken pieces over **indirect medium heat**. Drain and scatter the wood chips over the lit charcoal or put them in the smoker box of a gas grill, following manufacturer's instructions. Continue to grill the chicken, with the lid closed, for about 20 minutes. Then brush both sides with a thin layer of the sauce and cook until the juices run clear and the meat is no longer pink at the bone, about 15 minutes, occasionally turning and brushing with the sauce. Serve warm or at room temperature with the remaining sauce on the side.

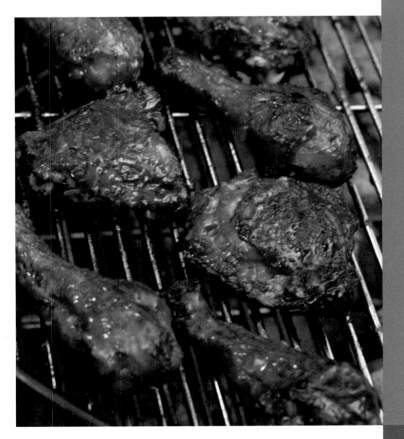

WAY TO CEDAR-PLANK BONE-IN CHICKEN THIGHS

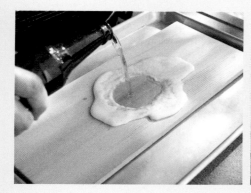

1. Soak the cedar plank in beer or water for at least 1 hour.

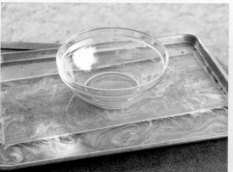

2. Weight the plank down with something heavy so it doesn't float.

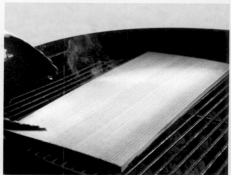

3. Place the soaked plank over direct medium heat and close the lid to start the plank smoking.

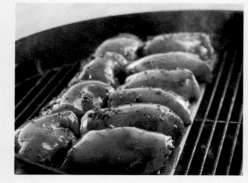

4. When the plank starts smoking, turn it over and arrange the marinated chicken thighs on top.

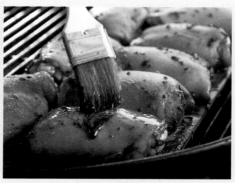

5. Finish cooking the chicken thighs with the plank over indirect heat, basting them occasionally with the reserved marinade. If you left the plank over direct heat for too long, it would ignite.

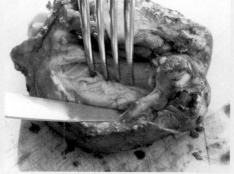

6. To check for doneness, pull one of the thickest thighs from the grill and cut into the underside. If the color of the meat near the bone is still pink, put it back on the plank until it is fully cooked.

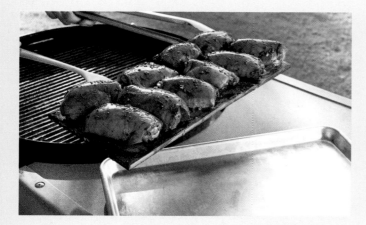

7. Using 2 pairs of tongs, carefully remove the plank and chicken thighs to a heat-proof surface.

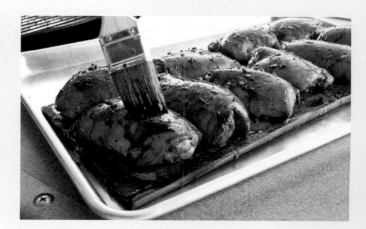

8. Before serving, glaze the chicken thighs one more time.

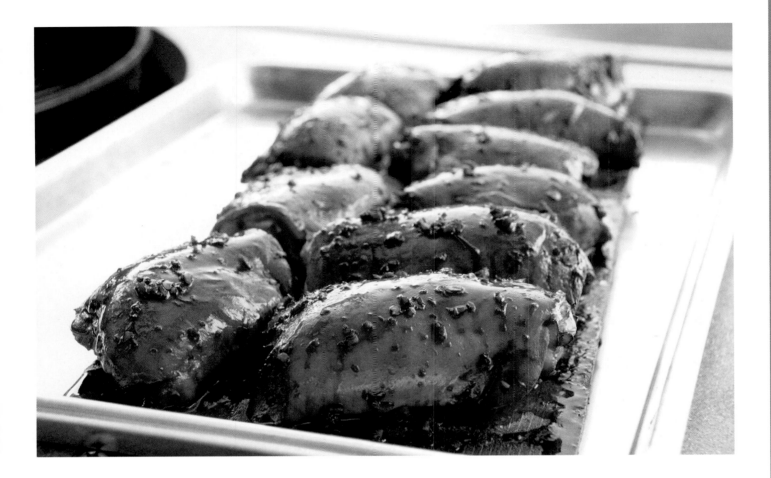

CEDAR-PLANKED CHICKEN THIGHS WITH SOY-GINGER GLAZE

SERVES: 4 TO 6
PREP TIME: 30 MINUTES

WAY TO GRILL: DIRECT AND INDIRECT MEDIUM HEAT
 (350° TO 450°F)
GRILLING TIME: 40 TO 50 MINUTES
SPECIAL EQUIPMENT: 1 UNTREATED CEDAR PLANK,
 12 TO 15 INCHES LONG AND ½ TO ¾ INCH THICK,
 SOAKED IN BEER OR WATER FOR AT LEAST 1 HOUR

GLAZE
 ¾ cup soy sauce
 ½ cup balsamic vinegar
 ½ cup brown sugar
 1 tablespoon minced garlic
 1 tablespoon minced fresh ginger
 1 teaspoon crushed red pepper flakes
 ¼ cup toasted sesame oil

10 skinless chicken thighs (with bone), 5 to 6 ounces each

1. In a small, non-reactive saucepan over medium-low heat, combine the soy sauce, vinegar, and sugar. Cook until reduced by half, about 20 minutes. Remove from the heat and add the garlic, ginger, and red pepper flakes. Cool slightly and then whisk in the oil. Reserve ½ cup of the glaze for basting the chicken.

2. Put the thighs in a large bowl, pour in the glaze, and toss to coat. Refrigerate until you are ready to grill.

3. Prepare the grill for direct and indirect cooking over medium heat. Place the soaked plank over **direct medium heat** and close the lid. After 5 to 10 minutes, when the plank begins to smoke and char, turn the plank over.

4. Remove the thighs from the bowl and discard the glaze. Arrange the thighs on the smoking plank and cook over **direct medium heat**, with the lid closed, for 5 to 10 minutes. Then move the plank over **indirect medium heat** and continue cooking, with the lid closed as much as possible, until the juices run clear, 35 to 40 minutes, basting occasionally with the reserved glaze during the last 10 to 15 minutes of grilling time. Remove from the grill and baste with the glaze once more before serving.

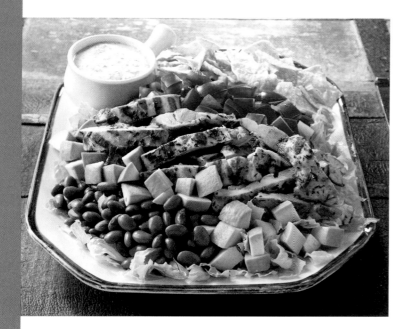

LAYERED MEXICAN CHICKEN SALAD

SERVES: 4 TO 6
PREP TIME: 35 MINUTES
MARINATING TIME: 30 MINUTES TO 1 HOUR

WAY TO GRILL: DIRECT MEDIUM HEAT (350° TO 450°F)
GRILLING TIME: 16 TO 20 MINUTES

MARINADE
- ¼ cup extra-virgin olive oil
- 2 tablespoons fresh lime juice
- 1 teaspoon dried thyme
- 1 teaspoon dried marjoram
- ½ teaspoon kosher salt
- ¼ teaspoon freshly ground black pepper

- 6 boneless, skinless chicken thighs, about 4 ounces each

DRESSING
- 1 large poblano chile pepper
- ½ cup sour cream
- ½ cup lightly packed fresh cilantro leaves and tender stems
- 1 tablespoon fresh lime juice
- 1 tablespoon extra-virgin olive oil
- 1 large garlic clove
- ½ teaspoon ground cumin
- ½ teaspoon kosher salt
- ¼ teaspoon freshly ground black pepper

SALAD
- 4 cups thinly sliced/shredded romaine lettuce
- 1½ cups crushed yellow or blue corn tortilla chips
- 1 cup medium-diced ripe tomato
- 2 Haas avocados, diced
- 1 can (15 ounces) pinto or black beans, rinsed

1. In a medium bowl whisk the marinade ingredients. Add the chicken thighs, turning several times to coat them evenly. Cover and refrigerate for 30 minutes to 1 hour.

2. Prepare the grill for direct cooking over medium heat. Brush the cooking grates clean. Grill the chile over **direct medium heat**, with the lid closed as much as possible, until the skin is blackened and blistered, 8 to 10 minutes, turning occasionally. Transfer the chile to a small bowl, cover with plastic wrap, and let steam for about 10 minutes. Gently peel the skin from the chile and remove the seeds. Put the chile in a blender with the remaining dressing ingredients and process until smooth. Refrigerate until ready to serve.

3. On a large platter arrange a bed of lettuce, and then add the chips, tomato, avocado, and beans in separate sections on top.

4. Grill the chicken over **direct medium heat**, with the lid closed as much as possible, until the meat is firm and the juices run clear, 8 to 10 minutes, turning once or twice. Transfer the chicken to a cutting board and cut into ½-inch strips. Place the chicken on a separate section of the platter. Four the dressing over the salad just before serving, and mix well.

WAY TO GRILL CHICKEN THIGHS

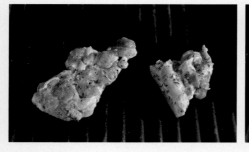

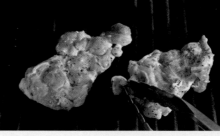

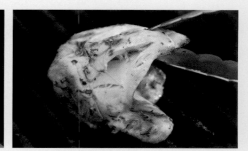

1. Lay chicken thighs, smooth side down first, over direct heat and resist the urge to turn them for at least 4 minutes. Otherwise, you might rip the meat.

2. However, if the meat is bunched on top of itself, unfold it so that it lies at flat as possible on the grate for better charred flavor.

3. You can check the doneness by bending back a thigh and opening up the meat. If there is no trace of pink, it's done.

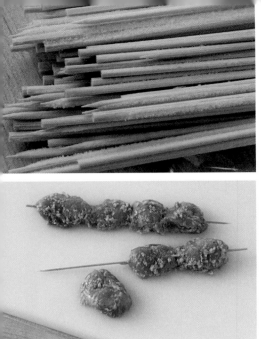

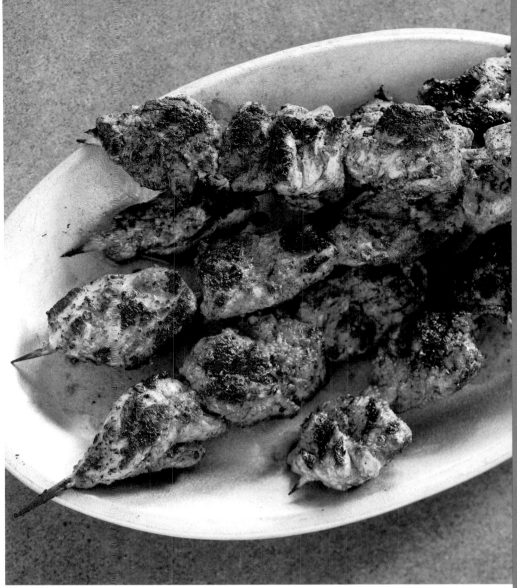

KEEPING FROZEN SKEWERS ON HAND

To avoid soaking bamboo skewers each time you need them, soak a big batch once for an hour or so, drain them, and then freeze them in a plastic bag. When it's time to grill, pull out as many skewers as you need.

Ingredients like chicken pieces will stay juicier longer if they are touching (but not crammed) on the skewers.

PERSIAN CHICKEN KABOBS

SERVES: 4 TO 6
PREP TIME: 15 MINUTES
MARINATING TIME: 30 MINUTES

WAY TO GRILL: DIRECT MEDIUM HEAT (350° TO 450°F)
GRILLING TIME: 8 TO 10 MINUTES
SPECIAL EQUIPMENT: BAMBOO SKEWERS,
   SOAKED IN WATER FOR AT LEAST 30 MINUTES

MARINADE
  1 large onion, coarsely chopped
  ½ cup fresh lemon juice
  2 tablespoons dried oregano
  2 teaspoons sweet paprika
  2 teaspoons minced garlic
  1 cup extra-virgin olive oil

  10 boneless, skinless chicken thighs, about 4 ounces each,
      cut into 1½-inch pieces

1. In the bowl of a food processor or blender, puree the onion, lemon juice, oregano, paprika, and garlic. With the motor running, slowly add the oil.

2. Place the chicken pieces in a large, resealable plastic bag and pour in the marinade. Press the air out of the bag and seal tightly. Turn the bag to distribute the marinade and let the chicken marinate at room temperature for 30 minutes.

3. Prepare the grill for direct cooking over medium heat.

4. Remove the chicken from the marinade and thread onto skewers, so that the pieces are touching (but not crammed together). Discard the marinade.

5. Brush the cooking grates clean. Grill the kabobs over **direct medium heat**, with the lid closed as much as possible, until the meat is fully cooked but not dry, 8 to 10 minutes, turning once. Serve warm.

WAY TO GRILL QUESADILLAS

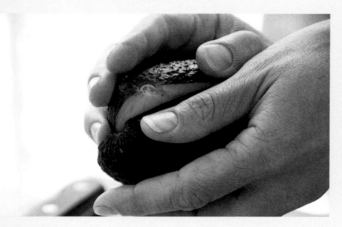

1. Of course most great quesadillas involve guacamole, and that means avocado. To pit one, cut lengthwise around the pit and then twist the halves in opposite directions.

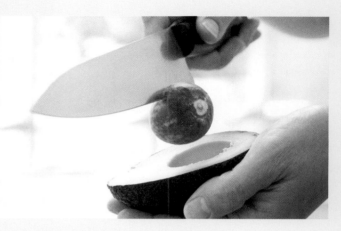

2. Tap the exposed pit with the heel of your knife. It will pull out easily from the avocado.

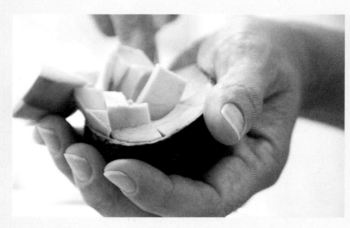

3. You can chop the avocado right in the skin by cross-hatching it and then scooping the little pieces into a bowl with a spoon. Then mash the avocado pieces with lime juice, garlic, and salt.

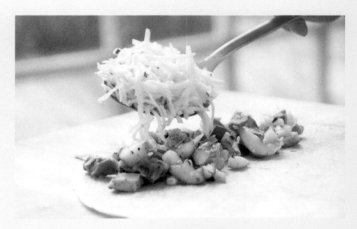

4. Load up one side of each tortilla with grilled chicken, vegetables, and some shredded cheese, but don't add so much that the filling might spill out the sides.

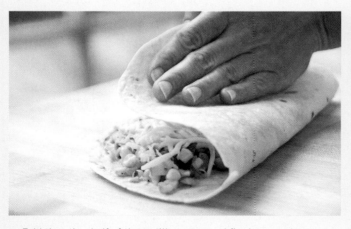

5. Fold the other half of the tortilla on top and firmly press down on it. At this point, you can set the quesadillas aside for a couple hours before grilling them.

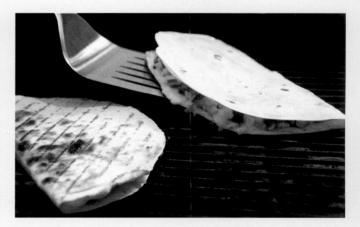

6. Grill the quesadillas over direct medium heat until toasted on each side. This is one time when it's best to leave the grill lid open, so you can keep an eye on the quesadillas and prevent them from burning.

CHICKEN AND VEGETABLE QUESADILLAS WITH GUACAMOLE

SERVES: 4 TO 6
PREP TIME: 30 MINUTES

WAY TO GRILL: DIRECT MEDIUM HEAT (350° TO 450°F)
GRILLING TIME: 10 TO 13 MINUTES

RUB
- 1 teaspoon pure chile powder
- 1 teaspoon kosher salt
- ½ teaspoon dried oregano
- ¼ teaspoon granulated garlic
- ¼ teaspoon granulated onion
- ¼ teaspoon freshly ground black pepper

- 4 boneless, skinless chicken thighs, about 4 ounces each
- 2 zucchini, trimmed and halved lengthwise
- 2 ears corn, husked
  Extra-virgin olive oil
- 2 teaspoons chopped fresh oregano
- 1 teaspoon minced garlic
- 1 tablespoon fresh lime juice
  Kosher salt
  Freshly ground black pepper

GUACAMOLE
- 2 medium Haas avocados, diced
- 2 teaspoons fresh lime juice
- 1 teaspoon minced garlic
- ¼ teaspoon kosher salt

- 10 flour tortillas (10 inches)
- 4 cups grated pepper jack cheese

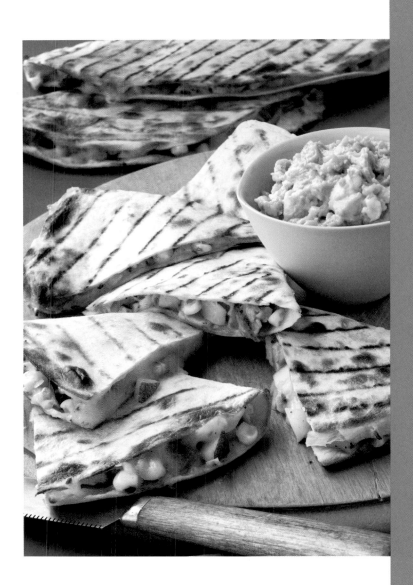

1. Prepare the grill for direct cooking over medium heat.

2. In a small bowl combine the rub ingredients. Lightly brush or spray the chicken, zucchini, and corn with oil. Season the chicken with the rub.

3. Brush the cooking grates clean. Grill the chicken and vegetables over **direct medium heat**, with the lid closed as much as possible, until the meat is firm and the juices run clear, the zucchini is barely tender, and the corn kernels are golden brown in spots, turning the chicken once and the vegetables occasionally. The chicken will take 8 to 10 minutes and the vegetables will take 6 to 8 minutes. Remove from the grill and allow to cool.

4. Cut the chicken and zucchini into ¼-inch chunks. Cut the kernels from the cobs. In a large bowl combine the zucchini and corn with the oregano, garlic and lime juice, and then season to taste with salt and pepper. Add the chicken to the vegetable mixture and stir to combine.

5. In a small bowl mash together the guacamole ingredients.

6. Lay the tortillas in a single layer on a work surface. Evenly divide the chicken and vegetable mixture, and then the cheese, over half of each tortilla. Fold the empty half of each tortilla over the filling, creating a half circle, and press down firmly.

7. Grill the quesadillas over **direct medium heat**, with the lid open, for 2 to 3 minutes, turning once. Transfer the quesadillas from the grill to a cutting board and cut into wedges. Serve warm with the guacamole.

WAY TO SPLIT CORNISH GAME HENS

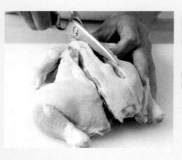 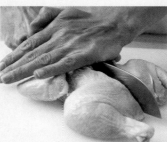 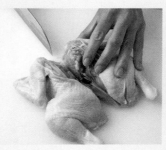 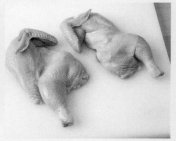

1. Use poultry shears to cut along both sides of the backbone. Then discard it.

2. Cut through the middle of the breast.

3. The breastbone will stay attached to one of the halves.

4. Hens cut into halves will absorb marinades more easily and cook faster than whole ones.

CORNISH HENS MARINATED IN BOURBON, HONEY, AND SOY

SERVES: 4
PREP TIME: 30 MINUTES
MARINATING TIME: 4 TO 8 HOURS

WAY TO GRILL: INDIRECT MEDIUM HEAT (350° TO 450°F)
GRILLING TIME: ABOUT 30 MINUTES

MARINADE
1½ cups soy sauce
¾ cup bourbon
6 garlic cloves, minced
2 tablespoons honey
1½ tablespoons grated fresh ginger

4 Cornish game hens, 1 to 1½ pounds each
   Extra-virgin olive oil
½ teaspoon freshly ground black pepper

1. In a medium bowl combine the marinade ingredients.

2. Remove and discard the giblets from each hen. Using poultry shears, cut along both sides of each backbone and discard it. Then cut through the middle of each breast.

3. Place the hens side by side in a shallow, non-reactive dish and cover with the marinade. Turn to coat the hens evenly, and then cover and refrigerate for 4 to 8 hours. (Do not marinate overnight or the ginger will cause the meat to break down and become mushy.)

4. Remove the hens from the dish and reserve the marinade. Lightly brush the hens with oil and season with the pepper. Allow to stand at room temperature for 20 to 30 minutes before grilling. Prepare the grill for indirect cooking over medium heat.

5. Pour the reserved marinade into a small saucepan and bring to a boil over high heat for about 30 seconds. Set aside to use as a basting sauce.

6. Brush the cooking grates clean. Grill the hens, skin side up, over **indirect medium heat**, with the lid closed, until the skin is golden brown and the internal temperature in the thickest part of the thigh reaches 170°F, about 30 minutes, basting the top of the hens with the sauce a couple of times during the last 10 minutes of cooking. Remove from the grill and serve warm.

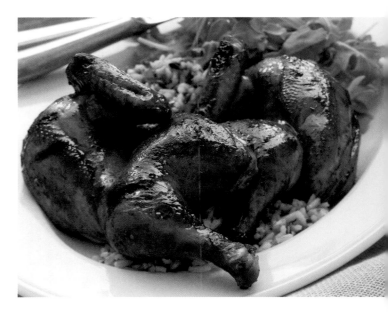

HULI-HULI CHICKEN

SERVES: 4 TO 6
PREP TIME: 15 MINUTES
MARINATING TIME: ABOUT 4 HOURS

WAY TO GRILL: INDIRECT MEDIUM HEAT (350° TO 450°F)
GRILLING TIME: 45 MINUTES TO 1 HOUR

MARINADE
- 1 cup thawed pineapple juice concentrate
- ½ cup soy sauce
- ¼ cup ketchup
- 2 tablespoons minced fresh ginger
- 2 teaspoons minced garlic

- 2 whole chickens, 3 to 4 pounds each
- 4 handfuls mesquite wood chips, soaked in water for at least 30 minutes

1. In a medium bowl whisk the marinade ingredients.

2. Place one of the chickens, breast side down, on a cutting board. Using poultry shears, cut along each side of the backbone and discard it. Open the chicken like a book, and then cut the chicken in half lengthwise along one side of the breastbone. Pull off and discard any lumps of fat. Remove and discard the wing tips. Repeat the process with the other chicken. Place the chicken halves in a 2-gallon, resealable plastic bag and pour in the marinade. Press the air out of the bag and seal it tightly. Turn the bag several times to coat the chicken evenly with the marinade. Place the bag in a bowl and refrigerate for about 4 hours, turning the bag occasionally.

3. Remove the chicken from the bag and discard the marinade.

4. Prepare the grill for indirect cooking over medium heat.

5. Drain half of the wood chips and toss them onto burning coals or into the smoker box of a gas grill, following manufacturer's instructions. Begin cooking the chicken when the wood starts to smoke.

6. Brush the cooking grates clean. Grill the chicken, skin side up first, over **indirect medium heat**, with the lid closed as much as possible, until the juices run clear and the internal temperature reaches 170°F in the thickest part of the thigh (not touching the bone), 45 minutes to 1 hour, turning every 15 minutes. Drain and add the rest of the wood chips after the first 15 minutes of grilling.

7. Remove from the grill and let the chicken rest for about 10 minutes before serving.

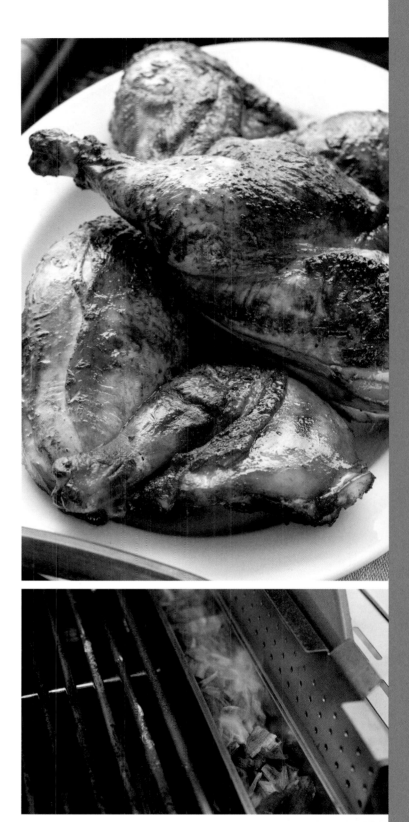

Huli-Huli is a Hawaiian term meaning turn-turn, which is exactly what you need to do here to prevent the sweet marinade from burning. That said, turn the chicken halves carefully with a spatula so they hold together. And don't forget the wood smoke. It is as important as any ingredient in the recipe.

WAY TO SMOKE BEER CAN CHICKEN

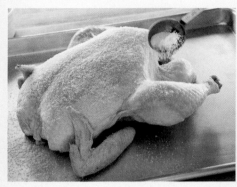

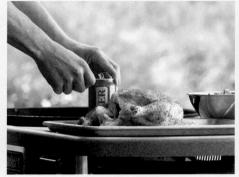

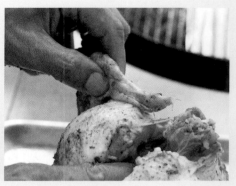

1. Blanketing a chicken with salt and refrigerating it for a couple hours will draw out some moisture and strengthen the chicken flavors. Don't worry; the chicken will not be salty. The next step is to rinse off the salt.

2. After you have rinsed and seasoned the chicken, open a beer can and pour out half of it (into a cold mug). With a can opener, make 2 more holes in the top to allow steam to escape.

3. Fold the wing tips behind the back of the chicken to shield the tips from the heat.

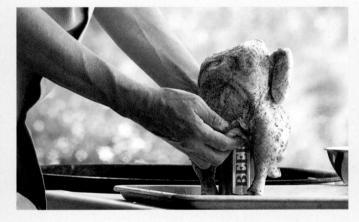

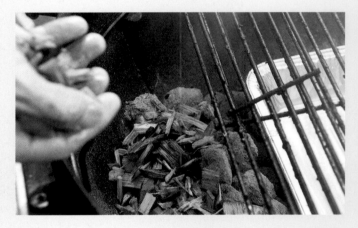

4. Working with a solid surface underneath, slide the chicken over the beer can as far as it will go.

5. Set up the grill with a water pan in the middle and coals on either side. Add a couple handfuls of damp chips to each pile of coals.

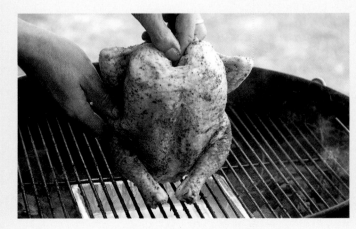

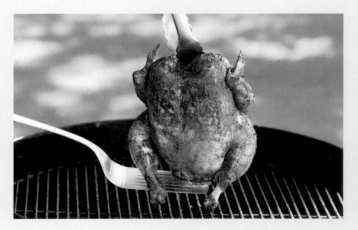

6. When the wood starts to smoke, place the chicken in the center of the cooking grate. Position the chicken legs toward the front so they balance the chicken with the can like a tripod.

7. When the chicken is fully cooked (170°F in the thickest part of the thigh), grab the back with tongs and slide a spatula under the can to lift it. Be careful; the beer will be very hot. Let the chicken rest and cool for about 10 minutes before sliding it off the can.

SMOKED BEER CAN CHICKEN

SERVES: 4
PREP TIME: 10 MINUTES
SALT-CURING TIME: 1½ TO 2 HOURS

WAY TO GRILL: INDIRECT MEDIUM HEAT (350° TO 450°F)
GRILLING TIME: 1¼ TO 1½ HOURS

- 1 whole chicken, about 5 pounds
- ¼ cup kosher salt

RUB
- 2 teaspoons granulated on on
- 2 teaspoons granulated garlic
- 1 teaspoon prepared chili powder
- ½ teaspoon freshly ground black pepper

- 1 can (12 ounces) beer, at room temperature
- 4 handfuls hickory wood chips, soaked in water for at least 30 minutes

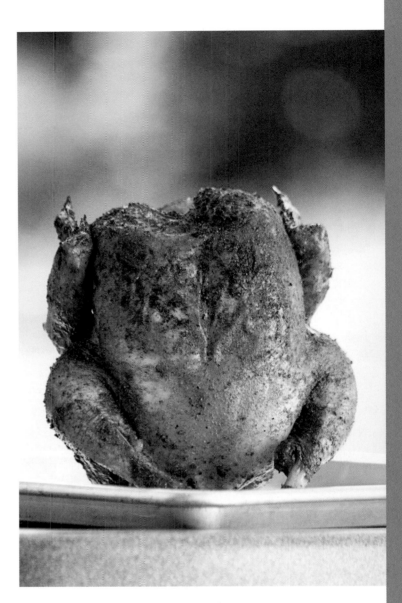

1. Remove and discard the neck, giblets, and any excess fat from the chicken. Sprinkle the salt over the entire surface and inside the cavity of the chicken, covering it all like a light blanket of snow. Cover the chicken with plastic wrap and refrigerate for 1½ to 2 hours.

2. In a small bowl mix the rub ingredients.

3. Rinse the chicken inside and out with cold water. Gently pat the chicken dry with paper towels. Season it all over with the rub. Fold the wing tips behind the chicken's back. Let the chicken stand at room temperature for 20 to 30 minutes before grilling. Prepare the grill for indirect cooking over medium heat.

4. Open the beer can and pour out about half the beer. Using a can opener, make 2 more holes in the top of the can. Place the beer can on a solid surface. Plunk the chicken cavity over the beer can.

5. Drain and add the wood chips directly onto burning coals or to the smoker box of a gas grill, following manufacturer's instructions. When the wood chips begin to smoke, transfer the bird-on-a-can to the grill, balancing the bird on its two legs and the can, like a tripod. Grill over ***indirect medium heat***, with the lid closed, until the juices run clear and the internal temperature registers 170°F in the thickest part of the thigh (not touching the bone), 1¼ to 1½ hours. Carefully remove the chicken and can from the grill (do not spill contents of the beer can, as it will be very hot). Let the chicken rest for about 10 minutes before lifting it from the beer can and cutting into serving pieces. Serve warm.

WAY TO COOK ROTISSERIE CHICKEN

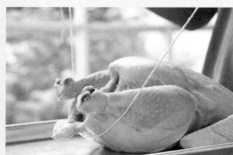 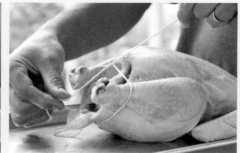 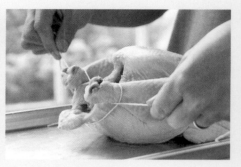

1. To truss the chicken, remove the wing tips and slide a 4-foot length of twine under the legs and back.

2. Lift both ends of the twine and cross it between the legs. Then run one end under one drumstick.

3. Run the other end under the other drumstick and pull both ends to draw the drumsticks together.

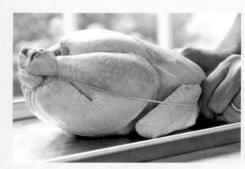 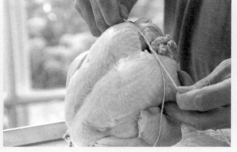 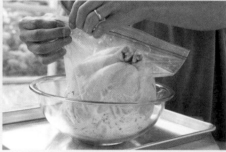

4. Bring the twine along both sides of the chicken so that it holds the legs and wings against the body.

5. Tie a knot in the ends between the neck and the top of the breast. If necessary, push the breast down a little to expose more of the neck.

6. Marinate the chicken in a bag with the buttermilk mixture for 2 to 4 hours in the refrigerator.

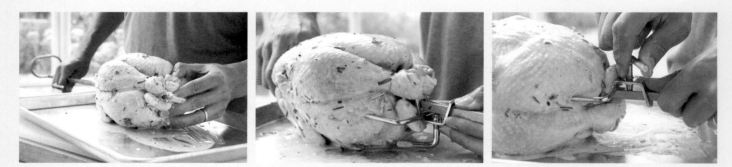

7. Position one set of fork prongs on the far end of the center rod (spit) and slide the spit into the opening between the neck and the knotted twine, though the chicken, and out the other side, just underneath the drumsticks. Slide the other set of fork prongs on the spit and drive the prongs into the back of the chicken. Make sure the chicken is centered on the spit before tightening the fork prongs into place.

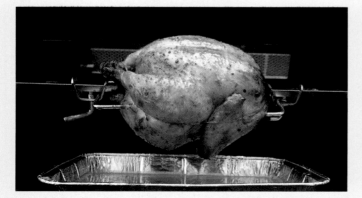 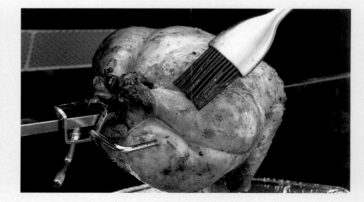

8. Position the chicken over a drip pan of water. Turn on the motor and let the chicken cook over indirect heat. Adjust the burners as necessary to maintain a cooking temperature of about 400°F. During the last 30 minutes of cooking, brush the chicken a few times with the glaze, but keep the lid closed as much as possible. For a crispier skin, turn on the infrared burner at the back of the grill during the final minutes of cooking.

ROTISSERIE BUTTERMILK CHICKEN WITH APRICOT GLAZE

SERVES: 4
PREP TIME: 25 MINUTES
MARINATING TIME: 2 TO 4 HOURS

WAY TO GRILL: INDIRECT MEDIUM HEAT (ABOUT 400°F)
GRILLING TIME: 1 TO 1¼ HOURS
SPECIAL EQUIPMENT: BUTCHER'S TWINE,
    ROTISSERIE, LARGE DISPOSABLE FOIL PAN,
    INSTANT-READ THERMOMETER

MARINADE
    2 cups buttermilk
    ¼ cup roughly chopped fresh rosemary leaves
    4 large garlic cloves, finely chopped
    2 tablespoons kosher salt
    1 teaspoon freshly ground black pepper

    1 whole chicken, 4½ to 5 pounds

GLAZE
    1 cup apricot nectar
    3 tablespoons maple syrup
    1 tablespoon Dijon mustard
    1 tablespoon white wine vinegar

1. In a large bowl combine the marinade ingredients.

2. Truss the chicken with butcher's twine (see preceding page). Place the chicken in a large, resealable plastic bag and pour in the marinade. Press the air out of the bag and seal it tightly. Turn the bag several times to coat the chicken evenly, place

in a large bowl, starting with the breast side facing down, and marinate in the refrigerator for 2 to 4 hours, turning the bag once or twice. Let the chicken stand at room temperature for about 30 minutes before grilling. Prepare the grill for indirect cooking at 400°F, with the outside burners on medium to high and the middle burners turned off.

3. In a small saucepan over medium-high heat, whisk the glaze ingredients. Bring to a boil and then gently simmer until you have about 1 cup remaining, about 5 minutes. Reserve half of the glaze to use as a sauce.

4. Remove the chicken from the bag. Wipe off most of the marinade and discard the marinade. Following the grill's instructions, secure the chicken in the middle of a rotisserie spit, put the spit in place, and turn on the motor. Place a large disposable foil pan under the chicken to catch drippings and pour about 1 cup of warm water into the pan. Grill the chicken over *indirect medium heat*, with the lid closed, until the internal temperature reaches 170°F in the thickest part of the thigh (not touching the bone), 1 to 1¼ hours. During the last 30 minutes of grilling, brush the chicken with the glaze a few times.

5. When the chicken is fully cooked, turn off the rotisserie motor and, wearing insulated mitts, carefully remove the spit from the grill. Tilt the chicken upright over the disposable foil pan so that the liquid that has accumulated in the chicken's cavity pours into the pan. Slice the chicken from the spit onto a cutting board. Let rest for about 10 minutes before carving into serving pieces. Serve warm with the reserved sauce.

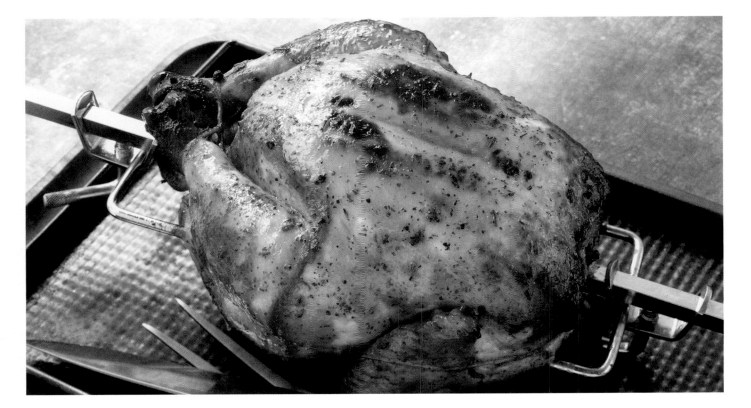

WAY TO ROAST CHICKEN

Most chickens in supermarkets today have been bred primarily for their appearance. Large-scale farmers select their breeds for plump breast meat and yellow skins, and raise the chickens in cramped cages, feeding them cheap diets that promote quick growth but contribute very little to flavor. One way around the blandness problem is to buy old-fashioned breeds instead. They might be a little harder to find, and they will cost you more, but they do taste better. Another way around the blandness problem is to roast mass-market chickens with plenty of butter, fresh herbs, and seasonings under the skin.

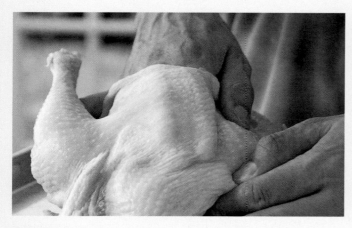

1. Starting at the bottom of the breast, work your fingertips gently under the skin and over the meat. Try not to tear the skin.

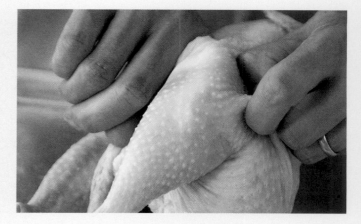

2. Use just one finger to reach down each drumstick and along the thigh meat.

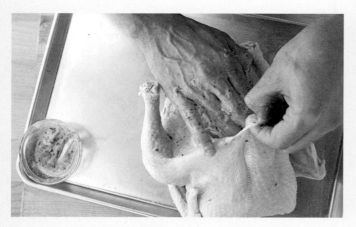

3. Smear the flavored butter over the breast meat and cover as much of the thigh meat as possible without tearing the skin. Use the remaining flavored butter to coat the outside of the chicken evenly.

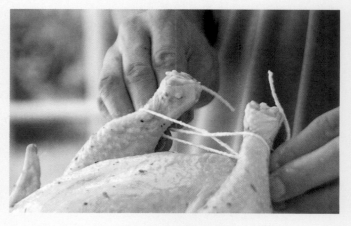

4. Wrap a piece of butcher's twine under and around the drumsticks, cross it in the middle, and pull the ends to draw the drumsticks together.

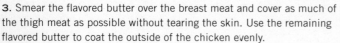

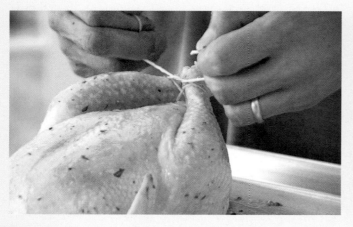

5. Cross the twine above the drumsticks and tie a knot. This will hold the chicken in a compact shape and help the meat cook more evenly.

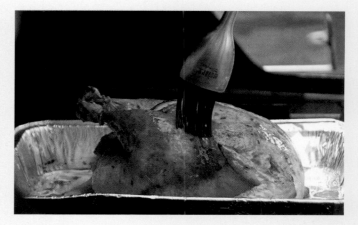

6. Roast the chicken inside a disposable foil pan to catch the melted butter and drippings. Baste the chicken occasionally with what's in the pan and rotate the pan as necessary for even browning.

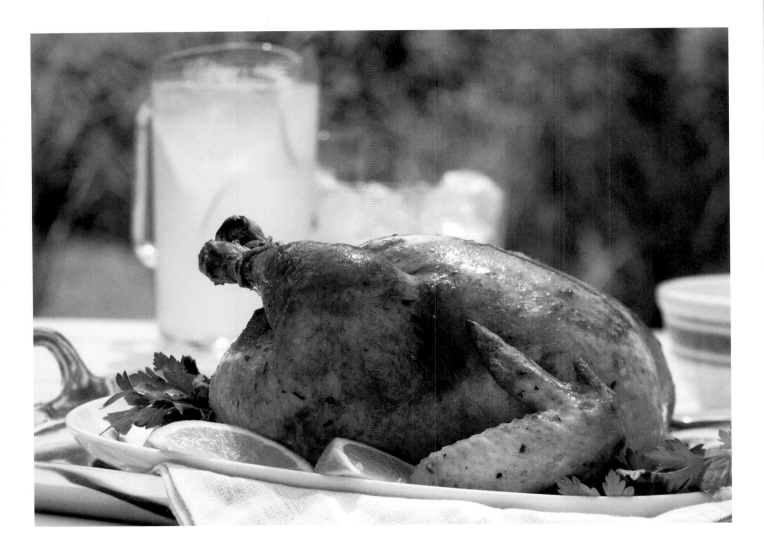

ORANGE-TARRAGON ROASTED CHICKEN

SERVES: 4
PREP TIME: 15 MINUTES

WAY TO GRILL: INDIRECT MEDIUM HEAT (350° TO 450°F)
GRILLING TIME: 1¼ TO 1½ HOURS
SPECIAL EQUIPMENT: LARGE DISPOSABLE FOIL PAN,
  BUTCHER'S TWINE

BUTTER

    4 tablespoons unsalted butter, softened
    1 tablespoon finely chopped fresh tarragon
    2 teaspoons finely grated orange zest
    ½ teaspoon kosher salt
    ¼ teaspoon freshly ground black pepper

    1 whole chicken, 5 to 5½ pounds
    1 teaspoon kosher salt
    ½ teaspoon freshly ground black pepper

1. In a small bowl, using the back of a fork, mix and mash the butter ingredients.

2. Remove and discard the neck, giblets, and any excess fat from the chicken. Loosen the chicken skin gently with your fingertips and spread the butter under the skin onto the breast meat and as much as you can reach on the drumsticks and thighs.

3. Season the chicken inside and out with the salt and pepper. Truss the chicken legs with butcher's twine. Place the chicken, breast side up, in a large disposable foil pan. Allow the chicken to stand at room temperature for 20 to 30 minutes before grilling. Prepare the grill for indirect cooking over medium heat.

4. Brush the cooking grates clean. Grill the chicken over ***indirect medium heat***, with the lid closed, until the juices run clear and the internal temperature in the thickest part of the thigh reaches 170°F, 1¼ to 1½ hours, rotating the pan as needed for even browning. Occasionally baste the chicken with the melted butter collected in the bottom of the pan. When fully cooked, transfer the chicken to a platter and loosely cover with aluminum foil. Let rest for about 10 minutes. Remove the twine and carve the chicken. Serve warm.

WAY TO GRILL BUTTERFLIED CHICKEN

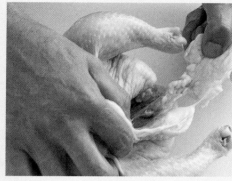

1. Pull out and discard the loose clumps of fat that are typically just inside the chicken. Otherwise they might drip into the grill and cause flare-ups.

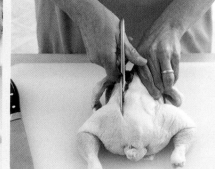

2. Turn the chicken over so that the back is facing up and the neck end is closest to you. Use poultry shears to cut along both sides of the backbone, and then discard it.

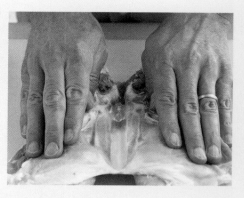

3. Open the chicken like a butterfly spreading its wings, and press down to flatten it.

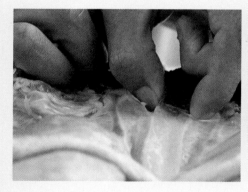

4. Run your fingertips along both sides of the breastbone to expose it.

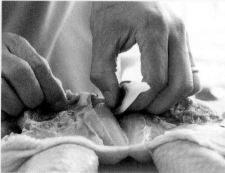

5. Dig your fingers down along the breastbone until it comes loose from the meat. Then pull it out and discard it.

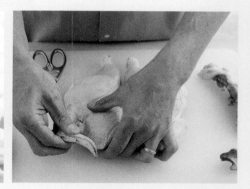

6. Fold the wing tips behind the chicken's back to prevent them from burning.

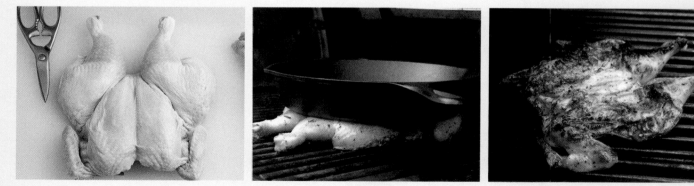
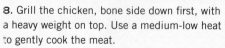

7. Now you have overcome one of the key cooking challenges of a whole chicken: an uneven shape. By butterflying (or spatchcocking) the bird, you have created a relatively even shape.

8. Grill the chicken, bone side down first, with a heavy weight on top. Use a medium-low heat to gently cook the meat.

9. After about 25 minutes, carefully turn the chicken over with a spatula and put the weight back on top. With the skin side down, flare-ups are more likely. If necessary, turn off the middle burners or move the chicken to finish cooking over indirect heat.

NUTMEG CHICKEN UNDER A CAST-IRON SKILLET

SERVES: 4
PREP TIME: 30 MINUTES
MARINATING TIME: 2 HOURS

WAY TO GRILL: DIRECT MEDIUM-LOW HEAT (ABOUT 350°F)
GRILLING TIME: 40 MINUTES TO 1 HOUR
SPECIAL EQUIPMENT: CAST-IRON SKILLET OR
    SHEET PAN AND 2 FOIL-WRAPPED BRICKS,
    INSTANT-READ THERMOMETER

MARINADE
  ¼ cup extra-virgin olive oil
  2 tablespoons minced fresh rosemary
  1 tablespoon minced fresh garlic
  1 tablespoon freshly grated nutmeg
  1 tablespoon kosher salt
  1 tablespoon granulated sugar
  1 teaspoon freshly ground black pepper

  1 whole chicken, about 5 pounds

1. In a large, shallow bowl or a 13x9-inch baking pan, combine the marinade ingredients.

2. Place the chicken, breast side down, on a cutting board. Using sturdy kitchen shears or a very sharp knife, cut from the neck to the tail end, along either side of the backbone, to remove it. Take special care if you are using a knife; you'll be cutting through small bones and will have to use some force.

3. Once the backbone is out, you'll be able to see the interior of the chicken. Make a small slit in the cartilage at the bottom end of the breastbone. Then, placing both hands on the rib cage, crack the chicken open like a book. Run your fingers along either side of the cartilage in between the breasts to loosen it from the flesh. Grab the bone and pull up on it to remove it along with the attached cartilage. The chicken should now lay flat.

4. Place the chicken inside the bowl or in the baking pan and turn to coat it evenly with the marinade. Cover with plastic wrap and refrigerate for about 2 hours.

5. Prepare the grill for direct cooking over medium-low heat.

6. Brush the cooking grates clean. Place the chicken, bone side down, over *direct medium-low heat* and put a heavy cast-iron skillet, or weight a sheet pan down with 2 foil-wrapped bricks, directly on top. Close the lid and cook for 20 to 30 minutes. Remove the skillet, turn the chicken over, replace the weight, close the lid, and cook until the juices run clear and an instant-read thermometer inserted into the thigh (not touching the bone) registers 170°F, 20 to 30 minutes. Remove from the grill and let rest for 3 to 5 minutes. Serve warm.

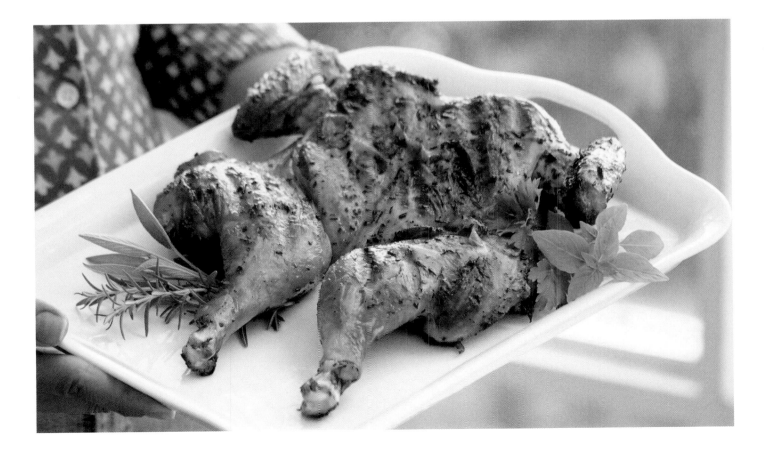

WAY TO GRILL BACON-WRAPPED TURKEY BREAST

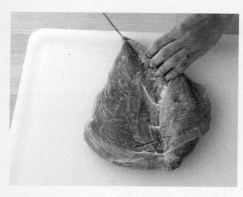

1. With the smooth side facing the board, open up the breast and cut down the center (but not all the way through) to make the breast as flat and even as possible.

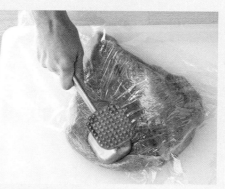

2. Lay the butterflied turkey breast between 2 large sheets of plastic wrap and pound it to a thickness of ¾ to 1 inch.

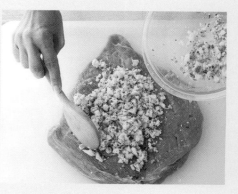

3. Spread the stuffing evenly over the turkey breast, but leave a margin all the way around the perimeter. Don't overstuff the breast.

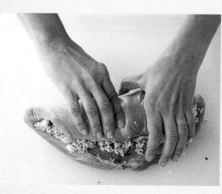

4. Roll up the breast lengthwise to create a cylinder. If any excess stuffing falls out, discard it.

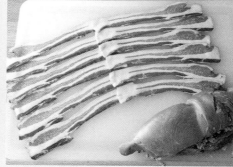

5. Arrange the bacon slices on a work surface in 6 tightly spaced parallel stripes, overlapping the ends of 2 slices to make each stripe.

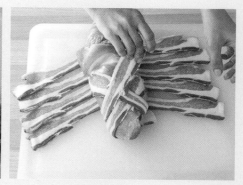

6. Place the rolled turkey breast in the center of the bacon and then crisscross the bacon around the turkey.

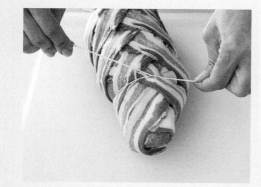

7. Tie the turkey crosswise with butcher's twine at 1-inch intervals.

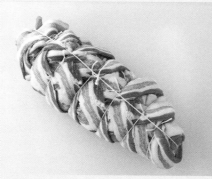

8. Thread a long piece of twine lengthwise, in and out of the crosswise pieces, and tie the ends together to create a uniform roast and to secure the bacon.

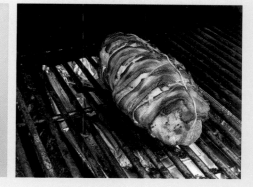

9. Set a disposable foil pan under the cooking grate to catch the bacon grease. Grill the roast over the pan, using indirect heat, until the internal temperature of the meat and stuffing reaches 165°F, turning to ensure even cooking.

BACON-WRAPPED TURKEY BREAST WITH HERB STUFFING

SERVES: 4 TO 6
PREP TIME: 30 MINUTES

WAY TO GRILL: INDIRECT HIGH HEAT (450° TO 550°F)
GRILLING TIME: 1 TO 1¼ HOURS
SPECIAL EQUIPMENT: BUTCHER'S TWINE, LARGE
    DISPOSABLE FOIL PAN, INSTANT-READ THERMOMETER

STUFFING
- 1½ cups fresh bread crumbs
- ¼ cup low-sodium chicken broth
- 1 tablespoon finely chopped garlic
- 2 teaspoons finely chopped fresh rosemary
- 2 teaspoons finely chopped fresh oregano
- 1 teaspoon finely grated lemon zest
- ½ teaspoon kosher salt
- ½ teaspoon freshly ground black pepper

- 1 pound sliced bacon
- 1 boneless, skinless turkey breast, about
    2 pounds, butterflied

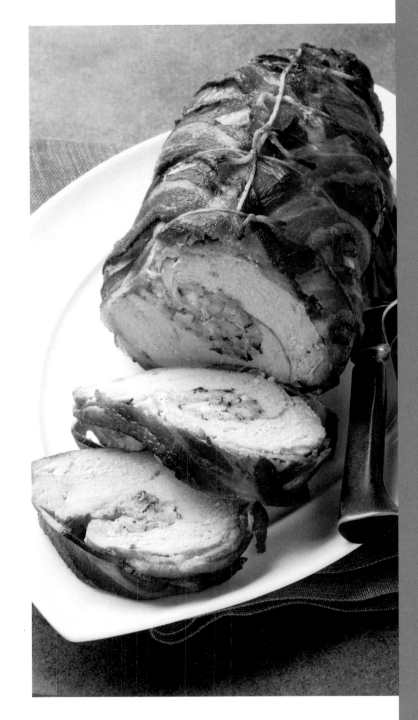

1. In a medium bowl combine the stuffing ingredients. The stuffing should be moist, mounding nicely on a spoon, but should not be sopping wet. Add more broth if needed.

2. Carefully place a large disposable foil pan underneath the cooking grate to catch the bacon grease. Prepare the grill for indirect cooking over high heat.

3. Place the butterflied turkey breast on a work surface between 2 sheets of plastic wrap and pound to an even thickness. Spread the stuffing evenly over the turkey breast and then roll up the breast lengthwise to create a cylinder. Arrange the bacon slices on a work surface in 6 tightly spaced parallel stripes, overlapping the ends of 2 slices to make each stripe. Place the rolled turkey breast in the center of the bacon and then crisscross the bacon around the turkey. Tie the turkey with butcher's twine to create a uniform roast and to secure the bacon.

4. Brush the cooking grates clean. Center the turkey over the drip pan and grill over **_indirect high heat_**, with the lid closed as much as possible, until the internal temperature reaches 165°F, 1 to 1¼ hours, turning occasionally to ensure the bacon gets crispy on all sides. Transfer to a carving board and let rest for 10 minutes (the internal temperature will rise 5° to 10°F during this time). Remove the twine and carve into 1-inch slices.

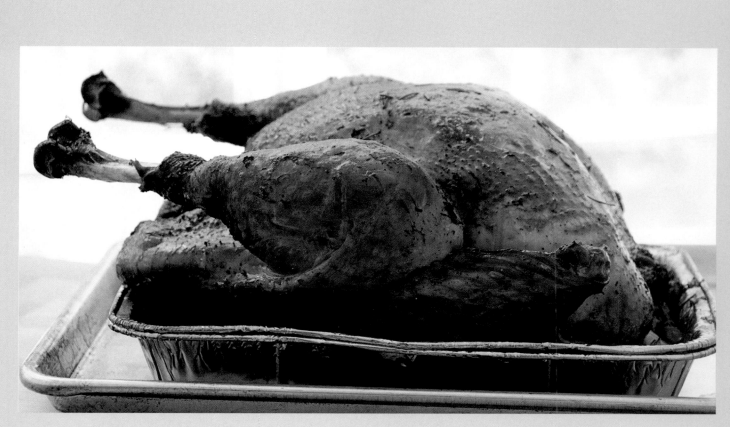

WAY TO COOK TURKEY

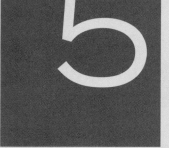 THINGS YOU NEED TO KNOW

Every November millions of Americans tighten up with stress at the thought of how to cook a golden, succulent turkey for Thanksgiving. Let me tell you; it's not that difficult. Focus on a handful of critical elements.

1 BRINING A DAY AHEAD

Because turkey meat is so lean and bland, some kind of brining is important. In the following recipe I call for a dry brine, which just means coating the turkey with kosher salt the day before cooking. Overnight, in the refrigerator, the salt will draw out some moisture, which will mix with the salt, and then the meat will reabsorb much of that flavorful moisture.

2 MAINTAINING AN EVEN TEMPERATURE

An even grilling temperature in the range of 350° to 400°F is also key here. That's easy enough to achieve on a gas grill, assuming there is plenty of gas in the tank. It's a bit more challenging with a charcoal grill. Before cooking your first turkey with charcoal, make sure you have had some good experiences maintaining a live fire over the course of several hours.

3 SHIELDING THE BREAST MEAT

Because the breast meat cooks faster than the leg meat, you should protect the breast and slow down its rate of cooking. I do that by facing the breast down inside a broth-and-vegetable-filled pan for the first hour of cooking.

4 CATCHING THE PERFECT DONENESS

In a very short period of time, a turkey can turn from moist and fabulous to dry and stringy, so it's imperative that you use an instant-read thermometer and remove the turkey from the grill when the internal temperature in the thickest part of the thigh reaches 170°F.

5 GETTING ENOUGH REST

Finally, don't skip the resting step after your turkey comes off the grill. During that period, the turkey will finish cooking and the juices will redistribute nicely.

WAY TO PREP TURKEY THE DAY BEFORE

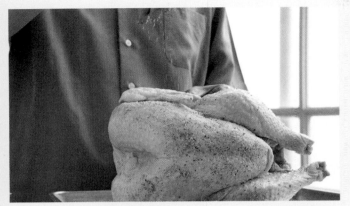

1. Generously season the turkey, inside and out, with kosher salt and freshly ground black pepper.

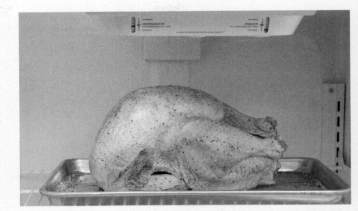

2. Refrigerate the seasoned turkey on a sheet pan, uncovered, for 12 hours. It's okay if the skin looks dry and tightened now.

WAY TO SMOKE TURKEY

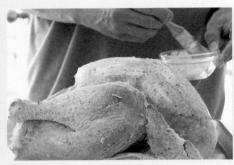

1. Remove the turkey from the refrigerator and let it sit at room temperature for 1 hour. Brush the legs, breast, and wings with butter.

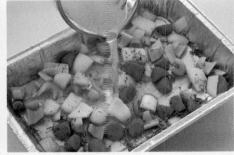

2. Place 1 large disposable foil pan inside the other and add the vegetables, herbs, and 2 cups of chicken broth.

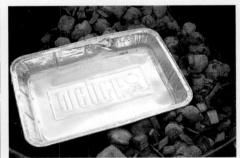

3. Arrange the charcoal in a half circle on one side of the charcoal grate. A drip pan filled with warm water will help you maintain the temperature of the fire.

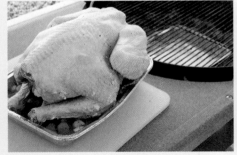

4. Place the turkey, breast side down, inside the foil pans and over the vegetables.

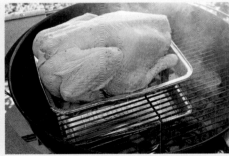

5. Add wood chips to the charcoal and set the pan over the water pan, with the legs facing the hottest side of the grill.

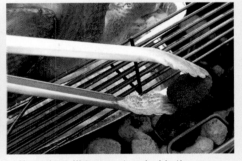

6. Keep the grill temperature inside the range of 350° to 400°F, adding charcoal as needed.

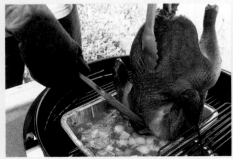

7. After grilling for 1 hour, flip over the turkey so that the breast side is facing up.

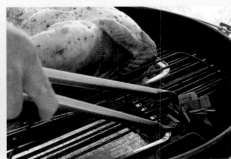

8. Continue grilling and smoking the turkey, occasionally adding damp wood chips.

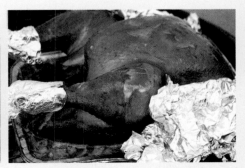

9. After the turkey has been on the grill for 1½ hours, cover any parts that are getting too dark.

WAY TO CARVE TURKEY

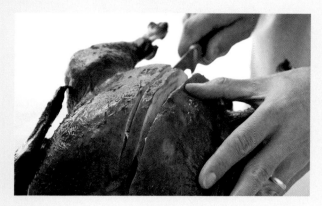

1. Remove each half of the turkey breast by cutting lengthwise along each side of the breastbone.

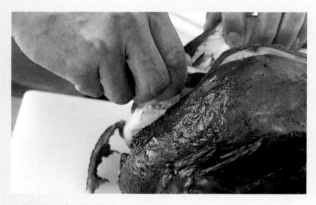

2. Pull the first half of the breast away from the breastbone, using a sharp knife to carefully release the meat from the rib cage.

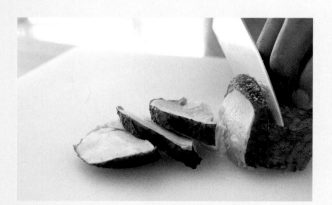

3. It is much easier to carve a half of a turkey breast into crosswise slices than it is to carve the breast while it is still attached to the body.

HICKORY-SMOKED TURKEY WITH BOURBON GRAVY

SERVES: 8 TO 12
PREP TIME: 20 MINUTES
DRY BRINING TIME: 12 HOURS

WAY TO GRILL: INDIRECT MEDIUM HEAT (350° TO 400°F)
GRILLING TIME: ABOUT 2½ HOURS
SPECIAL EQUIPMENT: 3 LARGE DISPOSABLE FOIL PANS, INSTANT-READ THERMOMETER

- 1 turkey, about 12 pounds
- 2 tablespoons kosher salt
- 2 teaspoons freshly ground black pepper
- 3 tablespoons unsalted butter, softened

AROMATICS
- 1 cup chopped yellow onion
- ½ cup chopped carrot
- ½ cup chopped celery
- 1 teaspoon dried rosemary
- 1 teaspoon dried thyme
- 1 teaspoon dried sage

- 2 cups chicken broth, plus more for gravy
- 4 handfuls hickory wood chips, soaked in water for at least 30 minutes

GRAVY
- ½ cup all-purpose flour
- 3 tablespoons bourbon
- ½ teaspoon kosher salt
- ¼ teaspoon freshly ground black pepper

1. The day before grilling, prepare the turkey. Remove the giblets from the turkey and set aside for another use. Rinse the turkey with cold water, shake off the excess water, but do not pat dry. In a small bowl combine the salt and pepper and season all over the turkey, inside and out. Place the turkey on a sheet pan. Refrigerate, uncovered, for 12 hours.

2. Remove the turkey from the refrigerator. The skin may look dry, and that's okay. Do not rinse the turkey. Let the turkey stand at room temperature for 1 hour. Brush the legs, breast, and wings with the butter.

3. Place one foil pan inside the other and combine the aromatics in the top pan. (Do not use a high-quality metal roasting pan, as the smoke may discolor it.) Add 2 cups of the chicken broth. Place the turkey, breast side down, inside the foil pans and over the aromatics.

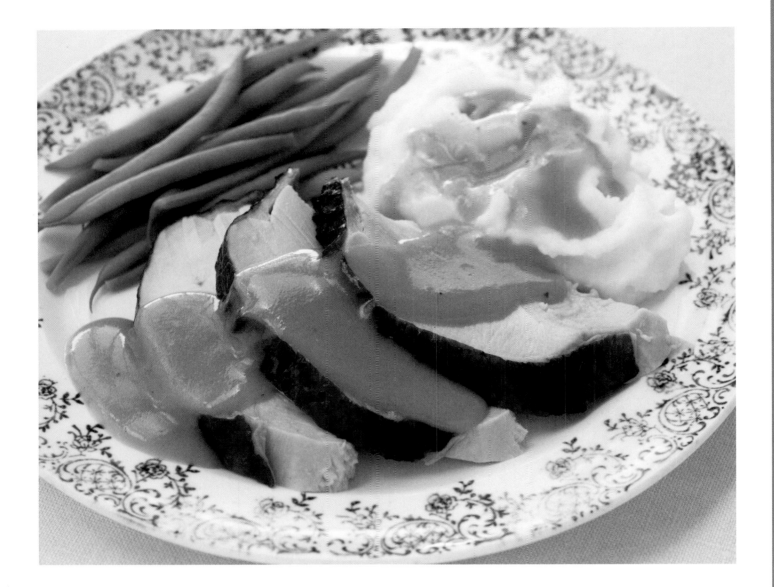

4. Drain and add 2 handfuls of the wood chips directly onto burning coals or to the smoker box of a gas grill, following manufacturer's instructions. Grill the turkey over _**indirect medium heat**_, with the lid closed, for 1 hour, keeping the grill's temperature between 350° to 400°F.

5. After grilling for 1 hour, wearing barbecue mitts and using a pair of tongs, flip over the turkey so that the breast side is facing up. For charcoal grilling, add 12 to 15 unlit briquettes to the coals to maintain the heat of the grill. Add the remaining 2 handfuls of the wood chips. Continue grilling and smoking the turkey until it is golden brown and a thermometer inserted in the thickest part of the thigh (not touching the bone) reaches 170°F, 1½ hours. After the turkey has been on the grill for 1½ hours, check to see if the wing tips or the ends of the drumsticks are getting too dark. If so, wrap them with foil.

6. Carefully remove the turkey and roasting pans from the grill. Transfer the turkey to a carving board and let rest for 20 to 30 minutes. Save the pan juices and vegetables to make the gravy.

7. Strain the pan juices into a fat separator, pressing the vegetables firmly with a wooden spoon to extract as much liquid as possible. Discard the vegetables left in the strainer. Let the pan juices stand until the fat rises to the surface, about 2 minutes. Pour the pan juices into a 1-quart measuring cup. Add more chicken broth, if needed, to make 3 cups. Measure the turkey fat; you should have ½ cup. Add melted butter, if needed.

8. In a medium, heavy-bottomed saucepan over medium heat, warm the fat. Whisk in the flour and let bubble until golden brown, about 2 minutes. Whisk in the stock mixture and the bourbon. Gently heat until lightly thickened, stirring often. Season with the salt and pepper.

9. Carve the turkey and serve with the gravy.

MAPLE-PLANKED TURKEY BURGERS

SERVES: 6
PREP TIME: 20 MINUTES

WAY TO GRILL: DIRECT MEDIUM HEAT (350° TO 450°F)
GRILLING TIME: 20 TO 30 MINUTES
SPECIAL EQUIPMENT: 2 UNTREATED MAPLE PLANKS,
    EACH 12 TO 15 INCHES LONG AND ½ TO ¾ INCH
    THICK, SOAKED IN BEER OR WATER FOR AT LEAST
    1 HOUR

SAUCE
  ½ cup ketchup
  ⅓ cup Worcestershire sauce
  3 tablespoons soy sauce
  1 tablespoon apple cider vinegar
  1 tablespoon brown sugar
 1½ teaspoons dry mustard
 1½ teaspoons ground cumin
  1 teaspoon hot sauce, or to taste

  2 pounds ground turkey thigh meat
  ¼ cup finely chopped shallot
  ¾ cup old-fashioned rolled oats
  1 teaspoon kosher salt
  ½ teaspoon freshly ground black pepper

  6 hamburger buns
 18 sweet pickle slices

1. In a medium bowl combine the sauce ingredients. Set aside about ½ cup of the sauce to serve with the burgers.

2. Mix the ground turkey with the shallot, oats, salt, and pepper and form into 6 patties, each about ¾ inch thick. With your thumb or the back of a spoon, make a shallow indentation about 1 inch wide in the center of each patty so the centers are about ½ inch thick.

3. Prepare the grill for direct cooking over medium heat.

4. Brush the cooking grates clean. Drain the planks and heat them over ***direct medium heat***, with the lid closed, until they begin to char and lightly smoke, 5 to 10 minutes. Turn the planks over and place 3 patties on each plank. Grill the burgers over ***direct medium heat***, with the lid closed as much as possible, for 15 to 20 minutes, turning and basting with the sauce once after 10 minutes.

5. During the last minute of grilling time, lightly toast the cut sides of the buns over ***direct medium heat***. Serve the burgers on buns with pickles, the reserved sauce, and rings of onion, if desired.

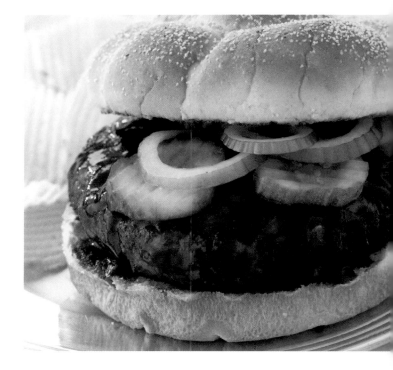

WAY TO SMOKE TURKEY BURGERS ON PLANKS

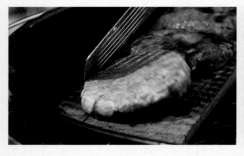

1. Cook the burgers for about 10 minutes on the planks, then begin basting them with sauce, and turn them over.

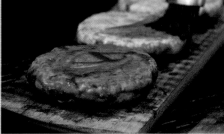

2. Cook them until there's no red left in the center and the internal temperature registers 165°F, 5 to 10 minutes, basting occasionally.

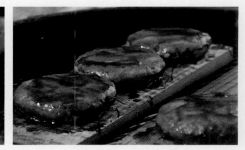

3. You will find that burgers made with dark thigh meat give you much juicer results than light breast meat.

WAY TO REMOVE CORN KERNELS

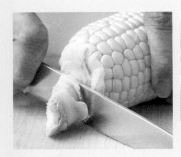

1. Cut off the stem end of an ear of corn to create a flat surface.

2. Stand the ear of corn, stem side down, in a dish or bowl. Cut from top to bottom so the kernels fall into the dish or bowl.

WAY TO SHRED CABBAGE

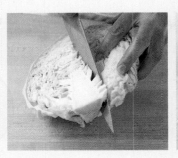
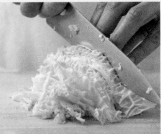

1. Split a head of cabbage in half lengthwise and cut out the tough, triangular core of each half.

2. Lay each half flat on a cutting board and slice as thinly as you can.

SOUTHWESTERN TURKEY BURGERS WITH SALSA SLAW

SERVES: 4
PREP TIME: 20 MINUTES

WAY TO GRILL: DIRECT MEDIUM HEAT (350° TO 450°F)
GRILLING TIME: 8 TO 10 MINUTES

SLAW
- 2 cups finely shredded savoy cabbage
- 1 cup fresh tomato salsa, drained
- ¼ cup finely chopped fresh cilantro
- 3 tablespoons sour cream

PATTIES
- 1½ pounds ground turkey thigh meat
- ⅓ cup fresh corn kernels
- ¼ cup finely chopped pickled jalapeño chile pepper, or to taste
- 1 tablespoon pure chile powder
- 2 teaspoons minced garlic
- 1½ teaspoons kosher salt
- 1 teaspoon ground cumin

- 4 whole-grain hamburger buns

1. In a medium bowl mix the slaw ingredients. Cover and refrigerate. Stir and then drain well just before serving.

2. Prepare the grill for direct cooking over medium heat.

3. In a large bowl gently mix the patty ingredients and shape into 4 patties, each about ¾ inch thick. With your thumb or the back of a spoon, make a shallow indentation about 1 inch wide in the center of each patty so the centers are about ½ inch thick. This will help the patties cook evenly and prevent them from puffing on the grill.

4. Brush the cooking grates clean. Grill the patties over **direct medium heat**, with the lid closed as much as possible, until fully cooked but still juicy, 8 to 10 minutes, turning once. During the last minute of grilling time, lightly toast the cut sides of the buns over **direct medium heat**. Top the patties with slaw and serve on the toasted buns.

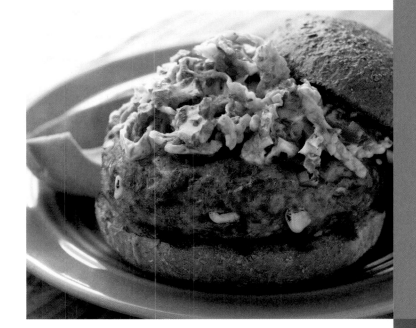

SEAFOOD

TECHNIQUES

RECIPES

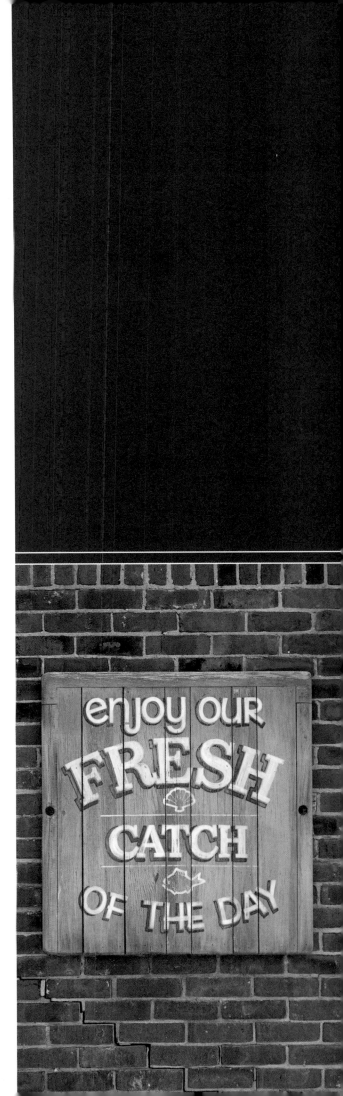

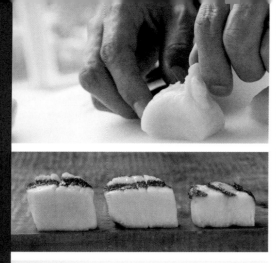

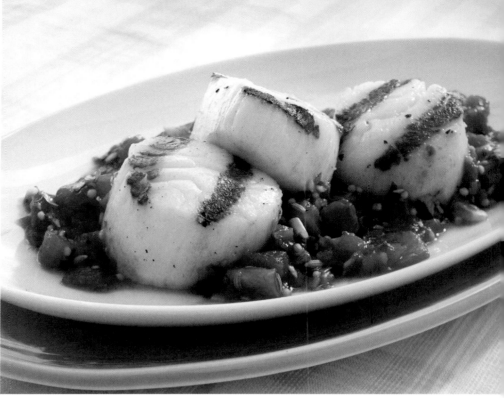

Before grilling, remove any tough little side muscles still attached to the scallops (top photo). After grilling, the interior of the scallops should be barely opaque, like the one in the center. The scallop on the left is a little underdone and the scallop on the right is overdone (bottom photo).

SCALLOPS WITH GRILL-ROASTED TOMATO SAUCE

SERVES: 4
PREP TIME: 25 MINUTES
MARINATING TIME: 10 TO 15 MINUTES

WAY TO GRILL: DIRECT MEDIUM HEAT (350° TO 450°F)
GRILLING TIME: 14 TO 16 MINUTES

SAUCE
- 1 pound plum tomatoes
- 3 scallions, tops and root ends trimmed
- 1 teaspoon finely grated lemon zest
- 2 tablespoons fresh lemon juice
- 1 tablespoon granulated sugar
- 1 teaspoon yellow mustard seed
- 1 teaspoon fennel seed
- ½ teaspoon kosher salt

- 12 jumbo sea scallops, about 2 ounces each

MARINADE
- 1 tablespoon unsalted butter, melted
- 1 tablespoon extra-virgin olive oil
- 1 teaspoon grated lemon zest
- 1 tablespoon fresh lemon juice
- ½ teaspoon kosher salt
- ¼ teaspoon freshly ground black pepper

- 1 tablespoon finely chopped fresh basil or Italian parsley

1. Prepare the grill for direct cooking over medium heat. Brush the cooking grates clean.

2. Grill the tomatoes and scallions over **direct medium heat**, with the lid closed as much as possible, until the tomato skins blister and brown and the scallions are lightly browned, turning

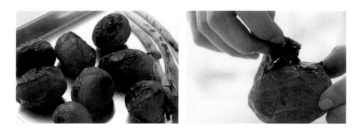

as needed. The tomatoes will take about 10 minutes and the scallions will take 4 to 5 minutes. Transfer the vegetables to a cutting board. Carefully pull off and discard the tomato skins and trim and discard the stem ends. Chop the tomatoes into ¼-inch pieces, and then transfer the tomatoes with their juices to a large skillet. Thinly slice the scallions, including the tops, and add to the tomatoes along with the rest of the sauce ingredients. Simmer the sauce over medium heat until the flavors blend, 5 to 6 minutes, stirring occasionally. Keep warm. (The sauce can be made a day ahead and reheated.)

3. Remove the small, tough side muscle that might be left on each scallop. In a small bowl combine the marinade ingredients. Toss the scallops in the marinade and let stand at room temperature for 10 to 15 minutes.

4. Brush the cooking grates clean. Lift the scallops from the bowl and lay slightly apart on the cooking grate. Discard the marinade. Grill over **direct medium heat**, with the lid closed as much as possible, until lightly browned and just opaque in the center, 4 to 6 minutes, turning once (check one by cutting it open).

5. Add the basil to the tomato sauce. Divide the sauce evenly on warm plates and top with hot scallops.

PROSCIUTTO-BELTED SCALLOPS WITH LENTIL SALAD

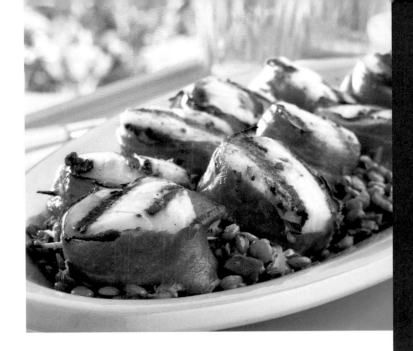

SERVES: 4
PREP TIME: 25 MINUTES
MARINATING TIME: 1 HOUR

WAY TO GRILL: DIRECT MEDIUM HEAT (350° TO 450°F)
GRILLING TIME: 4 TO 6 MINUTES

- 12 jumbo sea scallops, about 2 ounces each
- 6 thin slices prosciutto, cut in half lengthwise

MARINADE

- 3 tablespoons minced shallot
- 3 tablespoons fresh lemon juice
- 2 tablespoons extra-virgin olive oil
- 1½ tablespoons Dijon mustard
- ¾ teaspoon dried tarragon
- ¼ teaspoon freshly ground black pepper

LENTILS

- 6 thin slices prosciutto, finely chopped
- 2 tablespoons extra-virgin olive oil
- 1 cup finely chopped button mushrooms
- ⅓ cup minced shallot
- ½ teaspoon dried tarragon
- 1 cup green lentils
- 3 cups low-sodium chicken broth
- 1 teaspoon finely grated lemon zest
- ¼ cup chopped fresh Italian parsley
    Kosher salt
    Freshly ground black pepper

1. Remove the small, tough side muscle that might be left on each scallop.

2. Wrap one slice of prosciutto around each scallop and secure with a toothpick.

3. In a shallow dish mix the marinade ingredients. Gently turn the scallops in the marinade and then lay them flat in the dish. Cover with plastic wrap and refrigerate for 1 hour. Meanwhile prepare the lentils.

4. In a large saucepan over medium-high heat, combine the chopped prosciutto, oil, mushrooms, shallot, and tarragon. Stir often until the vegetables are limp and slightly browned, 5 to 7 minutes.

5. Sort through the lentils and discard any debris. Rinse and drain the lentils and add them to the saucepan along with the broth. Bring to a boil, reduce the heat, cover, and simmer until the lentils are tender, 40 to 55 minutes. Stir in the lemon zest and parsley. Season to taste with salt and pepper. Keep warm.

6. Prepare the grill for direct cooking over medium heat. Brush the cooking grates clean. Grill the scallops, unwrapped sides down, over **direct medium heat**, with the lid closed as much as possible, until the scallops are lightly browned and opaque in the center, 4 to 6 minutes, turning once. Remove from the grill and serve warm with the lentils.

WAY TO PREP SCALLOPS

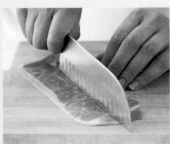

1. Cut each prosciutto slice to fit the scallops.

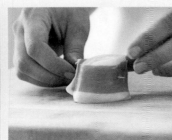

2. Wrap a strip of prosciutto around each scallop and secure it with a toothpick.

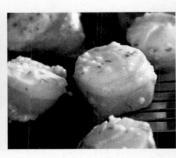

3. Brush the wrapped scallops with marinade and refrigerate for about 1 hour before grilling.

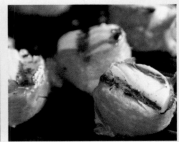

4. Grill so that the flat sides of each scallop lie flat on the hot grate.

CEDAR-PLANKED SCALLOPS WITH GRILLED CORN SALAD

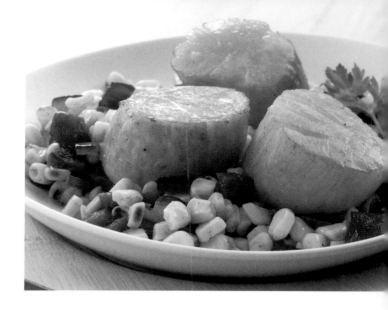

SERVES: 4 TO 6
PREP TIME: 25 MINUTES

WAY TO GRILL: DIRECT MEDIUM HEAT (350° TO 450°F)
GRILLING TIME: 23 TO 32 MINUTES
SPECIAL EQUIPMENT: 1 UNTREATED CEDAR PLANK,
   12 TO 15 INCHES LONG AND ½ TO ¾ INCH THICK,
   SOAKED IN WATER FOR AT LEAST 1 HOUR

MARINADE
   ⅓ cup extra-virgin olive oil
   ⅓ cup fresh lime juice
   1 tablespoon honey
   1 teaspoon kosher salt

   20 large sea scallops, each about 1¼ inches in diameter

SALAD
   ½ small red onion, cut into 3 wedges
   3 ears fresh sweet yellow corn, shucked
   1 red bell pepper
      Extra-virgin olive oil
      Kosher salt
      Freshly ground black pepper
   ½ teaspoon ground cumin
   1 teaspoon hot sauce, or to taste

1. In a medium bowl whisk the marinade ingredients. Transfer 3 tablespoons of the marinade to a large bowl to use for dressing the salad. Set the two bowls aside.

2. Remove the small, tough side muscle that might be left on each scallop. Refrigerate until ready to grill.

3. Prepare the grill for direct cooking over medium heat. Lightly brush or spray the onion, corn, and pepper with oil and season evenly with salt and pepper. Brush the cooking grates clean. Grill the vegetables over **direct medium heat**, with the lid closed as much as possible, until the onion has softened and started to collapse, the corn kernels are mostly brown, with some beginning to char, and the pepper is blackened and blistered all over, turning the vegetables as needed. The onion will take about 4 minutes, the corn will take 6 to 8 minutes, and the pepper, 10 to 12 minutes. Place the pepper in a bowl, cover with plastic wrap, and allow to cool.

4. When the vegetables are cool enough to handle, cut the onion into a small dice, cut the kernels off the cobs, and remove and discard the charred skin, stem, ribs, and seeds from the pepper. Cut the pepper into a medium dice, saving the juice. Combine the onion, corn, pepper with juice, cumin, and hot sauce into the large bowl with the 3 tablespoons of reserved marinade.

5. Place the soaked plank over **direct medium heat** and close the lid. After 5 to 10 minutes, when the plank begins to smoke and char, turn the plank over. Put the scallops in the bowl with the marinade and toss to coat. Place the scallops in a single layer on the plank. Close the grill lid and cook until they are slightly firm on the surface and opaque in the center, 8 to 10 minutes. Serve the scallops warm with the salad.

WAY TO CUT ONION WEDGES

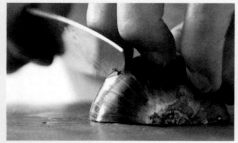

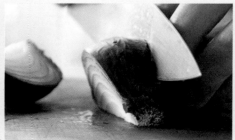

1. The layers of the onion wedges will hold together on the grill if you leave part of the root end attached.

2. After you have cut your wedges, peel off the papery skin.

CHECKING DONENESS

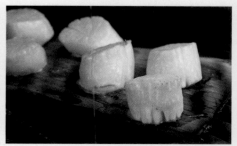

When smoked scallops are done, they will feel slightly firm on top and look lightly colored all over by the smoke.

THAI SHRIMP
WITH WATERMELON SALSA

SERVES: 4
PREP TIME: 25 MINUTES
MARINATING TIME: 30 MINUTES

WAY TO GRILL: DIRECT HIGH HEAT (450° TO 550°F)
GRILLING TIME: 3 TO 5 MINUTES
SPECIAL EQUIPMENT: 8 BAMBOO SKEWERS,
    SOAKED IN WATER FOR AT LEAST 30 MINUTES

SALSA
    2   tablespoons minced shallot
    2   teaspoons rice vinegar
    1   teaspoon granulated sugar
  1–2   tablespoons minced jalapeño chile pepper
    2   cups seedless watermelon, cut into ½-inch cubes
    1   three-inch section English cucumber, halved lengthwise,
        seeded, and thinly sliced into half-moons
    1   teaspoon minced fresh mint
    ¼   teaspoon kosher salt

MARINADE
    ½   cup lightly packed fresh cilantro leaves and tender stems
    ¼   cup lightly packed fresh mint leaves
    3   medium garlic cloves
    2   tablespoons coarsely chopped fresh ginger
    2   tablespoons rice vinegar
    2   tablespoons vegetable oil
    2   teaspoons granulated sugar
    1   teaspoon Thai red curry paste
    ¼   teaspoon kosher salt

  1¼   pounds extra-large shrimp (16/20 count), peeled and
        deveined, tails left on

1. In a large bowl mix the shallot, vinegar, sugar, and jalapeño.
Add the watermelon, cucumber, mint, and salt, and toss gently
to combine. To fully incorporate the flavors, let the salsa sit at
room temperature for 30 to 60 minutes.

2. In a food processor combine the marinade ingredients.
Process to create a coarse puree, occasionally scraping down
the sides of the bowl to incorporate the ingredients evenly.

3. Transfer the marinade to a medium bowl, add the shrimp,
and toss to coat them evenly. Cover the bowl and refrigerate for
30 minutes, turning the shrimp after 15 minutes. Prepare the
grill for direct cooking over high heat.

4. Remove the shrimp from the bowl and discard the marinade.
Thread the shrimp onto skewers. Brush the cooking grates
clean. Grill the skewers over **direct high heat**, with the lid
closed as much as possible, until the shrimp are firm to the
touch, lightly charred, and just turning opaque in the center,
3 to 5 minutes, turning once. Serve the shrimp warm or at room
temperature with the salsa.

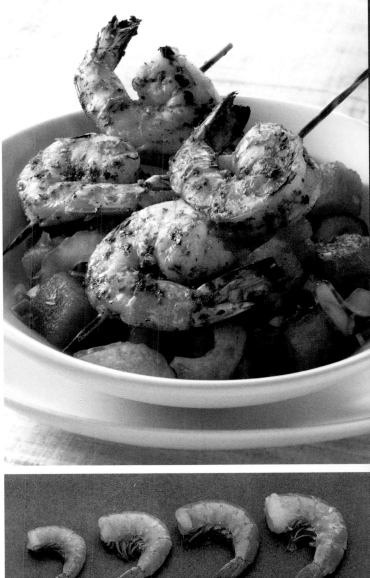

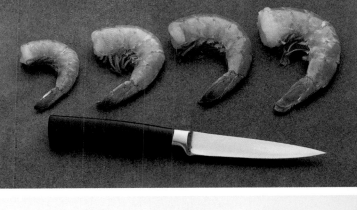

Terms like "small," "medium," and "large" are used inconsistently
where shrimp are sold. The best way to know for sure what you
are buying is to look for the number of shrimp per pound. A label
that reads "16/20" means that it takes sixteen to twenty of those
shrimp to make a pound. In the photo above, the shrimp on the
far left is an example of what you get when you buy "36/45."
Immediately to the right is an example of "31/35." The next
one is an example of "21/30." And the one on the far right is an
example of "16/20." Generally speaking, the two larger sizes are
the best choices for grilling, because they are easy to peel and
they don't dry out as quickly as the smaller shrimp.

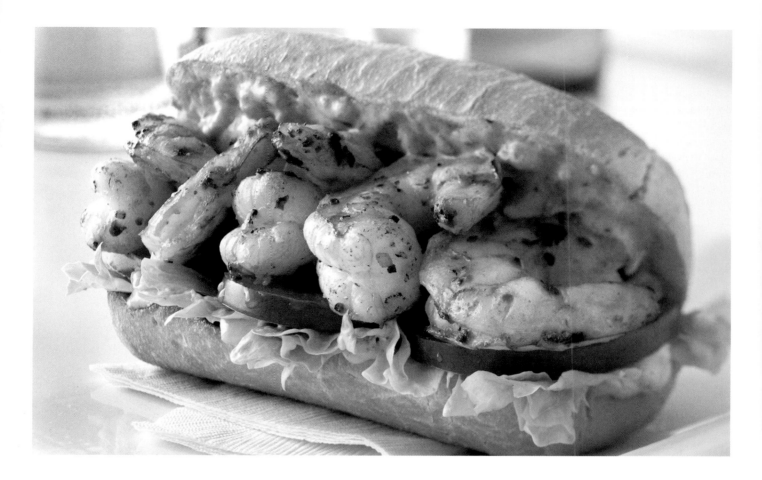

SHRIMP PO'BOYS WITH CREOLE RÉMOULADE

SERVES: 6
PREP TIME: 20 MINUTES

WAY TO GRILL: DIRECT HIGH HEAT (450° TO 550°F)
GRILLING TIME: 3 TO 5 MINUTES
SPECIAL EQUIPMENT: PERFORATED GRILL PAN

RÉMOULADE
- ½ cup mayonnaise
- 2 tablespoons Creole or Dijon mustard
- 2 tablespoons sweet pickle relish
- 1 tablespoon prepared horseradish
- 2 teaspoons minced fresh tarragon
- 1 teaspoon minced garlic
- ½ teaspoon hot sauce, or to taste
- ½ teaspoon sweet paprika
- ½ teaspoon kosher salt
- ¼ teaspoon freshly ground black pepper

- 2 pounds large shrimp (21/30 count), peeled and deveined, tails removed
- 2 tablespoons extra-virgin olive oil
- 1 tablespoon Creole seasoning
- 6 soft French sandwich rolls, split horizontally
- 4 cups chopped iceberg lettuce
- 18 ripe tomato slices

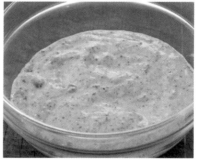

Rémoulade is a mayonnaise-based spread flavored with mustard and other condiments. Among mustards, Creole is one of the spiciest, thanks to its horseradish and vinegar-marinated brown mustard seeds.

1. In a small bowl combine the rémoulade ingredients. Cover and refrigerate until serving.

2. Prepare the grill for direct cooking over high heat. Preheat the grill pan for about 10 minutes.

3. Toss the shrimp with the oil and then evenly coat with the Creole seasoning. Spread the shrimp on the grill pan and grill over **direct high heat**, with the lid closed as much as possible, until firm to the touch and just turning opaque in the center, 2 to 4 minutes, turning once. Remove from the grill and keep warm.

4. Grill the rolls, cut sides down, over **direct high heat**, until lightly toasted, 30 seconds to 1 minute. Spread the rémoulade on the cut sides of the rolls and add lettuce, tomatoes, and shrimp. Serve warm.

SEAFOOD

ORANGE-FENNEL SHRIMP
OVER WATERCRESS

SERVES: 4
PREP TIME: 25 MINUTES
MARINATING TIME: 1 HOUR

WAY TO GRILL: DIRECT HIGH HEAT (450° TO 550°F)
GRILLING TIME: 2 TO 4 MINUTES
SPECIAL EQUIPMENT: PERFORATED GRILL PAN

MARINADE
       Grated zest of 2 oranges
  ½ cup fresh orange juice
  ⅓ cup extra-virgin olive oil
  2 tablespoons fresh lime juice
  1 tablespoon minced garlic
  1 teaspoon ground fennel
  1 teaspoon kosher salt
  ½ teaspoon ground cayenne pepper

1½ pounds large shrimp (21/30 count),
     peeled and deveined, tails left on
  2 cups watercress leaves and tender stems

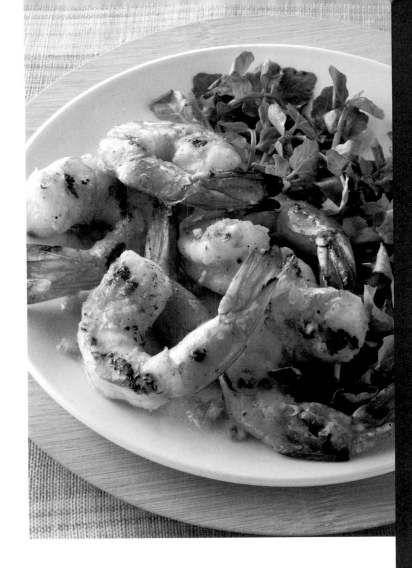

1. In a medium bowl mix the marinade ingredients. Set aside ½ cup of the marinade to use as a dressing for the salad.

2. Place the shrimp in a large, resealable plastic bag and pour in the marinade. Press the air out of the bag and seal tightly. Turn the bag several times to distribute the marinade, lay the bag flat on a plate, and refrigerate for 1 hour.

3. Prepare the grill for direct cooking over high heat. Preheat the grill pan for about 10 minutes.

4. Drain the shrimp in a sieve. Spread the shrimp in a single layer on the grill pan and cook over **direct high heat**, with the lid closed as much as possible, until the shrimp are slightly firm on the surface and completely opaque in the centers, 2 to 4 minutes, shaking the pan once or twice and turning the shrimp over for even cooking. Remove the pan from the grill and rest it on a sheet pan. Transfer the shrimp to a large bowl to stop the cooking.

5. Add the watercress to the shrimp in the large bowl. Spoon the reserved dressing over the watercress and shrimp (you may not need all of it). Toss to coat the ingredients evenly. Serve right away.

WAY TO PEEL AND DEVEIN SHRIMP

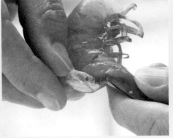

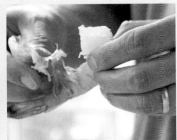

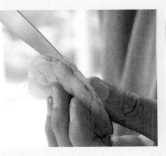

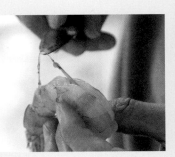

1. Grab the shell just above the tail and break it loose.

2. Peel off the shell along with all the little legs.

3. With a sharp paring knife, make a shallow slit along the back of each shrimp.

4. Lift any black vein out of the slit and discard it.

WAY TO GRILL SHRIMP POPS

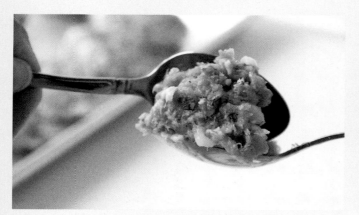

1. By using two spoons moving in opposite directions, you can make little football-shaped pieces called quenelles.

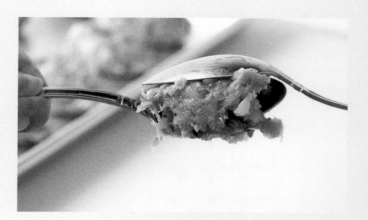

2. Move the top spoon over and behind the shrimp mixture while moving the bottom spoon under and in front.

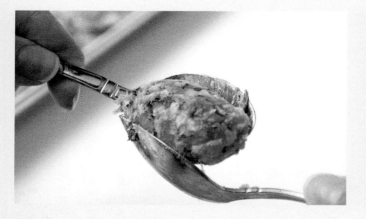

3. Continue to move the spoons over the surface of the mixture a few times to smooth it out and shape it.

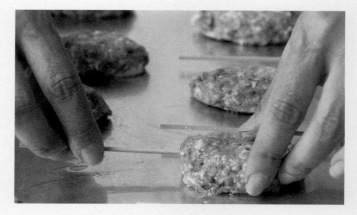

4. Slide a short bamboo skewer through the center of each quenelle, and turn the shrimp mixture on an oiled sheet pan to coat it with oil.

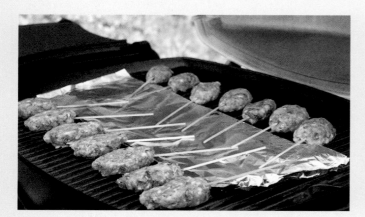

5. Grill the pops over high heat, with the bare ends of the skewers shielded by a folded sheet of aluminum foil.

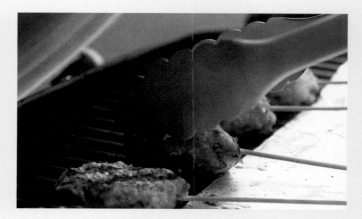

6. Cook them long enough on the first side that you can roll them over without any sticking, rather than picking them up with tongs and squeezing them.

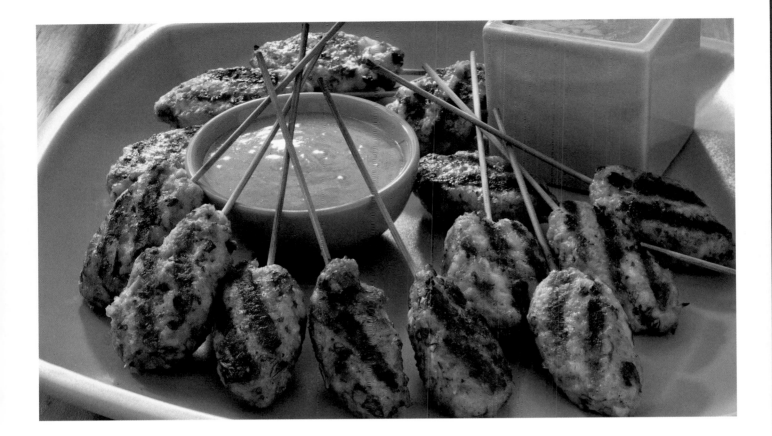

VIETNAMESE SHRIMP POPS WITH PEANUT SAUCE

SERVES: 4 TO 6
PREP TIME: 30 MINUTES
CHILLING TIME: 30 MINUTES TO 1 HOUR

WAY TO GRILL: DIRECT HIGH HEAT (450° TO 550°F)
GRILLING TIME: 4 TO 6 MINUTES
SPECIAL EQUIPMENT: BAMBOO SKEWERS,
   SOAKED IN WATER FOR AT LEAST 30 MINUTES

SAUCE
  1 cup unsweetened coconut milk, stirred
  ⅓ cup old-fashioned peanut butter, stirred
  1 teaspoon finely grated lime zest
  3 tablespoons fresh lime juice
  1 tablespoon soy sauce
  1 tablespoon brown sugar
  1 teaspoon hot chili sauce, such as Sriracha
  ½ teaspoon grated fresh ginger

SHRIMP POPS
  1 pound ground pork
  ¾ pound shrimp, peeled and deveined
  ½ cup coarsely chopped fresh basil
  ¼ cup panko bread crumbs
  2 large garlic cloves
  1 tablespoon soy sauce
  ½ teaspoon freshly ground black pepper

  ¼ cup vegetable oil

1. In a heavy-bottomed saucepan combine the sauce ingredients. Place over medium heat and cook (but do not simmer), whisking constantly, just until the sauce is smooth and slightly thickened, 2 to 3 minutes (the sauce will thicken further as it cools). Remove from the heat.

2. In a food processor or blender, pulse the shrimp pop ingredients and process until a chunky paste is formed. Pour the vegetable oil onto a sheet pan and brush it evenly all over the surface. Using 2 spoons shape the mixture into small ovals or quenelles, placing them on the oiled sheet pan as you make them. Turn them, making sure they are well coated with oil. Refrigerate for 30 minutes to 1 hour to firm up the texture.

3. Prepare the grill for direct cooking over high heat.

4. Place a quenelle on the end of each skewer. Brush the cooking grates clean. Grill the shrimp pops over **direct high heat**, with the lid closed as much as possible, until they are opaque throughout, 4 to 5 minutes, turning once or twice (cut one open with a sharp knife to test for doneness). Arrange the shrimp pops on a serving platter. Serve warm with the dipping sauce.

WAY TO MAKE ROASTED CHILE AND AVOCADO SAUCE

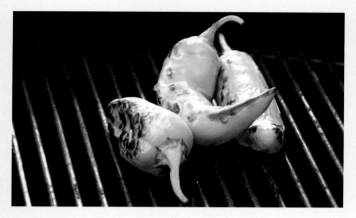

1. Roast mildly spicy Anaheim chiles over direct medium heat until the skins are blackened and blistered.

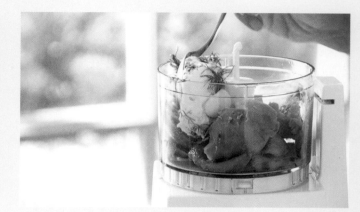

2. Discard the chile stems, skins, and seeds. Then combine the roasted chiles in a food processor with sour cream, mayonnaise, fresh dill, garlic, salt, and pepper.

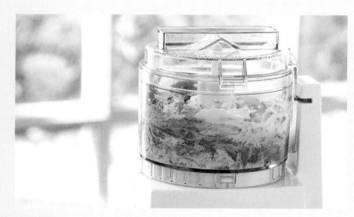

3. Give the sauce a whirl, stopping occasionally to scrape down the sides of the bowl.

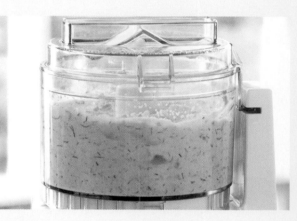

4. If the sauce seems a little thick, add a touch of water to thin it out. The sauce will keep well in the refrigerator for a couple of days.

WAY TO PREP THE SHRIMP

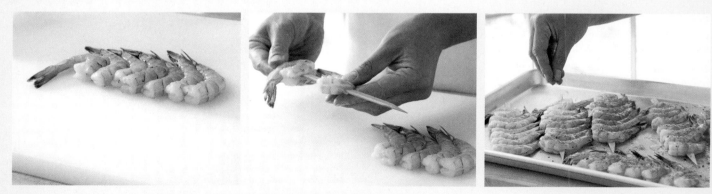

1. Choose shrimp that are the same size so that you can nestle them together with no empty spaces between them.

2. Begin by skewering one shrimp through both the head and tail ends. Skewer the next shrimp through the head end only, with the tail end pointing in the opposite direction. Skewer the remaining shrimp just like the second one, with all their tails facing the same way.

3. The shrimp are nestled closely together on the skewers, without spaces in between. This means they will stay juicy on the grill a little bit longer.

SEAFOOD

186

JUICY SHRIMP WITH ROASTED CHILE AND AVOCADO SAUCE

SERVES: 4 TO 6
PREP TIME: 20 MINUTES

WAY TO GRILL: DIRECT MEDIUM HEAT (350° TO 450°F)
AND DIRECT HIGH HEAT (450° TO 550°F)
GRILLING TIME: 10 TO 16 MINUTES
SPECIAL EQUIPMENT: 8 TO 10 FLAT-SIDED OR ROUND
BAMBOO SKEWERS, SOAKED IN WATER FOR AT LEAST
30 MINUTES

SAUCE
3   Anaheim chile peppers, each about 6 inches long
1   medium Haas avocado
¼   cup sour cream
¼   cup mayonnaise
2   tablespoons roughly chopped fresh dill
1   large garlic clove
½   teaspoon kosher salt
¼   teaspoon freshly ground black pepper

RUB
1   teaspoon granulated garlic
1   teaspoon paprika
¾   teaspoon kosher salt
½   teaspoon ground cumin
¼   teaspoon freshly ground black pepper

2   pounds large shrimp (21/30 count), peeled and
deveined, tails left on
Extra-virgin olive oil

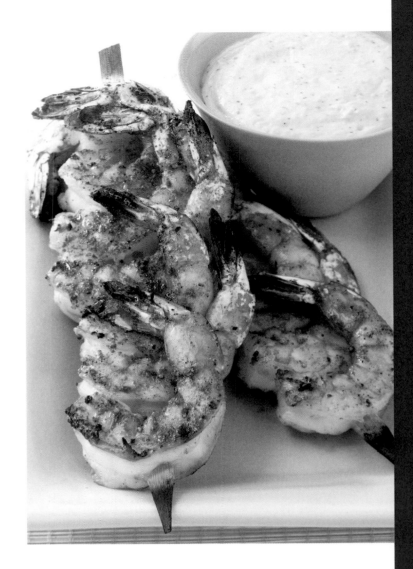

1. Prepare the grill for direct cooking over medium heat. Brush the cooking grates clean. Grill the chile peppers over **direct medium heat,** with the lid closed as much as possible, until they are blackened and blistered in spots all over, 8 to 12 minutes, turning occasionally. Put the chiles in a bowl, cover with plastic wrap, and let steam for 10 minutes. When cool enough to handle, remove and discard the stem ends, skins, and seeds. Drop the chiles into a food processor or blender. Add the remaining sauce ingredients. Process to create a smooth dipping sauce. If the sauce seems too thick, add a little water. Spoon the sauce into a serving bowl.

■■■

The "fresh" shrimp glistening on a bed of shaved ice at the market were almost certainly frozen previously, on the boat or at the harbor. Then they were thawed at the market. In fact, shrimp will be closer to "fresh" if you buy them frozen and thaw them yourself just before grilling.

■■■

2. In a small bowl mix the rub ingredients.

3. Lay 5 to 7 shrimp on a work surface and arrange them so that the shrimp on one end lays one way and all the rest lay in the same direction (see photo at left). Choose shrimp that are the same size so that you can nestle them together with no empty spaces between them. This will help to keep the shrimp from spinning and prevent them from drying out on the grill. Pick up and skewer each shrimp through the middle, pushing the shrimp together on each skewer. Repeat the process with the remaining shrimp and skewers. Lightly brush or spray the skewers with oil and then season them evenly with the rub.

4. Increase the temperature of the grill to high heat. Brush the cooking grates clean. Grill the shrimp over **direct high heat,** with the lid closed as much as possible, until slightly firm on the surface and opaque in the center, 2 to 4 minutes, turning once. Remove from the grill and serve warm with the dipping sauce.

WAY TO MAKE PAELLA

Paella is a rice dish that is traditionally cooked outdoors in a wide, shallow pan of the same name. Spreading the rice out in such a wide pan helps it to absorb the aromas of burning logs or charcoal. A big cast-iron skillet substitutes well for the pan, but there is no substitute for paella's quintessential spice: saffron.

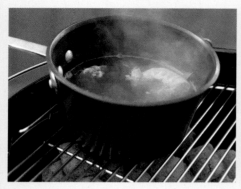

1. Heat the broth with shrimp shells, white wine, bay leaves, smoked paprika, salt, red pepper flakes, and saffron.

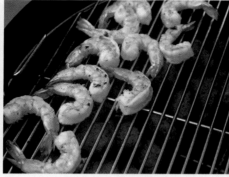

2. Grill the shrimp over direct high heat, but cook them only about halfway. They will finish cooking in the rice.

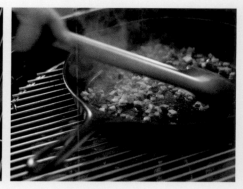

3. Cook the prosciutto ham in the skillet until it releases its fat and begins to crisp.

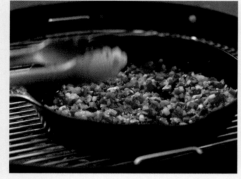

4. Cook the onions, bell pepper, and garlic with the prosciutto to create an aromatic base of flavors.

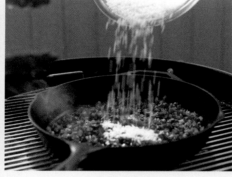

5. Add a medium- or round-grain rice, such as Arborio or Valencia, not a long-grain rice.

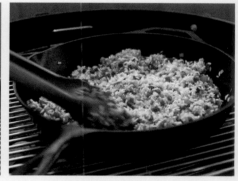

6. Stir to cook the rice lightly and to coat all the kernels in the pan juices.

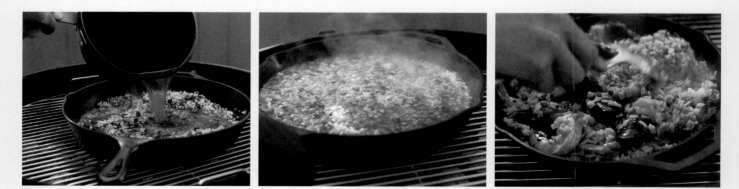

7. Add the hot, strained broth and close the lid of the grill so that the liquid gently simmers and the wood smoke does not escape.

8. At some point you may need to rotate the pan or move it to another part of the grill to even out the cooking.

9. The rice is done when it has absorbed most of the broth and the texture is tender but not mushy.

PAELLA

SERVES: 6 TO 8
PREP TIME: 40 MINUTES
SOAKING TIME FOR WILD MUSSELS: 30 MINUTES TO
    1 HOUR (SEE AUTHOR'S NOTE ON PAGE 190)

WAY TO GRILL: DIRECT HIGH HEAT (450° TO 550°F) AND
    DIRECT MEDIUM HEAT (350° TO 450°F)
GRILLING TIME: 35 TO 37 MINUTES
SPECIAL EQUIPMENT: 12-INCH CAST-IRON SKILLET

½ pound large shrimp (21/30 count), tails left on,
    shells reserved for broth
2 teaspoons extra-virgin olive oil
    Kosher salt
    Freshly ground black pepper

BROTH
    Shells from peeled shrimp
4 cups low-sodium chicken broth
¾ cup dry white wine
2 bay leaves
1½ teaspoons smoked paprika
1 teaspoon kosher salt
½ teaspoon crushed red pepper flakes
¼ teaspoon crushed saffron threads

12 live mussels, scrubbed and beards removed
3 tablespoons extra-virgin olive oil
4 ounces thick-sliced prosciutto, cut into ¼-inch dice
1 cup finely chopped red onion
¾ cup finely chopped red bell pepper
1 tablespoon minced garlic
2 cups medium-grain rice, such as Italian Arborio
1 cup frozen baby peas

1. Peel and devein the shrimp, reserving the shells to make the broth. In a large bowl toss the shrimp with the oil, and season evenly with salt and pepper. Cover and refrigerate until ready to grill.

2. In a medium saucepan over high heat, bring the shrimp shells and the broth ingredients to a simmer. Strain, discarding the shells and bay leaves, and reserve the broth. (The broth can be made up to 2 hours ahead.)

3. Check each mussel and discard those with broken shells, any that don't close up when you lightly tap on their shells, and any others that feel unusually heavy because of sand trapped inside.

4. Prepare the grill for direct cooking over high heat on one side and medium heat on the other side. Brush the cooking grates clean. Grill the shrimp over ***direct high heat*** until cooked halfway, about 2 minutes, turning once (the shrimp will finish cooking in the broth). Remove from the grill and set aside to cool.

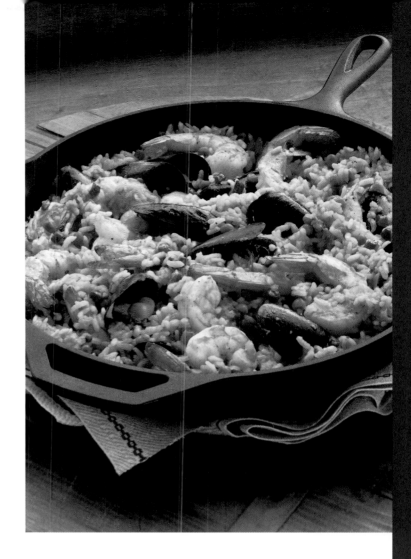

5. Place a 12-inch cast-iron skillet on the cooking grate over ***direct high heat.*** Heat the oil in the skillet. Add the prosciutto and cook, stirring occasionally, until it begins to crisp, about 3 minutes. Add the onion, bell pepper, and garlic. Cook, stirring occasionally, until the onion is translucent, about 5 minutes, rotating the pan for even cooking. Slide the pan away from the fire.

6. Place the skillet over ***direct medium heat***, stir in the rice, and cook until well coated with the pan juices, about 2 minutes. Stir in the shrimp broth and the frozen peas. Close the grill lid and let the rice cook at a brisk simmer until the rice is al dente, about 15 minutes. Nestle the shrimp into the rice. Add the mussels, hinged sides down. Cook, with the grill lid closed, until the mussels open, 8 to 10 minutes.

7. Remove from the heat, cover with aluminum foil, and let stand for 5 minutes. Serve hot from the skillet.

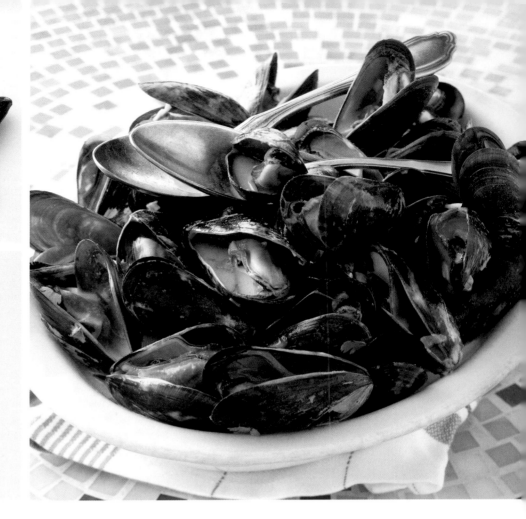

WILD VERSUS FARM-RAISED MUSSELS

Check each mussel and discard those with broken shells, any that don't close up when you lightly tap on their shells, and any others that feel unusually heavy because of sand trapped inside. Soak the mussels in cold, salted water for 30 minutes to 1 hour and then drain. The soaking is to remove sand, but that's only an issue with wild mussels (pictured at left) that grow in sandy places. If you use farm-raised mussels (pictured at right), you can skip the soaking step.

COCONUT-CURRY MUSSELS

SERVES: 4
PREP TIME: 15 MINUTES
SOAKING TIME FOR WILD MUSSELS: 30 MINUTES
    TO 1 HOUR

WAY TO GRILL: DIRECT MEDIUM HEAT (350° TO 450°F)
GRILLING TIME: 17 TO 22 MINUTES
SPECIAL EQUIPMENT: LARGE DISPOSABLE FOIL PAN

SAUCE
  1 can (13½ ounces) coconut milk, light or regular
  1 tablespoon Thai green curry paste
  1 tablespoon fresh lime juice
  2 teaspoons light brown sugar
  2 teaspoons fish sauce
  2 tablespoons peanut oil
  1 tablespoon finely chopped fresh ginger
  1 tablespoon finely chopped garlic

  2 pounds live mussels, scrubbed and beards removed
 ¼ cup loosely packed fresh cilantro leaves, finely chopped

1. Prepare the grill for direct and indirect cooking over medium heat.

2. In a medium bowl whisk the coconut milk, curry paste, lime juice, brown sugar, and fish sauce.

3. In a large disposable foil pan combine the peanut oil, ginger, and garlic. Place the pan over **direct medium heat**, close the grill lid, and let the aromatics cook for about 1 minute. Add the coconut milk mixture to the foil pan and gently stir to combine. Cook for 5 to 6 minutes to bring the sauce to a boil.

4. Add the mussels to the sauce. Cover the foil pan with a sheet pan (to trap the steam and cook the mussels), close the grill lid, and cook for 8 to 10 minutes. Check the mussels to see if they are open. If not, continue to cook 3 to 5 minutes more. Wearing barbecue mitts, carefully remove the sheet pan from the foil pan and carefully remove the foil pan from the grill. Remove and discard any unopened mussels. Sprinkle the cilantro on top. Serve the mussels and sauce in bowls with crusty bread, if desired.

CAJUN-STYLE CLAMBAKE

SERVES: 4
PREP TIME: 45 MINUTES

WAY TO GRILL: DIRECT MEDIUM HEAT (350° TO 450°F)
GRILLING TIME: 20 TO 25 MINUTES

- ½ cup (1 stick) unsalted butter, melted
- ⅓ cup fresh lemon juice
- 1 tablespoon Cajun seasoning
- 1 tablespoon minced garlic
- 2 teaspoons chopped fresh thyme leaves
- 4 medium red potatoes, halved and sliced into ⅛-inch half-moons
- ¾ pound jumbo shrimp (11/15 count), peeled and deveined, tails left on, *cold*
- 2 pounds littleneck clams, rinsed and scrubbed
- 1 package (12 ounces) andouille sausage, thinly sliced
- 2 ears fresh sweet corn, each shucked and cut into 4 pieces

1. In a small bowl combine the butter, lemon juice, seasoning, garlic, and thyme.

2. Prepare the grill for direct cooking over medium heat

3. Cut 8 sheets of aluminum foil, each about 12 by 20 inches. Line an 8x8-inch cake pan with 2 sheets of aluminum foil, arranged in a crisscross pattern. Layer the bottom of the foil-lined pan with the sliced potatoes (this will help insulate the shellfish and keep them from overcooking). Top the potatoes evenly with the shrimp, clams, sausage, and corn pieces. Drizzle each packet evenly with the butter mixture. Close the packet by bringing the ends of the two inner sheets together, folding them on top of the filling and then bringing the ends of the two outer sheets together, folding them down. Repeat this procedure with the remaining packets.

4. Grill the packets over **direct medium heat,** with the lid closed, until the clams have opened, the shrimp have turned opaque, and the potatoes are cooked, 20 to 25 minutes. To check for doneness, using tongs, gently unfold one of the packets and carefully remove a potato, being careful not to puncture the bottom of the foil. Using a knife, gently pierce the potato to ensure doneness. When everything is cooked remove the packets from the grill. Carefully open each packet to let the steam escape and then pour the contents into warm bowls and serve immediately.

WAY TO PREP FOR A CLAMBAKE

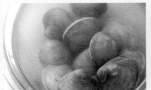
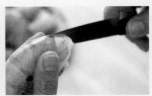

1. Rinse and scrub the clams under cold water. To remove sand and grit from inside the shells, soak the clams in ice-cold water mixed with salt (1 teaspoon of salt per cup of water) for a few hours.

2. You can peel and devein the shrimp ahead of time.

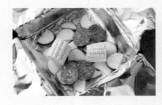
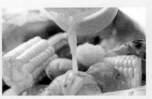

3. In a foil-lined pan, arrange the sliced potatoes on the bottom so that they will protect the other ingredients from the heat.

4. Be generous with the butter mixture.

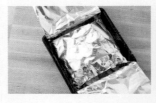
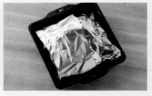

5. Fold up the ends of the foil tightly to prevent any liquid from escaping.

6. You will remove each packet from its pan and cook it directly on the grill so that all the ingredients steam and simmer inside.

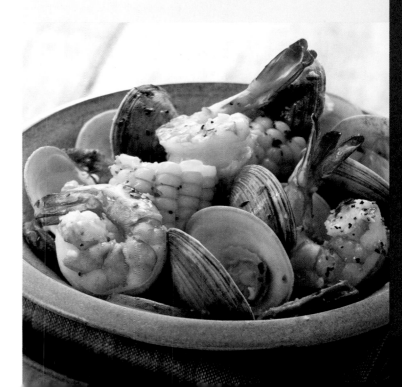

WAY TO CHAR-GRILL OYSTERS

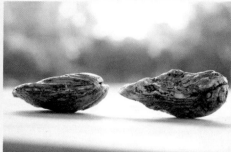

1. For grilling, choose oysters like these, with deep rounded shells to hold in their juices.

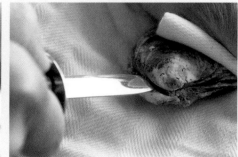

2. Holding each oyster in a towel with the flat side facing up, push the tip of an oyster knife into the small opening at the hinge of the shell.

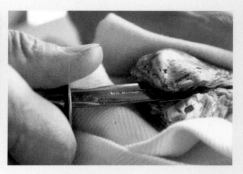

3. Twist the knife and wiggle it back and forth to pop open the shell.

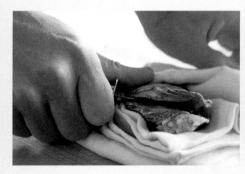

4. Drag the knife along the seam between the top and bottom shells.

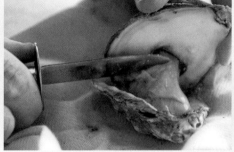

5. Use the side of the knife to cut the oyster meat loose from the top shell.

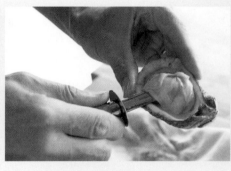

6. Slide the knife under the oyster meat to release it from the bottom.

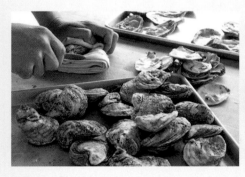

7. As you finish shucking each oyster, lay it flat on a sheet pan, keeping as much liquid as possible in the shells.

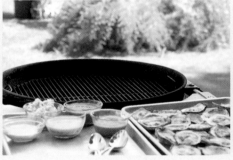

8. The grilling goes quickly, so have all your sauces and serving platters ready.

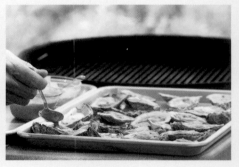

9. Spoon the sauces into the raw oysters, but don't overfill the shells.

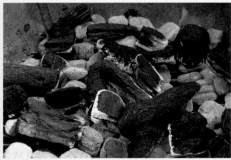

10. A very hot charcoal fire is crucial for cooking oysters in just a few minutes.

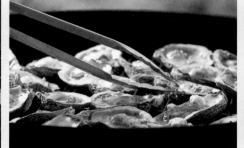

11. As soon as the juices start to bubble, remove the oysters from the grill.

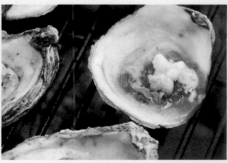

12. The meat of the oyster should be warm but not cooked all the way through.

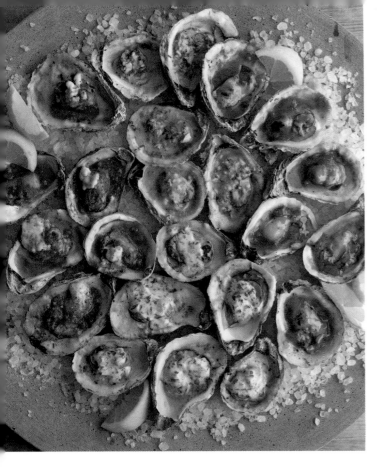

CHAR-GRILLED OYSTERS

SERVES: 4 TO 6
PREP TIME: 30 MINUTES

WAY TO GRILL: DIRECT HIGH HEAT (450° TO 550°F)
GRILLING TIME: 2 TO 4 MINUTES
SPECIAL EQUIPMENT: OYSTER KNIFE

    2 dozen large, fresh oysters
       Lemon wedges
       Hot sauce
       Cocktail sauce

1. Grip each oyster, flat side up, in a folded kitchen towel. Find the small opening between the shells near the hinge and pry it open with an oyster knife. Try not to spill the delicious juices, known as the "oyster liqueur," in the bottom shell. Cut the oyster meat loose from the top shell and then loosen the oyster from the bottom shell by running the oyster knife carefully underneath the body. Discard the top, flatter shell, keeping the oyster and juices in the bottom, deeper shell.

2. Prepare the grill for direct cooking over high heat.

3. Spoon some of your favorite dipping sauce on top of each oyster (recipes follow).

4. Brush the cooking grates clean. Grill the oysters, shell sides down, over **direct high heat**, with the lid closed as much as possible, until the oyster juices start to bubble and the edges curl, 2 to 4 minutes. Using tongs, carefully remove the oysters from the grill. Serve with lemon wedges, hot sauce, cocktail sauce, and your favorite dipping sauce.

GARLIC-THYME BUTTER
MAKES: ENOUGH FOR 2 DOZEN OYSTERS

    ¼ cup (½ stick) unsalted butter, divided
    1 tablespoon minced garlic
    2 teaspoons sherry vinegar
    ¼ cup white wine
    2 teaspoons minced fresh thyme
    ¼ teaspoon kosher salt

1. In a small skillet over medium heat, melt 1 tablespoon of the butter and sauté the garlic until it starts to brown, about 2 minutes. Add the vinegar and wine and simmer until the sauce reduces by half, about 2 minutes. Remove from the heat, whisk in the remaining butter, and stir in the thyme and salt.

GRAPEFRUIT-BASIL AIOLI
MAKES: ENOUGH FOR 2 DOZEN OYSTERS

    ¼ cup mayonnaise
    1 tablespoon chopped fresh basil
    1½ teaspoons finely grated grapefruit zest
    2 teaspoons fresh grapefruit juice
    1 teaspoon minced garlic
    ¼ teaspoon kosher salt

1. In a small bowl combine the ingredients and mix thoroughly.

ASIAN BUTTER SAUCE
MAKES: ENOUGH FOR 2 DOZEN OYSTERS

    1 tablespoon sesame oil
    2 teaspoons minced fresh ginger
    2 tablespoons oyster sauce
    1 teaspoon soy sauce
    ¼ teaspoon ground mustard
    ¼ cup (½ stick) unsalted butter, cut into small chunks

1. In a small skillet over medium heat, combine the oil and ginger and heat until the oil begins to foam. Remove from the heat; stir in the oyster sauce, soy sauce, and mustard. Whisk in the butter a few chunks at a time until completely incorporated.

GORGONZOLA-TOMATO SAUCE
MAKES: ENOUGH FOR 2 DOZEN OYSTERS

    1 tablespoon unsalted butter
    1 tablespoon minced shallot
    1 teaspoon minced garlic
    ½ cup vegetable juice
    2 teaspoons prepared horseradish
    ½ teaspoon kosher salt
    ¼ cup crumbled Gorgonzola cheese

1. In a small saucepan over medium heat, melt the butter and sauté the shallot and garlic for about 2 minutes. Add the vegetable juice, horseradish, and salt. Bring the sauce to a simmer and then remove it from the heat. After you've added the sauce to the oysters, sprinkle the cheese on top, and then grill.

WAY TO PREP AND GRILL LOBSTER TAILS

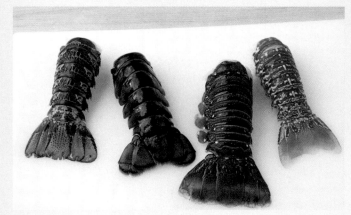

1. Different varieties and sizes of lobster tail are available. Shown here, left to right, are New Zealand, 6 to 8 ounces; Maine, 5 to 6 ounces; West Australian, 8 to 10 ounces; and South African, 4½ to 5 ounces. Adjust cooking times according to size.

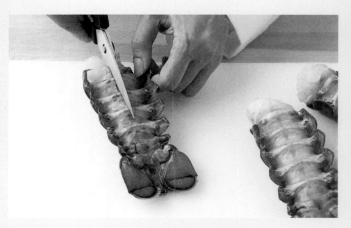

2. Use kitchen scissors to cut through the center of the shell on the underside of each tail.

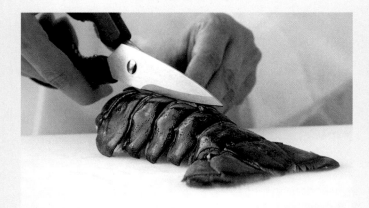

3. Turn each tail over and cut through the harder back shell all the way to the fins.

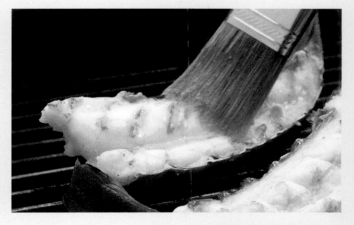

4. Use a sharp, heavy knife to cut each tail in half lengthwise, passing through the openings you have already made.

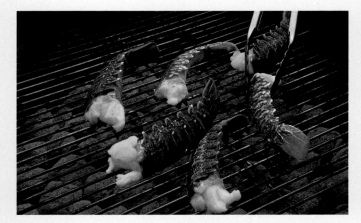

5. Grill the tails, meat side down, until the surface of the meat turns opaque.

6. Then turn the tails over onto their shells and brush with garlic butter while the meat turns opaque all the way to the center.

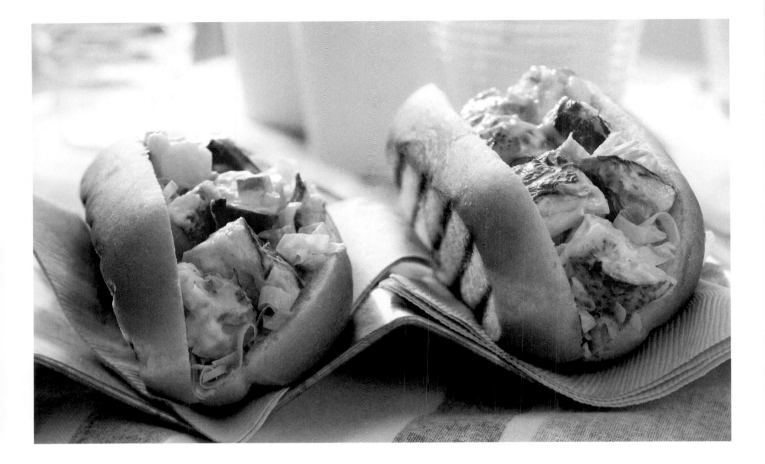

LOBSTER ROLLS

SERVES: 4
PREP TIME: 25 MINUTES

WAY TO GRILL: DIRECT MEDIUM HEAT (350° TO 450°F)
GRILLING TIME: 6 TO 7 MINUTES

3 large garlic cloves, lightly crushed
6 tablespoons salted butter
4 Maine lobster tails, about 6 ounces each
 Kosher salt
¼ cup mayonnaise
½ cup ¼-inch-diced plum tomato
2 tablespoons minced scallion, white and light green parts
2 teaspoons fresh lemon juice
 Hot sauce
2 teaspoons chopped fresh chervil
4 hot dog buns, sliced vertically from the top
1⅓ cups shredded romaine lettuce heart

1. In a small saucepan over medium-low heat, warm the garlic and butter until the butter melts. Set aside about 2 tablespoons for brushing on the buns.

2. Prepare the grill for direct cooking over medium heat. Carefully cut the lobster tails in half lengthwise. Season the meat with a little salt and brush some of the garlic butter over the surface of each one. Brush the cooking grates clean. Grill the tails, meat side down, over **direct medium heat**, with the lid open, until the meat is opaque, 2 to 3 minutes. Turn the tails over, brush with more garlic butter, and continue to grill until the meat is slightly firm, about 3 minutes. Set aside to cool.

3. In a large bowl combine the mayonnaise, tomato, scallion, and lemon juice. Season to taste with salt and hot sauce. Remove the lobster meat from the shells and cut into ½-inch pieces. Add the lobster meat to the mayonnaise mixture. For best flavor, chill at least 1 hour. Mix in the chervil just before serving.

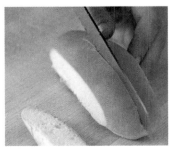

4. Using a serrated knife, trim some of the crust from the sides of the buns. Brush the remaining garlic butter on the cut sides (outside only) of the buns and toast over **direct medium heat** until golden brown on both sides, about 1 minute, turning once.

5. Place ⅓ cup romaine on the bottom of each roll and then top with the lobster mixture.

WAY TO PREP AND GRILL DUNGENESS CRABS

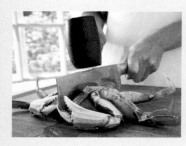

1. Lay each live crab flat on its back. Use a cleaver and mallet to cut right down the center and all the way through.

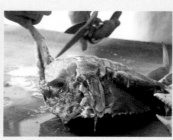

2. Cut off the dangling tail flap attached to the underside of one half.

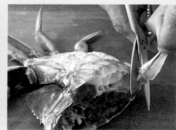

3. Also cut off the tail flap dangling on the other half.

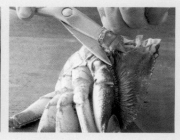

4. Find the parts of the mouth that protrude from the front of each half and cut those off.

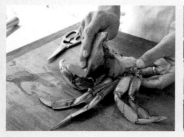

5. Turn each half over and pull off the top shell.

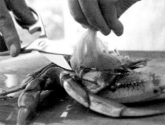

6. Remove the feathery gills, known as "dead man's fingers."

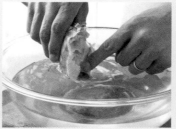

7. In a bowl of cold water, rinse out the brownish viscera.

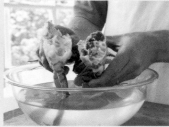

8. The half on the left is cleaned. The one on the right is not.

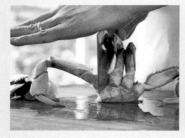

9. Cut through the shell between each leg with the cleaver or a sharp knife.

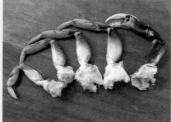

10. You should have five legs from each half crab.

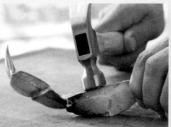

11. Use a clean hammer or a nutcracker to crack the shells prior to grilling.

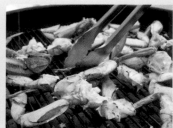

12. Grill the crab legs over direct high heat for a couple of minutes on each side to absorb the charcoal aromas.

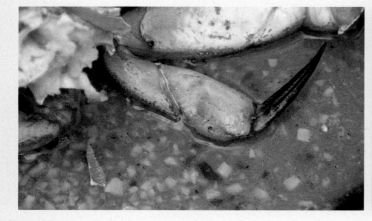

13. Move the crab legs to a skillet with butter, garlic, wine, lemon, and chiles.

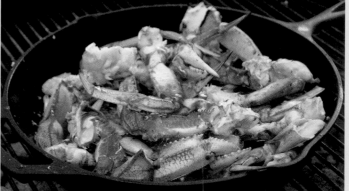

14. Turn and coat the crab legs in the buttery mixture as they finish cooking.

DUNGENESS CRABS WITH WHITE WINE-GARLIC BUTTER

SERVES: 2 AS A MAIN COURSE OR 4 APPETIZERS
PREP TIME: 30 MINUTES

WAY TO GRILL: DIRECT HIGH HEAT (450° TO 550°F)
GRILLING TIME: 9 TO 11 MINUTES
SPECIAL EQUIPMENT: 12-INCH CAST-IRON SKILLET

- 2 large live Dungeness crabs
- ½ cup (1 stick) unsalted butter, cut into 8 equal pieces
- 2 tablespoon minced garlic
  Finely grated zest and juice of 1 lemon
- ½ teaspoon crushed red pepper flakes
- ½ teaspoon kosher salt
- ¼ teaspoon freshly ground black pepper
- ⅔ cup dry white wine
- 1 baguette, torn into bite-sized pieces

1. Prepare the grill for direct cooking over high heat.

2. To kill each crab, place it on its back and hold it down with a large cleaver. Use a hammer to tap the top edge of the cleaver and cut the crab in half lengthwise all the way through. Remove and discard the dangling tail flaps and mouth parts. Turn the crab over. Pull off and discard the top shell. Remove and discard the gills. Rinse each half of the crab under cold running water and use your finger to scoop out and discard the dark viscera. Slice each half into 5 pieces by cutting between each leg and through the body. Using the hammer again (or a nutcracker or crab cracker), crack each section of each leg to make eating easier after the crabs are cooked.

3. In a 12-inch cast-iron skillet combine the butter, garlic, lemon zest, lemon juice, red pepper flakes, salt, and pepper. Mix well.

4. Place the skillet over **_direct high heat_** and cook, with the lid open, until the butter melts and the garlic turns golden, 2 to 3 minutes. Add the wine and cook until it comes to a boil. Remove the skillet from the grill and set it down on a heat-proof surface.

5. Grill the crab pieces over **_direct high heat_**, with the lid open, for about 4 minutes, turning once, and then move them to the skillet. Return the skillet over **_direct high heat_** and gently turn the crab pieces with tongs to coat them with the sauce. Cook until the liquid boils and the crab is fully cooked, 2 to 3 minutes. Serve warm with pieces of bread to dip into the liquid remaining in the skillet.

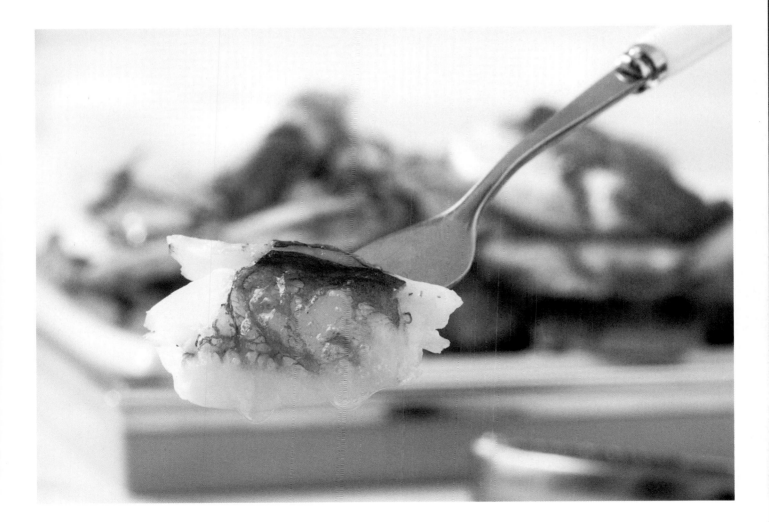

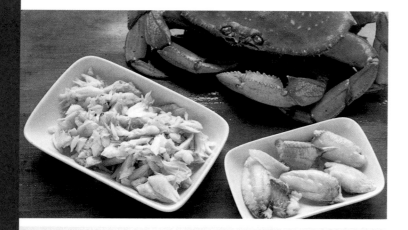

The difference in quality between fresh and canned crabmeat is striking. While crabmeat hand-picked from freshly caught, seasonal crabs is sweet and luscious, what you often find in cans is pasteurized and metallic in flavor. Even the crabmeat from previously frozen crabs can't compete with the truly fresh stuff. For this recipe, the variety of crab (such as Dungeness, rock, or Pacific blue) is far less important than freshness. However, don't bother spending high prices on "jumbo" crab, the big unbroken pieces of meat. "Backfin" or broken pieces of crabmeat will work just great.

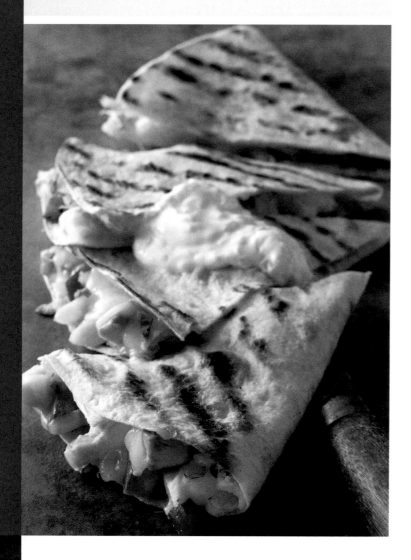

CRAB AND AVOCADO QUESADILLAS

SERVES: 4 TO 6
PREP TIME: 20 MINUTES

WAY TO GRILL: DIRECT MEDIUM HEAT (350° TO 450°F)
GRILLING TIME: 2 TO 4 MINUTES

- 1 pound fresh crabmeat
- ⅓ cup finely chopped fresh basil
  Finely grated zest of 2 lemons, divided
  Juice of 2 lemons
- 1 tablespoon minced jalapeño chile pepper
- ½ teaspoon kosher salt
- ¼ teaspoon freshly ground black pepper
- ½ cup sour cream
- 6 flour tortillas (8 inches)
- 2 ripe Haas avocados, seeded, peeled, and cubed
- 1 cup finely diced tomatoes
- 2 cups grated Monterey Jack cheese
  Extra-virgin olive oil

1. In a medium bowl combine the crabmeat, basil, half of the lemon zest, the lemon juice, jalapeño, salt, and pepper. Mix well.

2. In a small bowl combine the sour cream with the remaining half of the lemon zest. Set aside.

3. Prepare the grill for direct cooking over medium heat.

4. Lay the tortillas in a single layer on a work surface. Evenly divide the crabmeat mixture, avocados, tomatoes, and cheese over half of each tortilla. Fold the empty half of each tortilla over the filling, creating a half circle, and press down firmly. Lightly brush the tortillas with oil. Brush the cooking grates clean. Grill the quesadillas over **direct medium heat**, with the lid closed as much as possible, until the cheese melts and the tortillas are well marked, 2 to 4 minutes, carefully turning once. Cut each quesadilla into wedges. Serve with the sour cream mixture.

SEAFOOD ZUPPA

SERVES: 4
PREP TIME: 30 MINUTES

WAY TO GRILL: DIRECT MEDIUM HEAT (350° TO 450°F)
    AND DIRECT HIGH HEAT (450° TO 550°F)
GRILLING TIME: 17 TO 19 MINUTES
SPECIAL EQUIPMENT: PERFORATED GRILL PAN

ZUPPA
    2 small fennel bulbs
    1 lemon, ends trimmed, cut in half
    2 red bell peppers, cut into flat pieces
  4–5 shallots, about 1/2 pound, peeled
       Extra-virgin olive oil
    1 cup clam juice
    1 cup vegetable broth
    ½ teaspoon paprika
    ⅛ teaspoon crushed red pepper flakes
    ⅛ teaspoon saffron threads
       Kosher salt
       Freshly ground black pepper

    4 large or jumbo scallops, 1½ to 2 ounces each
    8 jumbo shrimp (11/15 count), peeled and deveined
    1 skinless sea bass fillet, about ½ pound,
       cut into 4 pieces
    1 skinless swordfish fillet, about ½ pound,
       cut into 4 pieces
    2 tablespoons extra-virgin olive oil

    4 thick slices bread
    ¼ cup finely chopped fresh Italian parsley

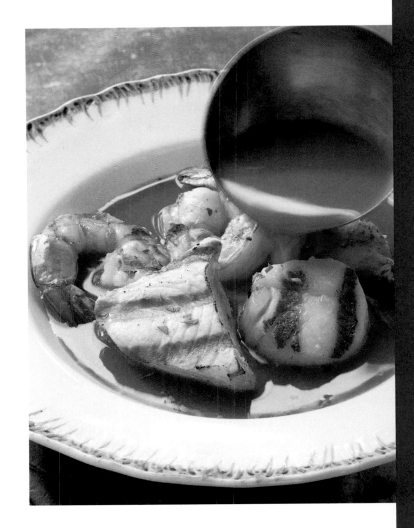

1. Prepare the grill for direct cooking over medium heat.

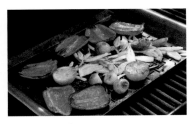

2. Preheat the grill pan over **direct medium heat** for about 10 minutes. While the pan preheats, prepare the vegetables. Cut off the thick stalks above the fennel bulbs and save for another use. Cut each fennel bulb into quarters and then remove the thick triangular-shaped core. Slice the fennel vertically into ¼-inch-thick slivers. Lightly brush the lemon halves, peppers, and shallots with oil. Place the vegetables on the grill pan and grill over **direct medium heat**, with the lid closed as much as possible, until the vegetables are tender, about 10 minutes, turning as needed.

3. Place the vegetables in a large bowl and cover the bowl with aluminum foil. Let them steam for 10 minutes. Remove and discard any charred skin from the shallots. Coarsely chop the shallots along with the red peppers. In a blender combine the

fennel, peppers, shallots, and the juice of one grilled lemon half. Puree until smooth. Then add the clam juice and vegetable broth and puree again (the blender will be very full). Pour the *zuppa* through a strainer into a medium saucepan and discard any bits left in the strainer. Season with the paprika, red pepper flakes, and saffron. Keep warm over low heat. Add additional grilled lemon juice, salt, and pepper to taste.

4. Increase the temperature of the grill to high heat. Remove the small, tough side muscle that might be left on each scallop. Lightly coat the shellfish and fish fillets with the oil and season with salt and pepper. Brush the cooking grates clean. Grill over **direct high heat**, with the lid closed as much as possible, until the shrimp is lightly charred on the outside and just turning opaque in the center, the scallops are slightly firm on the surface and opaque in the center, and the fish fillets are just beginning to separate into layers and the color is opaque at the center, turning once. The shrimp will take 3 to 5 minutes, the scallops will take 4 to 6 minutes, and the fillets will take 6 to 8 minutes.

5. Toast the bread over direct heat for about 1 minute, turning once. Evenly divide the shellfish and fish among individual bowls. Ladle ½ cup of the *zuppa* into each bowl. Garnish with parsley and serve with the bread.

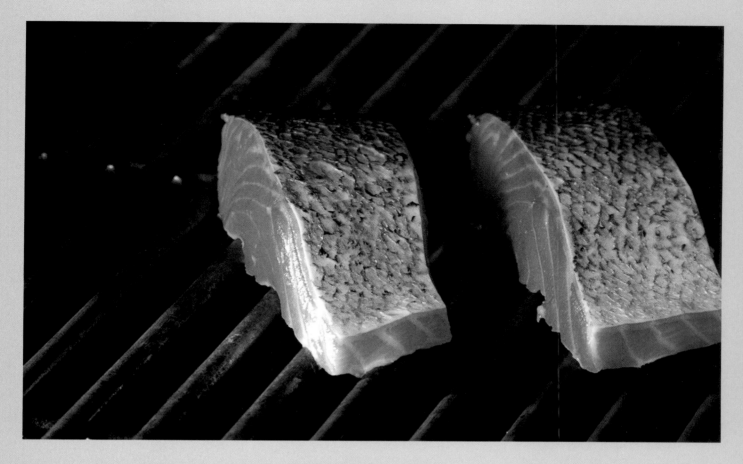

WAY TO GRILL FISH
5 THINGS YOU NEED TO KNOW

1 PRACTICE MAKES PERFECT

Many grillers consider fish fillets and steaks their biggest challenge. They remember the times when fish stuck to the grate and fell to pieces when they tried to take it off the grill. To greatly improve your chances of success, learn to grill firm fish first, especially the ones that are a bit oily, including salmon, swordfish, and tuna.

2 DON'T OVERDO IT

Fish and seafood don't have the muscle structure and firmness that many four-legged creatures have. Therefore marinades work more quickly to break down the structure of fillets and steaks. So, to prevent mushy textures, limit marinating times to just a few hours. And, above all else, don't overcook fillets and steaks.

3 FEED THE FIRE

Don't be afraid of high heat. It creates a bit of a crust on the surface of fish, and the crust helps the fish release from the cooking grate. The thinner the fillets or steaks you have, the higher the heat should be.

4 NO FLIP-FLOPPING

Every time you turn fish on the grill, you create a new possibility for sticking, so turn it only once.

5 QUICK FINISH

Grill the first side longer than the second. This assures you a nicely developed crust on the first side. Plus, if you are grilling with the lid closed (as you should), the second side will begin to cook while the first side is on the grate. So the second side will not need as long on the grate.

SALMON WITH NECTARINE SALSA

SERVES: 4
PREP TIME: 20 MINUTES

WAY TO GRILL: DIRECT HIGH HEAT (450° TO 550°F)
GRILLING TIME: 8 TO 11 MINUTES

SALSA
- 2 nectarines, about 1 pound, cut into ½-inch dice
- ½ cup ¼-inch-diced red bell pepper
- ¼ cup ¼-inch-diced red onion
- ¼ cup finely chopped fresh chervil
- 1 jalapeño chile pepper, seeded and finely diced
- 2 tablespoons finely chopped fresh mint
- 1 tablespoon honey
- 1 tablespoon fresh lime juice
- ¼ teaspoon crushed red pepper flakes
- ¼ teaspoon kosher salt

- 4 salmon fillets (with skin), 6 to 8 ounces each and about 1 inch thick
- ½ teaspoon kosher salt
- ¼ teaspoon crushed red pepper flakes
- 2 tablespoons fresh lime juice
- 1 tablespoon extra-virgin olive oil

1. In a medium bowl combine the salsa ingredients. Cover and refrigerate until ready to serve.

2. Prepare the grill for direct cooking over high heat.

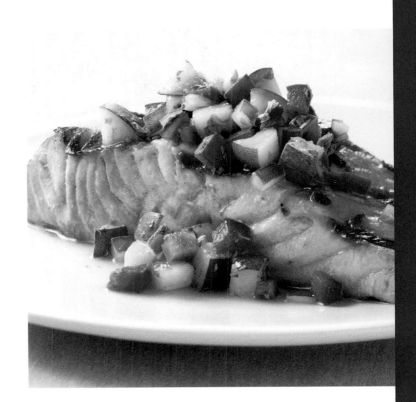

3. Season the salmon on both sides with the salt and red pepper flakes and then drizzle with the lime juice and oil. Brush the cooking grates clean. Grill the salmon, flesh side down, over **direct high heat**, with the lid closed as much as possible, until you can lift the fillets off the grate with tongs without sticking, 6 to 8 minutes. Turn the fillets and cook them to your desired doneness, 2 to 3 minutes for medium rare. Slip a spatula between the skin and the flesh, and transfer the fillets to serving plates. Serve warm with the salsa.

WAY TO GRILL SALMON

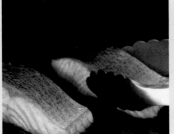

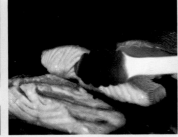

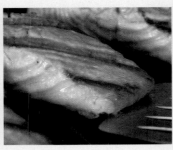

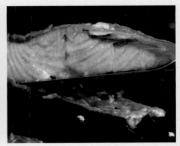

1. Start with generously oiled fillets, flesh side down, on a clean, hot grate.

2. Grill them over high heat and roll them over when the flesh side releases easily.

3. When the salmon is done, wiggle a spatula into the seam between the flesh and skin.

4. Scoop the flesh off the skin and pat yourself on the back. Serving the skin is optional.

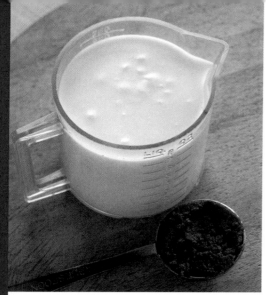

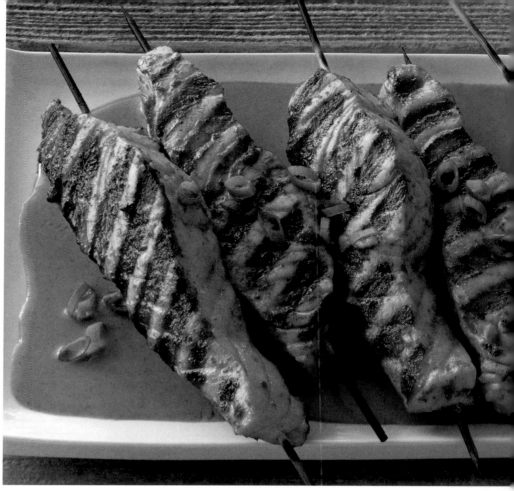

The sauce for this recipe features some classic Thai ingredients, including coconut milk and red curry paste. The cream that rises to the top of chilled coconut milk contains a good amount of oil, so use it to fry the curry paste, releasing its spicy flavors, before adding the rest of the milk and the other sauce ingredients.

SALMON WITH RED CURRY-COCONUT SAUCE

SERVES: 4 TO 6
PREP TIME: 25 MINUTES

WAY TO GRILL: DIRECT HIGH HEAT (450° TO 550°F)
GRILLING TIME: 3 TO 6 MINUTES
SPECIAL EQUIPMENT: 12 BAMBOO SKEWERS,
    SOAKED IN WATER FOR AT LEAST 30 MINUTES

1¼   cups chilled coconut milk, divided
3½   tablespoons Thai red curry paste, divided
1   tablespoon fish sauce
1   tablespoon soy sauce
1½   teaspoons light brown sugar
1   skinless salmon fillet, about 2 pounds
2   tablespoons vegetable oil
2   tablespoons finely chopped scallion

1. Scoop ¼ cup coconut cream from the top of the chilled coconut milk and transfer it to a small saucepan. Place over medium heat and bring to a boil. Add 2 tablespoons of the curry paste and cook, stirring constantly, until very fragrant, 3 to 5 minutes. Stir the remaining 1 cup coconut milk to achieve a smooth consistency, and then slowly incorporate it into the curry paste mixture. Add the fish sauce, soy sauce, and sugar. Bring to a boil, stirring constantly, and then adjust the heat to maintain a simmer. Cook, stirring frequently, until thickened to a thin sauce consistency, 5 to 10 minutes. Set aside.

2. Prepare the grill for direct cooking over high heat.

3. Remove any remaining pin bones from the salmon fillet. Cut the fillet into ¾-inch-thick slices. Thread them onto skewers.

4. In a small bowl, combine the remaining 1½ tablespoons curry paste with the oil and generously brush the salmon with the mixture. Brush the cooking grates clean. Grill the skewers over **direct high heat**, with the lid closed as much as possible, until you can lift them off the cooking grate with tongs without sticking, 2 to 4 minutes. Turn the skewers and cook them to your desired doneness, 1 to 2 minutes for medium. Reheat the sauce and pool it onto a serving dish or divide evenly among individual plates, top with the salmon, and scatter the scallions over the top. Serve warm.

CEDAR-PLANKED SALMON
WITH TARATOR SAUCE

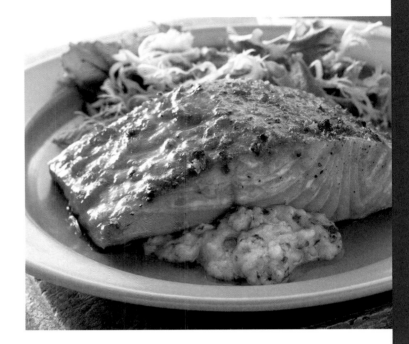

SERVES: 4
PREP TIME: 20 MINUTES

WAY TO GRILL: DIRECT MEDIUM HEAT (350° TO 450°F)
GRILLING TIME: 20 TO 30 MINUTES
SPECIAL EQUIPMENT: 1 UNTREATED CEDAR PLANK,
    12 TO 15 INCHES LONG AND ½ TO ¾ INCH THICK,
    SOAKED IN SALTED WATER FOR AT LEAST 1 HOUR

SAUCE
    2 pieces firm white bread, crusts removed
    2 garlic cloves
    ½ cup hazelnuts, lightly toasted and skinned
    3 tablespoons fresh lemon juice
    ½ cup extra-virgin olive oil
    ¼ cup fresh Italian parsley leaves
       Kosher salt
       Freshly ground black pepper

    1 salmon fillet (skin on), about 2 pounds
    ½ cup brown sugar

1. Soak the bread briefly in water, squeeze dry, and set aside.
In the bowl of a food processor combine the garlic and
hazelnuts and process until the nuts are finely ground. Add
the bread and lemon juice and process until smooth. With the
motor running, add the oil in a slow, steady stream. Add the
parsley, ½ teaspoon salt, and ¼ teaspoon pepper and pulse
quickly. Season to taste with additional salt, pepper, and lemon
juice, if desired.

2. Prepare the grill for direct cooking over medium heat.
Remove any remaining pin bones from the fillet. Cut the fillet
crosswise to make 4 servings. but do not cut through the skin.
Generously season with salt and pepper.

3. Place the soaked plank over *direct medium heat* and
close the lid. After 5 to 10 minutes, when the plank begins to
smoke and char, turn the plank over and then lay the fillet on
the plank. Carefully sprinkle the brown sugar over the entire
surface of the fillet. Close the lid and let the salmon cook until
lightly browned on the surface and cooked to your desired
doneness, 15 to 20 minutes for medium rare. Cooking time will
vary according to the thickness of the fillet. Serve warm with the
sauce on the side.

WAY TO PLANK SALMON

Cooking salmon on a cedar plank prevents the fish from sticking to the cooking grate and imbues it with delicious smoky flavors.

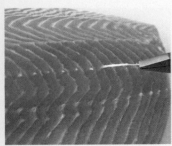

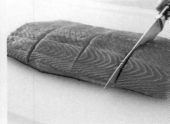

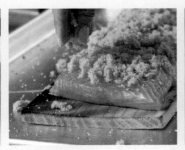

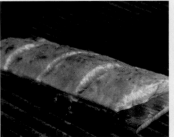

1. Run your fingertips over the
salmon to feel for any bones.
Use needle-nose pliers to grab
the ends of any tiny pin bones
and pull them out.

2. Cut the raw fish into individual
portions, right down to the skin
but not through it, to make it
easier to serve later.

3. Lay the salmon on a lightly
charred, smoldering plank and
sprinkle brown sugar over the top.

4. The sugar will melt and
caramelize on the surface
while the cedar smoke permeates
the flesh.

WAY TO PREP FENNEL

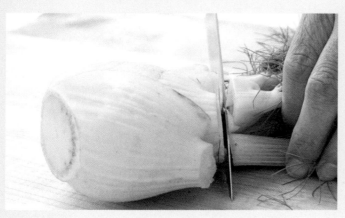

1. Cut off the thick stalks above the bulb, leave the root end attached to hold the bulb together, and then cut the bulb in half through the root end.

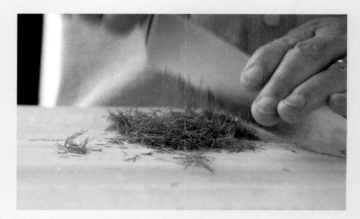

2. Chop some of the flavorful fronds to season the salad.

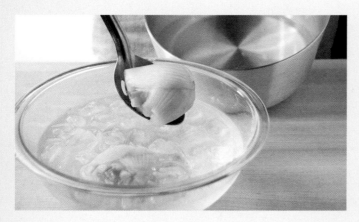

3. Simmer the fennel halves in salted water until just tender. Plunge the fennel into an ice bath to stop the cooking.

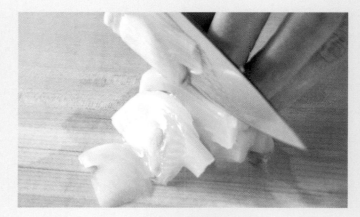

4. Trim off the root end and thinly slice the fennel.

WAY TO BONE SALMON STEAKS

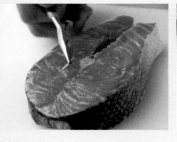 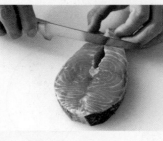 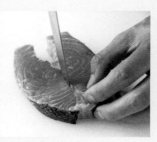 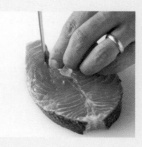

1. Find any pin bones and remove them with needle-nose pliers.

2. Trim off any thin, dangling flaps of flesh.

3. Starting at the top of the steak, cut alongside the bone.

4. Continue to cut all along the bone and rib sections.

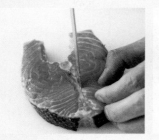 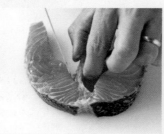 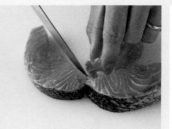 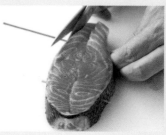

5. Cut along the other side of the bones, too.

6. The goal is to isolate the bones only, without cutting away much of the flesh.

7. Cut the bones free near the top, leaving just a little bit of bone attached to hold the flesh together.

8. Bring the sides together and secure the ends with a shortened bamboo skewer.

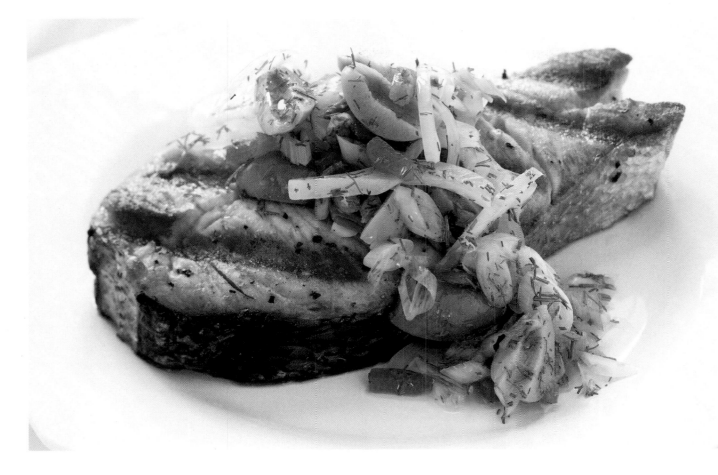

SALMON WITH FENNEL AND OLIVE SALAD

SERVES: 4
PREP TIME: 30 MINUTES

WAY TO GRILL: DIRECT HIGH HEAT (450° TO 550°F)
GRILLING TIME: 8 TO 11 MINUTES
SPECIAL EQUIPMENT: 8 BAMBOO SKEWERS,
   SOAKED IN WATER FOR AT LEAST 30 MINUTES

SALAD
  1 medium fennel bulb
 ½ cup green olives with pimentos, quartered
  3 scallions, white and light green parts, finely chopped
  2 tablespoons chopped fennel fronds
  1 tablespoon extra-virgin olive oil
 ½ teaspoon finely grated lemon zest

  4 salmon steaks or fillets, each 6 to 8 ounces
     and 1 to 1½ inches thick
  2 tablespoons extra-virgin olive oil
 ½ teaspoon kosher salt
 ¼ teaspoon freshly ground black pepper

1. If the fennel stalks have the fronds attached, trim off the fronds and chop enough to make 2 tablespoons; set aside. Cut off the thick stalks above the bulb and save the stalks for another use. Leave the root end attached to hold the bulb together. Cut the fennel bulb in half. Fill a small saucepan with water. Lightly salt the water and bring to a boil over medium-high heat. Reduce the heat to medium and gently simmer the fennel bulb for 3 minutes. Remove from the water and plunge into an ice bath to rapidly cool it. Remove the bulb from the ice bath, trim off the root end, and thinly slice.

2. In a medium bowl combine the salad ingredients. Toss to coat and set aside to let the flavors marinate while you grill the salmon.

3. Prepare the grill for direct cooking over high heat.

4. Prepare the salmon steaks as detailed at left. Brush the salmon with the oil and season with the salt and pepper. Brush the cooking grates clean. Grill the salmon over *direct high heat*, with the lid closed as much as possible, until you can lift the steaks off the grate with tongs without sticking, 6 to 8 minutes. Turn and cook to your desired doneness, 2 to 3 minutes for medium. If using fillets, to easily remove the skin, just slip a spatula between the skin and the flesh, and lift the salmon flesh from the grill. Transfer the salmon to plates and top with the salad.

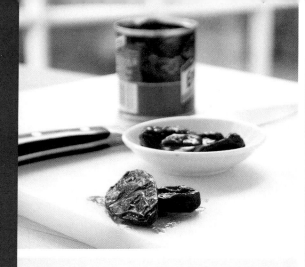

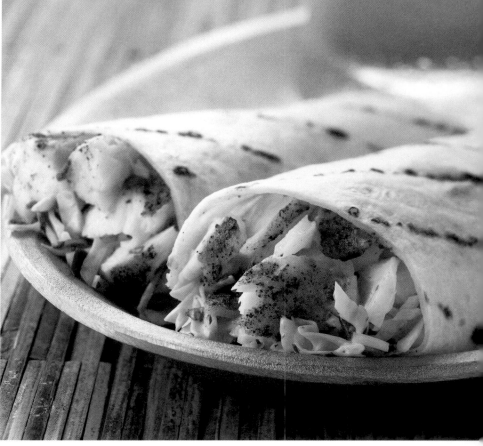

A potent ingredient in any griller's pantry, chipotles are dried and smoked jalapeno chiles. They are often found packed in adobo, which is a tomato-based sauce with vinegar, onions, garlic, and spices. Way to freeze leftover chiles: Spoon one chile, with a little of the sauce, into each space of an ice cube tray. After they have frozen, pop them out of the tray, tightly wrap them with plastic wrap, and place them in a resealable freezer bag.

BAJA FISH WRAPS WITH CHIPOTLE-LIME SLAW

SERVES: 6
PREP TIME: 20 MINUTES

WAY TO GRILL: DIRECT HIGH HEAT (450° TO 550°F)
GRILLING TIME: 7 TO 8 MINUTES

RUB
- ½ teaspoon pure chile powder
- ½ teaspoon ground cumin
- ½ teaspoon kosher salt
- ¼ teaspoon ground cayenne pepper
- ¼ teaspoon ground cinnamon

- 4 halibut or salmon fillets or 2 of each (with skin), about 6 ounces each and 1 to 1½ inches thick
  Vegetable oil

SLAW
- 3 cups very thinly sliced green cabbage
- ¼ cup coarsely chopped fresh cilantro
- ¼ cup mayonnaise
- 2 tablespoons fresh lime juice
- 2 teaspoons granulated sugar
- 1 teaspoon canned chipotle chile in adobo, minced
- ½ teaspoon kosher salt

- 6 flour tortillas (10 to 12 inches)

1. In a small bowl mix the rub ingredients. Lightly brush the fillets with oil and then apply the rub evenly. Cover and set aside in the refrigerator.

2. In a large bowl combine the slaw ingredients and toss to coat. Set aside until ready to assemble the wraps. Prepare the grill for direct cooking over high heat.

3. Brush the cooking grates clean. Grill the fillets over **direct high heat**, with the lid closed as much as possible, until you can lift them with a spatula off the cooking grate without sticking, about 4 minutes. Turn the fillets over and cook them until they are opaque in the center, 2 to 3 minutes. Transfer to a plate. Warm the tortillas over **direct high heat** for 30 seconds to 1 minute, turning once.

4. To assemble the wraps, break a fillet into large chunks and arrange on one half of a warm tortilla, then top with some of the slaw. Roll the tortilla to enclose the fillings, fold in the sides, and continue rolling to the end. Cut the wrap in half. Serve warm or at room temperature.

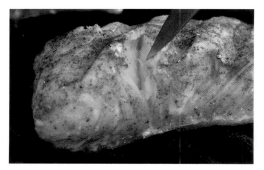

Halibut has a nice, mild, sweet flavor, but the flesh is quite lean, so it dries out quickly if it's overcooked. The key is to remove it from the grill before it begins to flake apart. Check each fillet first with a paring knife to make sure the flesh is no longer translucent at the center.

HALIBUT FILLETS
WITH BOMBAY TOMATO SAUCE

SERVES: 4
PREP TIME: 30 MINUTES

WAY TO GRILL: DIRECT MEDIUM HEAT (350° TO 450°F)
    AND DIRECT HIGH HEAT (450° TO 550°F)
GRILLING TIME: 19 TO 23 MINUTES
SPECIAL EQUIPMENT: 12-INCH CAST-IRON SKILLET

SAUCE

    3 tablespoons peanut oil
    1 medium yellow onion, halved and thinly sliced
    1 tablespoon minced garlic
    2 teaspoons finely grated fresh ginger
    1 teaspoon ground coriander
    1 teaspoon paprika
    ½ teaspoon turmeric
    ½ teaspoon kosher salt
    ¼ teaspoon ground cayenne pepper
    1 large can (28 ounces) peeled, chopped tomatoes
       with juice
    ¾ cup unsweetened coconut milk, stirred

    ¼ cup peanut oil
    1 teaspoon finely grated fresh ginger
    1 teaspoon kosher salt
    ½ teaspoon freshly ground black pepper
    ¼ teaspoon turmeric
    4 halibut fillets, 6 to 8 ounces each and about 1 inch thick
    2 tablespoons torn fresh basil leaves, optional

1. Prepare the grill for direct cooking over medium heat on one side and high heat on the other side. Brush the cooking grates clean. In a 12-inch cast-iron skillet over **direct medium heat**, warm the oil. Add the onion and cook until it softens and begins to brown, about 5 minutes, stirring often. Add the garlic, ginger, coriander, paprika, turmeric, salt, and cayenne. Mix well and cook for 2 to 3 minutes, stirring often to avoid burning. Add the tomatoes and coconut milk. Taste and adjust the seasoning, if needed. Allow the sauce to simmer for 5 minutes or so while you prepare the halibut.

2. In a small bowl mix the oil, ginger, salt, pepper, and turmeric. Generously brush the halibut on both sides with the oil mixture.

3. Grill the fillets over **direct high heat**, with the lid closed, until they release easily from the cooking grate, 4 to 5 minutes, without turning. Lift the fillets, one at a time, with a wide spatula and turn them over into the pan with the sauce, so that the grilled side is facing up. Nestle the fillets into the sauce, close the lid, and let the fillets cook over **direct medium heat** until they just begin to flake when you poke them with the tip of a knife, 3 to 5 minutes.

4. Remove the skillet from the grill. Scatter the basil on top. Serve warm.

WAY TO PREP HALIBUT

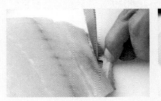

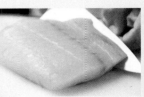

1. The first step is to skin the fish. Along one end of the fillet, cut a slit all the way through the skin large enough to get your finger though it.

2. Holding the skin steady with your finger in the slit, angle the blade of a large, sharp knife inside the seam between the flesh and skin.

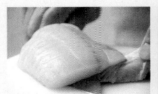

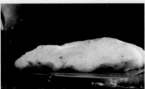

3. Cut away from you and over the top of the skin, always with the knife angled slightly downward.

4. Grill the fillets on one side only until they release easily from the grate.

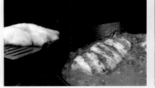

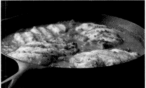

5. Move the fillets to a skillet with warm tomato sauce, grilled sides facing up.

6. The sauce helps to keep the fillets moist as they finish cooking.

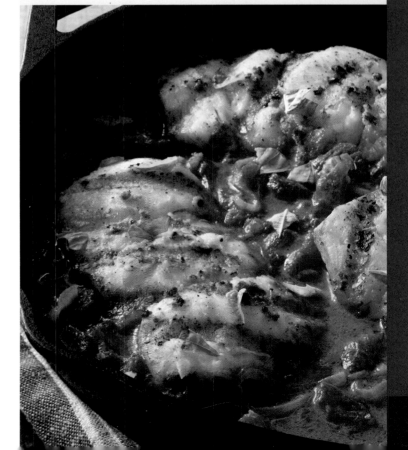

WAY TO SKIN MAHI-MAHI FILLETS

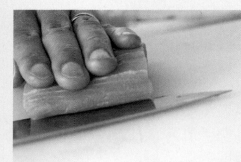 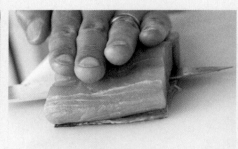 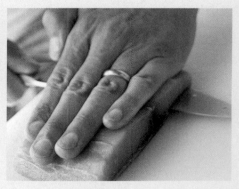

1. Angle the blade of a large, sharp knife into the seam between the flesh and skin on one end of a fillet.

2. Hold the fillet steady with your other hand and slide the knife right over the skin.

3. For safety's sake cut away from your body, in case the knife slips, and tilt the blade downward so that you don't cut into the flesh of the fillet.

WAY TO MAKE CORN AND MUSHROOM SALSA

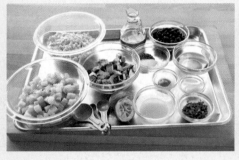 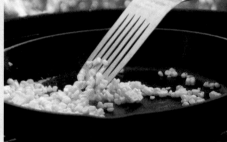 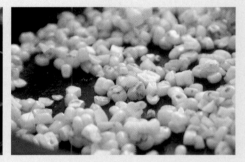

1. The cooking goes quickly, so have all your ingredients chopped and measured beforehand. Chefs refer to this as their *mise en place*.

2. Cook the corn in a smoking-hot skillet, stirring occasionally to prevent the kernels from popping right out of the pan.

3. The goal is to caramelize the natural sugars in the corn, turning the kernels golden brown and super-sweet.

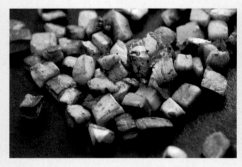 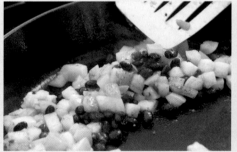 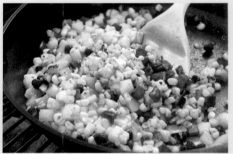

4. Cook the mushrooms in the same hot skillet. The less you stir them, the browner and more delicious they will be.

5. Cook the tomatillos, black beans, and garlic just until the garlic begins to brown, too.

6. Combine all the vegetables in the skillet, adjust the seasonings, and cook just long enough to marry the flavors.

WAY TO CHECK FOR DONENESS

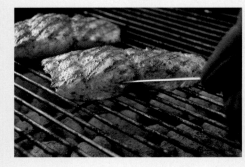 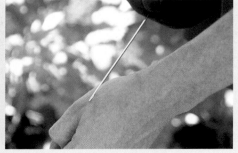

When you insert the end of a metal skewer into the center of a fillet and then quickly and carefully touch the end of the skewer on the outside of the base of your thumb, it should feel warm. If it feels less than warm, the fish is under cooked. If it feels hot, the fish is overcooked.

SEAFOOD

MAHI-MAHI
WITH CORN AND MUSHROOM SALSA

SERVES: 4
PREP TIME: 25 MINUTES
MARINATING TIME: UP TO 1 HOUR

WAY TO GRILL: DIRECT HIGH HEAT (450° TO 550°F)
GRILLING TIME: 13 TO 15 MINUTES
SPECIAL EQUIPMENT: 12-INCH CAST-IRON SKILLET

RUB
- 1 teaspoon pure chile powder
- 1 teaspoon granulated garlic
- 1 teaspoon paprika
- 1 teaspoon kosher salt
- ½ teaspoon ground coriander
- ½ teaspoon ground cumin
- ½ teaspoon freshly ground black pepper

- 4 skinless mahi-mahi fillets, each about 8 ounces and ¾ inch thick
- ¼ cup extra-virgin olive oil

SALSA
- 2 ears fresh sweet yellow corn, husked
- 1 large portabello mushroom, stemmed and cleaned
- 3–4 medium tomatillos
- 3 tablespoons extra-virgin olive oil, divided
- ½ cup cooked black beans
- 2 teaspoons minced garlic
- 2 tablespoons roughly chopped fresh cilantro
- 2 teaspoons fresh lime juice
- ½ teaspoon kosher salt
- ¼ teaspoon freshly ground black pepper
  Hot chile sauce

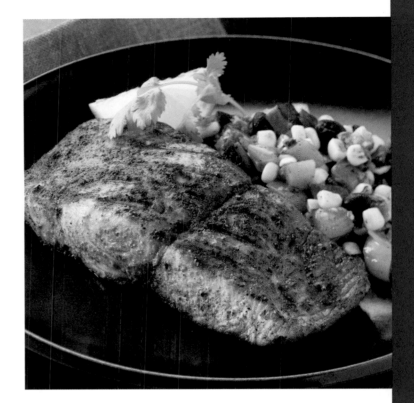

1. In a small bowl mix the rub ingredients. Generously coat the mahi-mahi fillets on both sides with the oil. Season evenly with the rub. Cover and refrigerate for up to 1 hour.

2. Cut the corn kernels from the cobs. Cut the mushroom into ¼-inch slices and then cut the slices into ¼- to ½-inch pieces. Cut the tomatillos into ¼- to ½-inch pieces. Measure and set aside the remaining salsa ingredients so that everything is ready for quick cooking.

3. Prepare the grill for direct cooking over high heat.

4. In a 12-inch cast-iron skillet over **direct high heat**, warm 1 tablespoon of the oil. When it is smoking hot, add the corn and spread the kernels in an even layer. Cook until most of the kernels are golden brown and crisp-tender, about 2 minutes, stirring 2 or 3 times. Transfer to a medium bowl. Add another tablespoon of oil, and when the oil begins to smoke add the mushrooms and spread them out in a single layer. Cook without

touching them for 30 seconds, then give them a stir and cook until the mushrooms are browned and tender, about 3 minutes. Add the mushrooms to the bowl with the corn. Add another tablespoon of the oil to the skillet and immediately add the tomatillos, black beans, and garlic. Mix well and cook until the garlic begins to brown, about 30 seconds. Then add the corn kernels and the mushrooms from the bowl. Add the remaining salsa ingredients. Heat for about 1 minute. Taste and adjust the seasonings, if necessary. Pour the salsa into the medium bowl and let cool while you grill the fish.

5. If cooking over charcoal, you'll probably need to add more briquettes to the fire so it is hot enough to grill the fish properly. Grill the mahi-mahi fillets over **direct high heat**, with the lid closed as much as possible, until the fish is fully cooked but still moist, 6 to 8 minutes, turning once.

6. Serve the fish fillets warm with the salsa served on the side.

■ ■ ■

Recipe from the chefs at Weber Grill® Restaurant

■ ■ ■

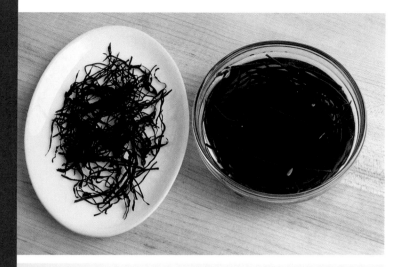

Poke is a beloved Hawaiian dish of finely chopped raw fish tossed with edible seaweed, seeds or nuts, and a dressing. In this recipe, the flavor and texture of the fish benefit from a quick sear on the grill. If you use dried seaweed, be sure to rehydrate it in water for about 15 minutes.

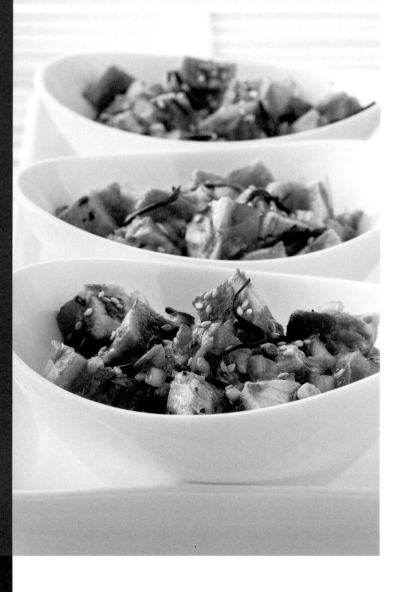

GRILLED AHI POKE

SERVES: 4 AS AN APPETIZER
PREP TIME: 15 MINUTES

WAY TO GRILL: DIRECT HIGH HEAT (450° TO 550°F)
GRILLING TIME: ABOUT 2 MINUTES

- 2 tablespoons dried Japanese *arame* or other thin edible seaweed
- ¼ cup finely chopped sweet onion
- ¼ cup thinly sliced scallion, white and light green parts
- 2 tablespoons soy sauce
- 1 tablespoon dark sesame oil
- 1 teaspoon grated fresh ginger
- ½ teaspoon minced serrano chile pepper

- 2 sushi-grade ahi tuna fillets, 6 to 8 ounces each and ¾ to 1 inch thick
  Vegetable oil
  Coarse sea salt or *alaea* (Hawaiian sea salt)
  Freshly ground black pepper
- 2 tablespoons toasted sesame seed
- 1 lemon, cut into wedges, optional

1. If using dried seaweed, place the seaweed in a small bowl, add enough water to cover, and set aside to soften for 15 minutes. Drain and coarsely chop before using.

2. Prepare the grill for direct cooking over high heat.

3. In a medium bowl mix the onion, scallion, soy sauce, sesame oil, ginger, and chile. Add the seaweed.

4. Brush the tuna with oil and lightly season with salt and pepper, patting the seasoning into the fish. Brush the cooking grates clean. Grill the tuna over **direct high heat**, with the grill lid open, just until seared on both sides but still rare inside, about 2 minutes, turning once.

5. Transfer the tuna to a cutting board and cut into ½- to ¾-inch cubes. Add to the bowl containing the onion mixture and toss to combine. Divide equally into individual bowls. Sprinkle with the sesame seeds. Serve warm with lemon wedges, if desired.

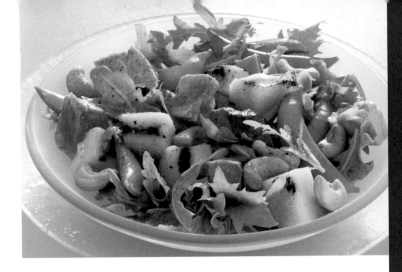

SMOKED TUNA SALAD WITH GRILLED MANGO

SERVES: 4 TO 6
PREP TIME: 30 MINUTES

WAY TO GRILL: DIRECT MEDIUM HEAT (350° TO 450°F)
GRILLING TIME: ABOUT 10 MINUTES
SPECIAL EQUIPMENT: 4 TO 6 CEDAR PAPERS, SOAKED IN
    WATER FOR 10 MINUTES; BUTCHER'S TWINE

DRESSING
⅓ cup honey
3 tablespoons Dijon mustard
2 tablespoons rice wine vinegar
2 tablespoons mayonnaise
½ teaspoon kosher salt
¼ teaspoon prepared chili powder

2 mangoes, firm but ripe
   Vegetable oil
2 cups sugar snap peas
¼ teaspoon kosher salt
2 tuna steaks, each about 1 pound and 1 inch thick
5 ounces mixed baby greens, rinsed and crisped
1 cup roasted and salted cashews
   Freshly ground black pepper

1. In a small bowl whisk the dressing ingredients until thoroughly combined. Set aside ⅓ cup of the dressing for the tuna.

2. Slice the sides from the mangoes, cutting along either side of the pit. Carefully, without cutting through the skin, slice 3 to 4 short lines along the inside of the flesh. Using the point of the knife, cut 3 to 4 lines in the opposite direction of the first set of cuts to create mango cubes. Brush the mango halves with oil.

3. Place the snap peas just off the center on a 12x12-inch sheet of aluminum foil and season them with the salt. Fold the foil over the snap peas and seal to create a pouch.

4. Slice each tuna steak to create equal strips that will fit on the cedar papers. Liberally brush the tuna with the reserved dressing and roll up in the cedar paper, using butcher's twine to keep the paper secure.

5. Prepare the grill for direct cooking over medium heat. Brush the cooking grates clean. Grill the cedar bundles over **direct medium heat**, with the lid closed as much as possible, until the tuna is pink but still juicy, about 6 minutes, turning once. Keep an eye on the cedar paper. If it catches on fire, use a spray bottle to mist out the flames. Remove the cedar bundles from the grill, cut the twine, remove the tuna from the cedar paper, and let cool. Gently flake the tuna.

6. Place the mangos and the foil pouch with the snap peas over **direct medium heat** and cook with the lid closed as much as possible, for about 4 minutes, turning once. Remove from the grill. Open the foil pouch to let the steam escape so the peas do not overcook. When the mangoes are cool enough to handle, hold each mango slice in both hands and press up on the skin side to expose the cubes. Slice the cubes off the skin.

7. Divide the salad greens evenly on serving plates. Top with grilled mango, snap peas, flaked tuna, and cashews. Drizzle with some dressing and finish with a grinding of pepper.

WAY TO SMOKE TUNA IN CEDAR PAPERS

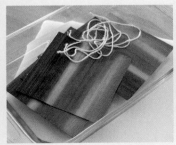

1. Submerge the cedar papers and twine in water for 10 minutes.

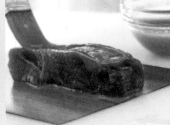

2. Cut thick tuna steaks into strips that will fit inside the papers. Lay a strip of tuna on each paper parallel to the grain of the wood. Brush the tuna with some of the dressing.

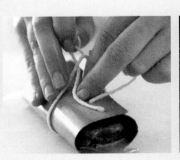

3. Roll up the sides of the paper over the tuna and secure with twine.

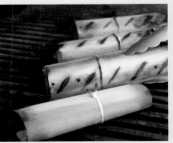

4. Grill for a few minutes on each side to produce some smoke while the fish cooks.

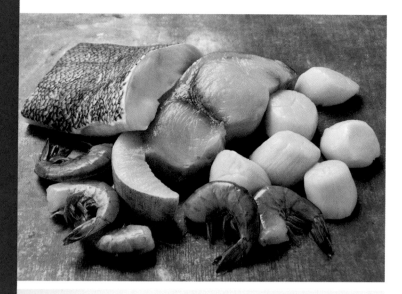

A cardinal rule for grilling seafood is that freshness and firmness always matter more than a particular type of fish. Don't go to the store thinking, for example, that only grouper will work for this recipe. If the grouper is not fresh that day, choose whatever else is firm and fresh. Good options here are swordfish, scallops, shrimp, and sea bass.

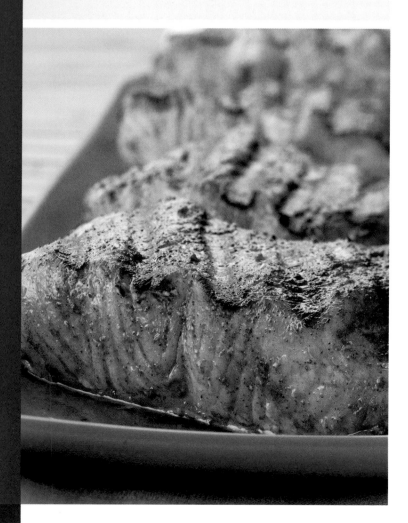

GRILLED FISH
IN A CARIBBEAN CITRUS MARINADE

SERVES: 6
PREP TIME: 15 MINUTES
MARINATING TIME: 3 HOURS

WAY TO GRILL: DIRECT HIGH HEAT (450° TO 550°F)
GRILLING TIME: 8 TO 10 MINUTES (FILLETS) OR
4 TO 6 MINUTES (SHELLFISH)

MARINADE
- 2 teaspoons grated orange zest
- ½ cup fresh orange juice
- 1 teaspoon grated lime zest
- ¼ cup fresh lime juice
- ¼ cup extra-virgin olive oil
- ¼ cup pure chile powder
- 1½ tablespoons finely minced garlic
- 1½ teaspoons ground coriander
- 1 teaspoon finely minced jalapeño chile pepper
- ¾ teaspoon ground allspice
- ¾ teaspoon freshly ground black pepper
- ¼ teaspoon ground cayenne pepper

- 6 fish fillets, grouper, sea bass, flounder, cod, or halibut (with skin), each 5 to 6 ounces and about 1 inch thick or 1½ pounds large prawns or scallops
  Extra-virgin olive oil
  Kosher salt

1. In a medium bowl combine the marinade ingredients. Reserve ⅓ cup of the marinade to serve with the grilled fish.

2. Place the fillets or shellfish side by side in a non-reactive dish, such as an 8x8-inch glass dish. Pour the remaining marinade over the fish or shellfish and turn to coat them. Cover and refrigerate the fish and reserved marinade for 3 hours.

3. Prepare the grill for direct cooking over high heat.

4. Remove the fillets or shellfish from the dish and discard the marinade. Lightly brush with oil and season with some salt.

5. Brush the cooking grates clean. Grill the fillets, skin side up, over **direct high heat**, with the lid closed as much as possible, until just opaque in the center, 8 to 10 minutes, turning once after 6 to 7 minutes when they release easily from the cooking grate. If using prawns or scallops, grill over **direct high heat** for 4 to 6 minutes, turning once. Serve with the reserved marinade spooned over the fillets or shellfish.

SWORDFISH ESCABÈCHE

SERVES: 4
PREP TIME: 30 MINUTES
MARINATING TIME: UP TO 2 HOURS

WAY TO GRILL: DIRECT MEDIUM HEAT (350° TO 450°F)
GRILLING TIME: 14 TO 18 MINUTES

MARINADE

- ½ cup extra-virgin olive oil
- 3 tablespoons sherry vinegar
- 1 tablespoon minced garlic
- 1 teaspoon dried oregano
- ¾ teaspoon kosher salt
- ½ teaspoon crushed red pepper flakes
- ¼ teaspoon freshly ground black pepper

- 8 button mushrooms
- 2 plum tomatoes, cored and halved lengthwise
- 1 large Anaheim chile pepper
- 1 small yellow squash, halved lengthwise
- 4 swordfish steaks, 8 to 10 ounces each and about 1 inch thick

ESCABÈCHE

- 1 cup low-sodium chicken broth
- 1 tablespoon sherry vinegar
- ¼ teaspoon dried oregano
- ⅛ teaspoon freshly ground black pepper

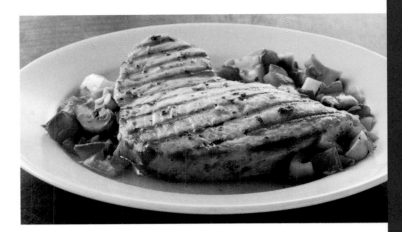

1. In a small bowl whisk the marinade ingredients. Transfer ¼ cup of the marinade to a medium bowl. Add the vegetables to the medium bowl and mix to coat them evenly.

2. Place the swordfish steaks flat on a plate large enough to fit them in a single layer. Spoon the remaining marinade over the steaks, turning them over to coat them evenly. Cover with plastic wrap and refrigerate for as long as 2 hours.

3. Prepare the grill for direct cooking over medium heat. Brush the cooking grates clean. Grill the vegetables over ***direct medium heat***, with the lid closed as much as possible, until the vegetables are lightly marked and tender, 6 to 8 minutes, turning occasionally. Remove the vegetables from the grill.

4. Place the pepper in a bowl and cover with plastic wrap. When cool enough to handle, remove and discard the stem, seeds, and skin. Roughly chop all the vegetables.

5. In a medium skillet over medium-high heat, combine the escabèche ingredients and bring the liquid to a boil. Add the chopped vegetables, and spread them out in the skillet. Cook until the vegetables are tender, 3 to 5 minutes. Remove the skillet from the heat, cover, and keep warm.

6. Lift the swordfish steaks off the plate and let the excess marinade drip onto the plate. Discard the marinade. Brush the cooking grates clean. Grill the steaks over ***direct medium heat***, with the lid closed as much as possible, until the center is opaque but the flesh is still juicy, 8 to 10 minutes, turning once. Serve the swordfish warm with the vegetable mixture.

WAY TO MAKE SWORDFISH ESCABÈCHE

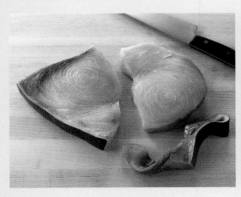

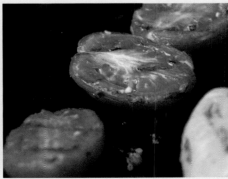

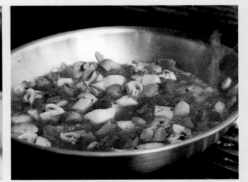

1. Swordfish steaks work well here, as would any firm-flesh fish. Remove the tough outer skin before marinating and grilling the swordfish.

2. Grilling the tomatoes and chile pepper (squash and mushrooms, too) will add depth and complexity to the final dish.

3. Escabèche is a preparation involving fish and hot vinegar-based liquid poured over the top. Grilled vegetables enliven the savory liquid.

WAY TO GRILL FISH FILLETS IN BANANA LEAVES

As you get closer and closer to the equator, you will find more and more grillers in the tropics using banana leaves to wrap and steam fish, vegetables, rice, and tamales. These inexpensive leaves, which are now available frozen in most Asian and Latino markets, trap moisture and add a subtle tea-like fragrance to the food. Thaw them in the refrigerator for a few hours or pour boiling water over them to make them pliable quickly.

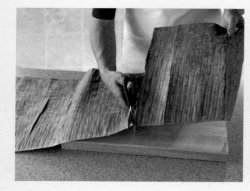

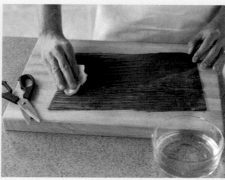

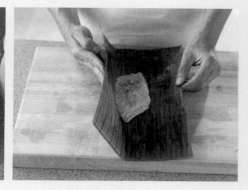

1. Cut the leaves into rectangles large enough to wrap around each fish fillet. Leave the sturdy fibrous vein along one edge intact, which holds the leaves together.

2. Wipe both sides with a damp towel to clean the leaves, moving in the same direction as the grain so you don't split them open.

3. Fold one side over the marinated fish, and then overlap the first side with the opposite side.

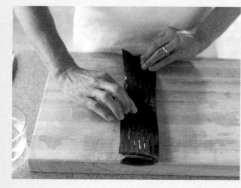

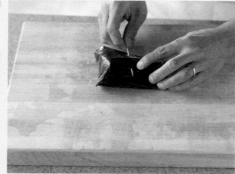

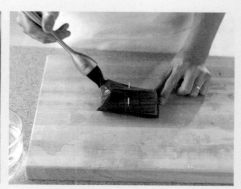

4. Fold down the top and bottom sides so that they overlap in the middle. If the leaf splits, use a second leaf to double-wrap the fish.

5. Thread a toothpick in and out of the overlapping leaves but not into the fish itself.

6. Brush each packet generously with water to prevent drying out. Assemble the packets on a sheet pan and cover with damp towels until ready to grill.

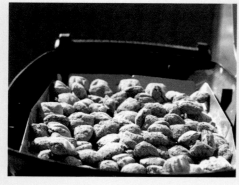

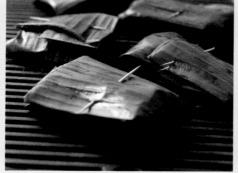

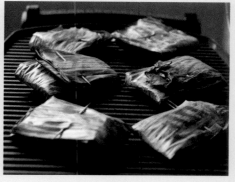

7. Let the charcoal burn down to medium heat.

8. Grill the packets with the toothpicks on top most of the time so the wood does not burn.

9. When the fish is fully cooked, you can unwrap the leaves and use them as serving plates.

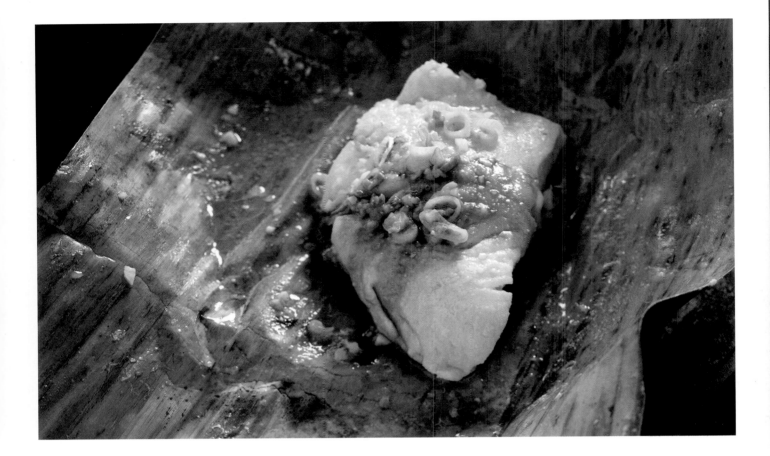

GINGER AND MISO BLACK COD IN BANANA LEAVES

SERVES: 6
PREP TIME: 20 MINUTES
MARINATING TIME: 2 HOURS

WAY TO GRILL: DIRECT MEDIUM HEAT (350° TO 450°F)
GRILLING TIME: 8 TO 10 MINUTES

MARINADE
⅓ cup white miso paste
¼ cup unsweetened coconut milk, stirred
2 teaspoons minced garlic
2 teaspoons granulated sugar
1 teaspoon finely grated fresh ginger

6 skinless black cod (sable fish) fillets, 5 to 6 ounces
    each and about ½ inch thick
6 banana leaves, each about 12 inches square
6 scallions, white and light green parts, thinly sliced
1½ teaspoons low-sodium soy sauce
4–6 cups steamed rice, optional

1. In a small bowl whisk the marinade ingredients into a smooth paste. Smear the paste all over the fillets. Cover with plastic wrap and refrigerate for 2 hours.

2. Rinse the banana leaves under cool running water or carefully wipe them clean with a soft, damp cloth.

3. Prepare the grill for direct cooking over medium heat.

4. Remove the excess marinade from the fillets, discard the marinade, and place each fillet on the center of a banana leaf. Place some scallions on top. Fold the leaf over to completely enclose the fillet and make a packet. Secure with a toothpick, being careful not to pierce the fish. Brush each packet on both sides with water.

5. Brush the cooking grates clean. Grill the packets over **direct medium heat**, with the lid closed as much as possible, until the leaves are blackened in some parts, 8 to 10 minutes, turning once. (If the leaves begin to burn through, move the packet[s] over *indirect medium heat*.) Remove one of the packets from the grill to check the fish for doneness. If it is opaque all the way through, the fish is done. If not, return to the grill for a few more minutes.

6. Carefully open each packet, remove any pin bones from the fillets, drizzle each with ¼ teaspoon of soy sauce, or more to taste, and serve with steamed rice, if desired.

WAY TO FILLET RED SNAPPER

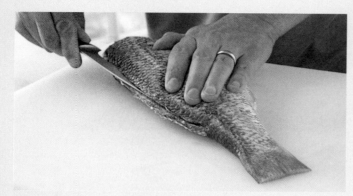

1. Scale the fish, remove the head, and make a shallow cut all along one side of the backbone.

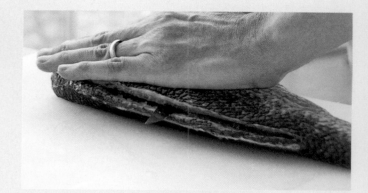

2. Run the knife under the top fillet and over the fish bones.

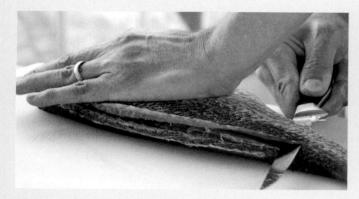

3. Use your other hand to steady the fish as you slide the knife toward the tail. Remove the top fillet.

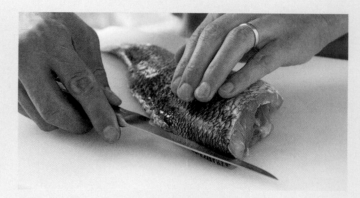

4. Turn the fish over and make a second shallow cut, this time on the other side of the backbone.

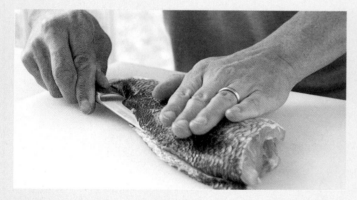

5. Use the tip of the knife to make deeper and deeper cuts along the tops of the bones.

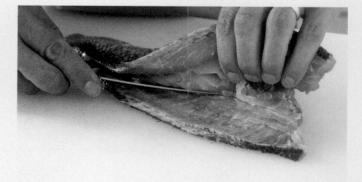

6. Use your other hand to pull the fillet gently upward so you can see where to cut.

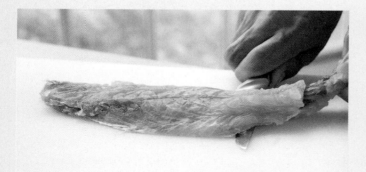

7. To skin the fillets, hold the end of the skin with your fingertips and run the knife just under the flesh.

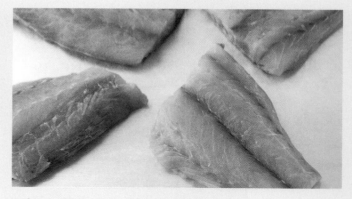

8. Cut the fillets into individual portions.

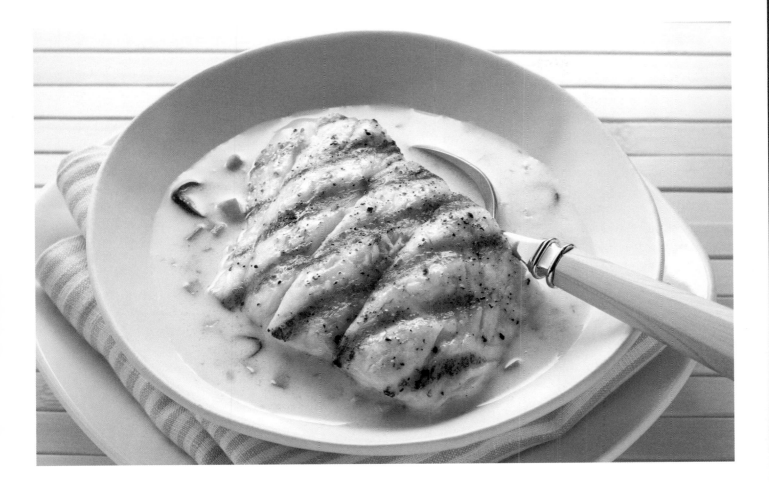

RED SNAPPER IN COCONUT BROTH

SERVES: 8

PREP TIME: 20 MINUTES

WAY TO GRILL: DIRECT HIGH HEAT (450° TO 550°F)

GRILLING TIME: 4 TO 5 MINUTES

BROTH
- 3 tablespoons peanut oil
- 1 cup finely diced carrot
- ¼ cup finely chopped shallot
- 1 teaspoon freshly grated ginger
- 1 teaspoon finely grated lime zest
- 1 can (13½ ounces) unsweetened coconut milk stirred
- ½ cup water
- 3 tablespoons fresh lime juice
- 1 tablespoon granulated sugar
- 2 teaspoons minced or thinly sliced red Thai chile pepper
- 1 teaspoon fish sauce

- 8 skinless red snapper fillets, each 4 to 6 ounces and about ½ inch thick
  Peanut or canola oil
  Kosher salt
  Freshly ground black pepper

1. In a small saucepan over medium heat, warm the oil. Add the carrot, shallot, ginger, and lime zest. Mix well and cook until the carrots are softened, 3 to 5 minutes, stirring often. Add the remaining broth ingredients, mix well, and let simmer for 2 to 3 minutes.

2. Prepare the grill for direct cooking over high heat. Lightly brush each fillet on both sides with oil Season evenly with salt and pepper. Brush the cooking grates clean. Grill over **direct high heat**, with the lid closed as much as possible, until the fish

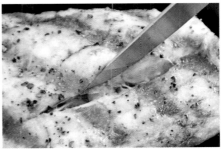

just barely begins to flake when you poke it with the tip of a knife, 4 to 5 minutes, turning once with a spatula. Meanwhile, warm the broth over medium heat.

3. Spoon equal portions of the broth, about ⅓ cup, into 8 shallow bowls. Lay a fillet in the center of each bowl. Serve warm.

WAY TO USE A GRILL PAN FOR VEGETABLES AND FISH

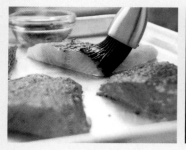
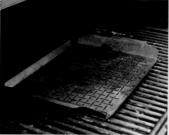
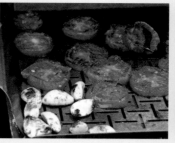
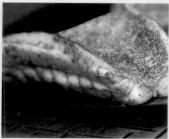

1. Coat the fillets generously with the marinade on both sides.

2. Preheat the grill pan over medium heat for about 10 minutes to prevent food from sticking.

3. Place the vegetables on the grill pan and cook until they soften and begin to brown.

4. Grill each fillet flesh side down first, turning with a spatula only when it releases easily from the grill pan.

SOUTH-OF-THE-BORDER GRILL PAN FISH

SERVES: 4
PREP TIME: 15 MINUTES
MARINATING TIME: 30 MINUTES

WAY TO GRILL: DIRECT MEDIUM HEAT (450° TO 550°F)
GRILLING TIME: 16 TO 20 MINUTES
SPECIAL EQUIPMENT: PERFORATED GRILL PAN

MARINADE
- ¼ cup extra-virgin olive oil
- 4 teaspoons fresh lime juice
- 2 teaspoons pure chile powder
- 1½ teaspoons kosher salt
- ½ teaspoon ground cumin
- ½ teaspoon granulated garlic
- ½ teaspoon dried Mexican oregano
- ½ teaspoon paprika

- 4 rock cod, grouper, or red snapper fillets (with skin), 6 to 8 ounces each and about ¾ inch thick
  Kosher salt

- 2 poblano chile peppers, stems and seeds removed, cut into ½-inch rings
- 4 plum tomatoes, cored and cut into ½-inch slices
- 8 garlic cloves, peeled
- 4 large scallions, rinsed and trimmed

1. In a small bowl combine the marinade ingredients. Transfer 2 tablespoons of the marinade to a large bowl.

2. Arrange the fillets in a single layer on a platter, pour the marinade from the small bowl over the fillets to coat each piece evenly, and season with some salt. Cover with plastic wrap and marinate at room temperature for 30 minutes.

3. Place the chiles, tomatoes, garlic, and scallions in the large bowl with the reserved marinade and toss to coat them evenly.

4. Prepare the grill for direct cooking over medium heat. Brush the cooking grates clean. Preheat the grill pan over *direct medium heat* for about 10 minutes. When hot, grill the vegetables on the pan, with the lid closed as much as possible, until the chiles and tomatoes soften and the garlic and scallions begin to brown, 6 to 8 minutes, turning occasionally. Remove the vegetables from the grill pan and set aside. Grill the fish, skin side up, on the grill pan, over *direct medium heat*, with the lid closed as much as possible, until the fish is opaque and still juicy, 10 to 12 minutes, carefully turning once when the fish releases easily from the grill pan.

5. Transfer the fish to a serving platter and arrange the vegetables all around. Serve warm.

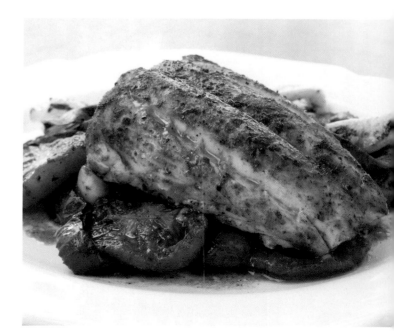

WHOLE STRIPED BASS
IN MOROCCAN MARINADE

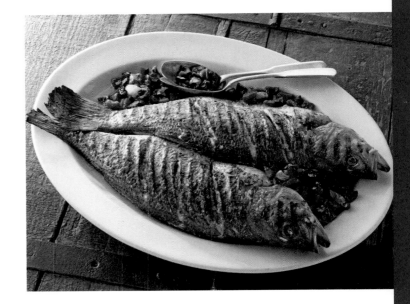

SERVES: 4 TO 6
PREP TIME: 10 MINUTES
MARINATING TIME: 2 TO 3 HOURS

WAY TO GRILL: DIRECT MEDIUM HEAT (350° TO 450°F)
GRILLING TIME: 12 TO 15 MINUTES

MARINADE
⅓ cup extra-virgin olive oil
¼ cup fresh lemon juice
¼ cup chopped fresh Italian parsley
¼ cup chopped fresh cilantro
1 tablespoon minced garlic
1½ teaspoons sweet paprika
1 teaspoon ground cumin
1 teaspoon kosher salt
½ teaspoon freshly ground black pepper
¼ teaspoon ground cayenne pepper

2 whole striped bass, 1½ to 2 pounds each, scaled, cleaned, and fins removed

1. In a medium bowl combine the marinade ingredients. Set aside ⅓ cup to spoon over the fish after grilling.

2. Cut 3 or 4 slashes about ½ inch deep and 1 inch apart on each side of the fish.

3. Place the fish on a sheet pan. Spread the marinade over the fish, inside and out, working it well into the cuts. Cover with plastic wrap, and refrigerate the fish and the reserved marinade for 2 to 3 hours.

4. Prepare the grill for direct cooking over medium heat.

5. Remove the fish from the refrigerator and brush with a little more olive oil. Grill over **direct medium heat**, with the lid closed

as much as possible, until the flesh is opaque near the bone but still juicy, 12 to 15 minutes, carefully turning once. Transfer to a platter and spoon the reserved marinade over the top. If desired, serve with Roasted Pepper, Lemon, and Olive Relish (see recipe below).

ROASTED PEPPER, LEMON, AND OLIVE RELISH
PREP TIME: 10 MINUTES

2 roasted red bell peppers, peeled, seeded, and cut into ¼-inch dice
1 whole lemon peeled, white pith removed, segmented, seeded, and coarsely chopped
½ cup oil-cured black olives, pitted and coarsely chopped
⅓ cup extra-virgin olive oil
2 tablespoons fresh lemon juice
2 tablespoons chopped fresh cilantro
Kosher salt
Freshly ground black pepper

1. In a medium bowl combine the relish ingredients, including salt and pepper to taste. Keep at room temperature.

WAY TO PREP WHOLE FISH

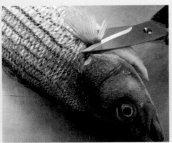

1. Scale the fish and cut off the pectoral fins with kitchen scissors.

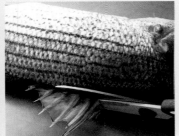

2. Cut the spiny dorsal fins off the backbone.

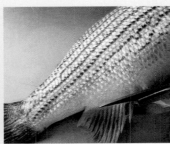

3. Also cut off the fins along the belly (ventral) side of the fish.

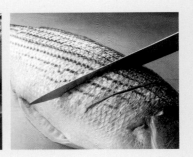

4. Cut 3 or 4 slashes about ½ inch deep and 1 inch apart on each side of the fish.

WAY TO GRILL TROUT IN A BASKET

Whole fish can be difficult to grill without their skins sticking to the grate. A fish basket allows you to turn the fish easily. Just be sure to oil the basket itself so the skins of the fish pull away cleanly after they are cooked.

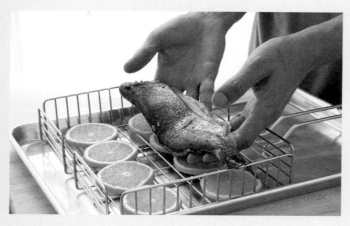

1. Lining the fish basket with orange slices, lettuce leaves, or thick scallions prevents the skins of the fish from sticking to the basket.

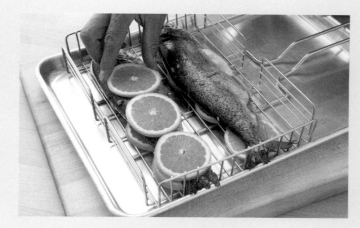

2. In this recipe, the juice of the orange also complements the sake marinade on the fish.

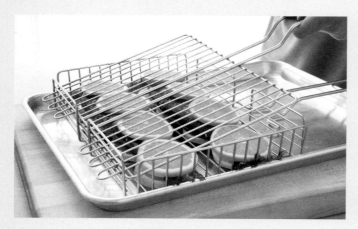

3. Lower the moveable section of the basket so that it rests snugly on the top layer of orange slices, preventing the ingredients from shifting.

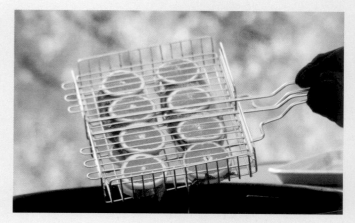

4. You can grill the fish without the cooking grate. Just wear barbecue mitts and hold the basket over the coals, turning it over as needed for even cooking.

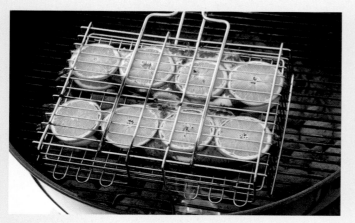

5. If flare-ups occur, move quickly to rotate the basket away from the flames.

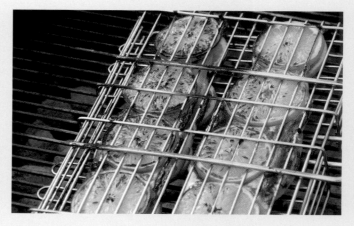

6. The goal is to lightly char the orange and cook the fish all the way to the bone without burning the skins.

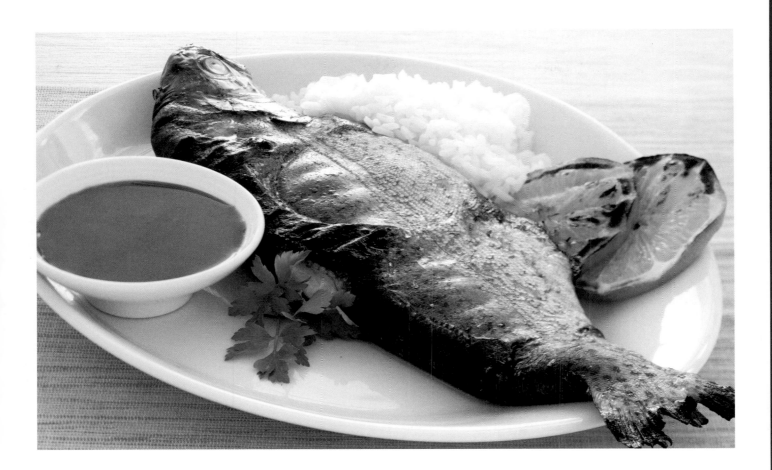

SAKE-MARINATED TROUT

SERVES: 4
PREP TIME: 25 MINUTES
MARINATING TIME: 15 TO 30 MINUTES

WAY TO GRILL: DIRECT MEDIUM HEAT (350° TO 450°F)
GRILLING TIME: ABOUT 8 MINUTES
SPECIAL EQUIPMENT: FISH BASKET

MARINADE
⅓ cup sake or dry sherry
¼ cup soy sauce
¼ cup mirin (sweet rice wine)
2 tablespoons peeled and finely chopped fresh ginger
2 tablespoons unseasoned rice vinegar
2 garlic cloves, finely chopped
¼ teaspoon crushed red pepper flakes

4 whole boneless trout, each about ¾ pound, cleaned
   and gutted
   Vegetable oil
4–6 oranges, cut into 32 slices, each about ¼ inch thick

1. In a medium bowl whisk the marinade ingredients. Place the trout in a large, resealable plastic bag and pour in the marinade. Press out the air and seal the bag tightly. Turn to distribute the marinade. Refrigerate for 15 to 30 minutes. Take care not to over marinate the fish. (Although this marinade isn't highly acidic, the delicate flesh could become overwhelmed by the sake, soy sauce, and mirin.)

2. Remove the trout from the bag and transfer to a sheet pan. Strain the marinade into a medium saucepan. Bring to a boil over medium-high heat. Cook until syrupy and reduced to about ¼ cup, 10 to 15 minutes. Set aside.

3. Prepare the grill for direct cooking over medium heat.

4. Lightly brush the inside of the grill basket with oil. Lay 4 orange slices in the basket and place 1 trout on top of them. Then place 4 more orange slices on top of the fish in the same manner. Repeat with the remaining trout, and then close and secure the grill basket (if your grill basket is not large enough to hold 4 whole trout, you will need to grill the fish in 2 batches). Grill the trout over **direct medium heat**, with the grill lid open, until the flesh is opaque in the center and the skin and oranges are lightly charred, about 8 minutes, turning every 2 minutes and rotating the basket when needed for even cooking. Using a spatula, carefully remove the trout from the grill basket and transfer each fish to a dinner plate. Serve hot with the reduced marinade on the side.

WAY TO TRIM TROUT

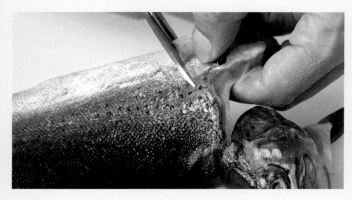

1. Trim off the collarbone with scissors and cut off the head.

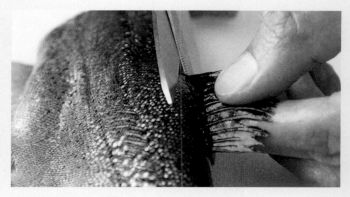

2. Cut off the dorsal fin.

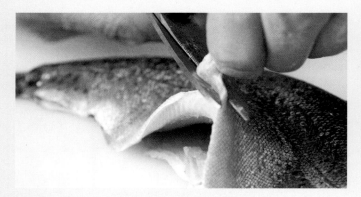

3. Cut off the fins attached to each side of the belly.

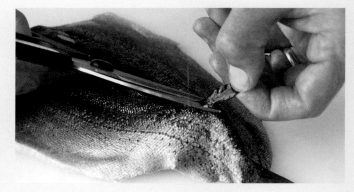

4. Cut off the fin near the tail.

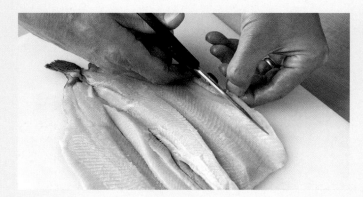

5. Trim the very thin edges of the belly.

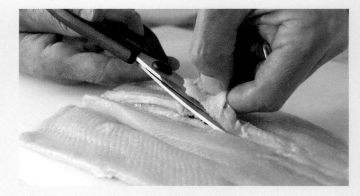

6. Remove the bit of backbone between the fillets.

WAY TO SEGMENT AN ORANGE

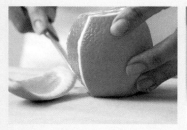

1. Slice off the ends of each orange and stand it upright. Following the curve of the sides, slice off the peel, leaving as much flesh as possible.

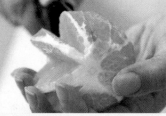

2. Cut out the individual segments by slicing as close as possible to the membrane on both sides of each segment.

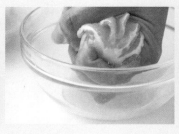

3. Squeeze the remaining orange "skeleton" to capture all the juices.

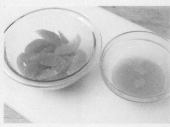

4. Use the segments for the salad and the juice for the dressing.

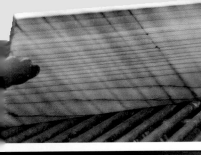

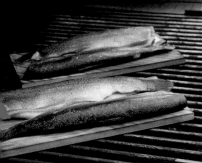

Heat the soaked cedar planks by themselves until they begin to smoke and char. Then turn them over and set the trout on top to cook and smoke simultaneously.

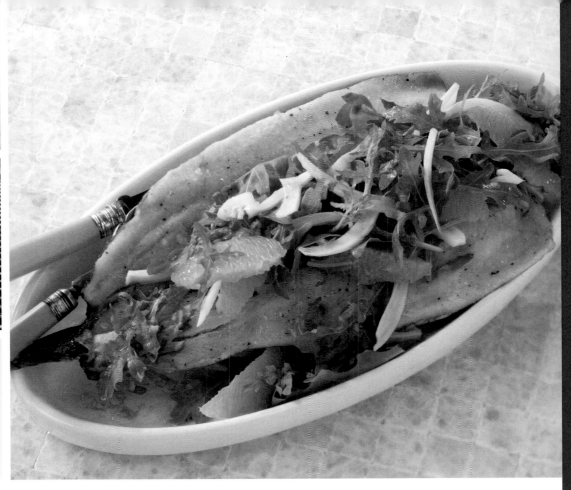

CEDAR-PLANKED TROUT WITH ARUGULA, FENNEL, AND ORANGE

SERVES: 4 TO 6
PREP TIME: 20 TO 25 MINUTES

WAY TO GRILL: DIRECT MEDIUM-HIGH HEAT
   (375° TO 450°F)
GRILLING TIME: 11 TO 18 MINUTES
SPECIAL EQUIPMENT: 2 UNTREATED CEDAR PLANKS,
   EACH 12 TO 15 INCHES LONG AND ½ TO ¾ INCH
   THICK, SOAKED IN WATER FOR AT LEAST 1 HOUR

   2 tablespoons red wine vinegar
   1 small shallot, finely chopped
   2 medium oranges
   ¼ cup grapeseed oil
      Kosher salt
      Freshly ground black pepper

   4 whole boneless trout, each about ¾ pound, cleaned
      and gutted with head, tails, and fins removed
      Extra-virgin olive oil

   3 cups arugula
   1 medium fennel bulb, cored and thinly sliced

1. In a small, non-reactive bowl combine the vinegar and shallot. Zest 1 of the oranges, and then peel and segment both oranges, reserving the juice. Set aside the orange segments. Whisk the orange juice (there should be about ¼ cup) into the vinegar and shallot. Drizzle in the oil, whisking constantly, and then season to taste with salt and pepper.

2. Prepare the grill for direct cooking over medium-high heat. Rinse the trout under cold water and pat dry with paper towels. Lightly brush the inside of the trout with oil and generously season with salt and pepper.

3. Place the soaked planks over ***direct medium-high heat*** and close the lid. After 5 to 10 minutes, when the planks begin to smoke and char, turn them over and then place two trout, slightly overlapping, on each plank. Grill over ***direct medium-high heat***, with the lid closed, until the fish are firm to the touch and cooked through, 5 to 8 minutes.

4. Using a spatula, carefully lift each fish onto an individual serving plate, skin side down and open like a book.

5. Put the arugula in one bowl and the orange segments and fennel in another. Season both with salt and pepper and toss with vinaigrette. Spoon some of the orange-fennel mixture over each fish, top with the dressed greens, and garnish with the remaining orange and fennel mixture.

WAY TO PREP SQUID

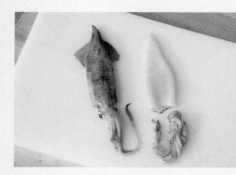

1. Cleaning a whole squid (left) will leave you with a tube-like body and separate tentacles (right).

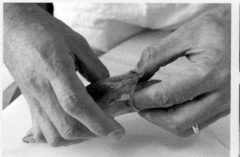

2. To start, pull the tentacles away from the body (tube) of each squid. Then reach inside to grab the end of the hard quill.

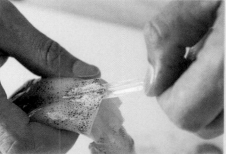

3. Pull the plastic-like quill out of the tube and discard.

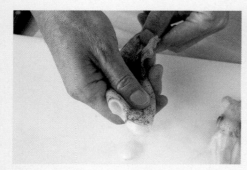

4. Squeeze the tube to push out and discard the mushy innards.

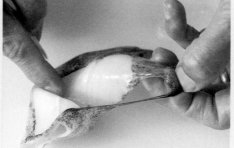

5. Scratch the surface of the brownish skin and peel it off the tubes. Discard the skin.

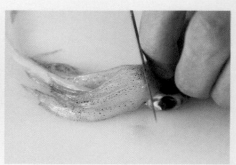

6. Cut the tentacles from the head just above the eyes. Discard the eyes.

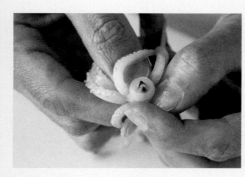

7. Squeeze the hard mouth (beak) from the tentacles and discard it.

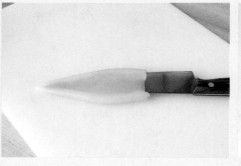

8. Slide a knife into each tube.

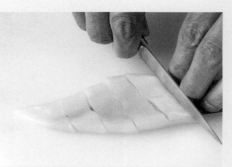

9. The knife inside the tube allows you to score each tube without cutting all the way through.

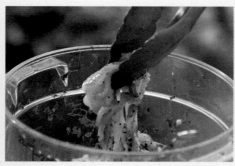

10. As you remove the squid from the marinade, shake off the excess liquid to help browning.

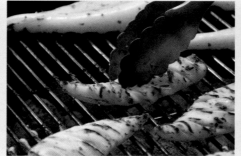

11. Grill the tubes as quickly as possible over very high heat.

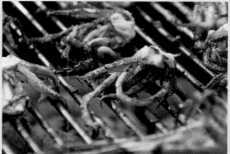

12. The tentacles will cook a little faster. Be careful not to lose them through the cooking grate.

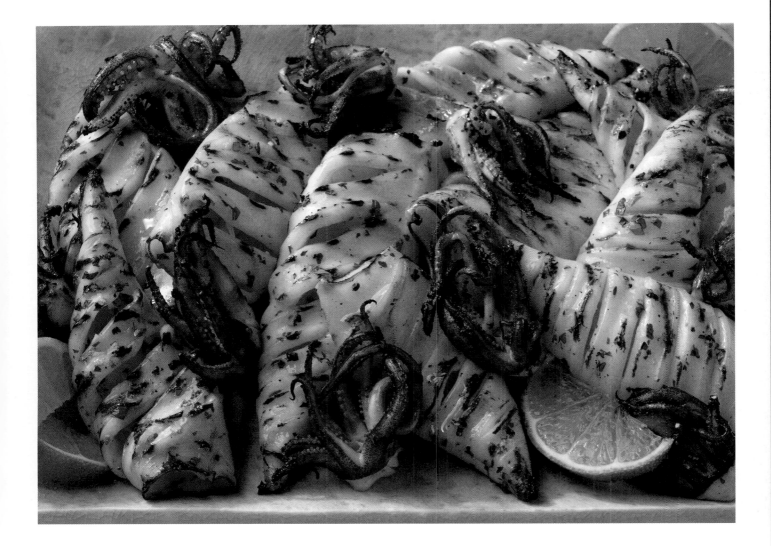

THAI SQUID

SERVES: 4
PREP TIME: 45 MINUTES
MARINATING TIME: 20 MINUTES

WAY TO GRILL: DIRECT HIGH HEAT (450° TO 550°F)
GRILLING TIME: 2 TO 3 MINUTES

  12 whole, small squid

MARINADE
  ¼ cup finely chopped fresh cilantro
  ¼ cup fresh lime juice
  ¼ cup fish sauce
  2 tablespoons granulated sugar
  1 tablespoon minced garlic
  ½ teaspoon freshly ground black pepper

1. Hold each squid and gently pull to separate the tube from the tentacles. Pull out and discard any remaining contents from inside the tube, including the plastic-like quill. Peel off the brownish skin that covers the tube. Rinse the inside of the tube and set aside. Slice off the tentacles portion just above the eyes and discard everything except the tentacles. Squeeze out and discard the hard peak found at the base of the tentacles. Remove the gritty "teeth" on the tentacles (you can feel them) by rubbing them between your fingers under cold running water.

2. In a large bowl combine the marinade ingredients. Add the squid and toss to coat them evenly. Cover and refrigerate for 20 minutes. Prepare the grill for direct cooking over high heat.

3. Remove the squid from the bowl and discard the marinade. Brush the cooking grates clean. Grill the squid over **direct high heat**, with the lid open, until they are just turning opaque and no longer look wet, 2 to 3 minutes, turning once. Serve warm.

WAY TO GRILL CALAMARI UNDER BRICKS

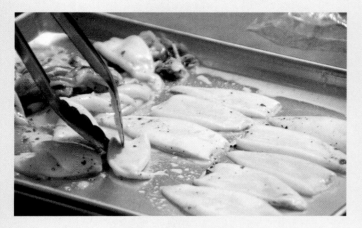

1. On a sheet pan, divide the tubes from the tentacles. Everything should be well coated with the marinade.

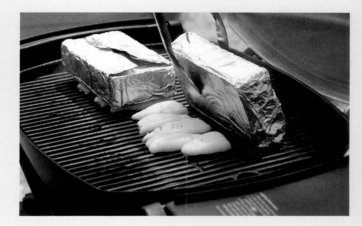

2. Line up the tubes on the grill in groups of 4. Immediately set a brick on top of each group, with the smooth side of the foil facing down.

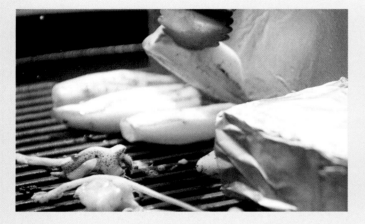

3. Grill the tubes for about 2 minutes. Then carefully roll the bricks over onto their sides so you can turn the tubes over.

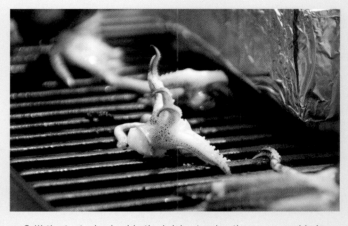

4. Grill the tentacles beside the bricks, turning them once and being careful not to lose them through the grate.

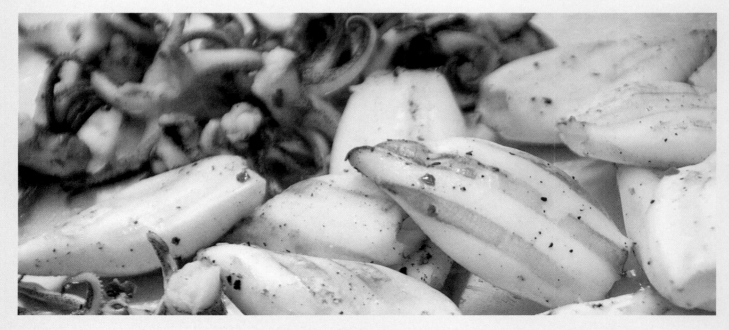

5. For the most flavorful and tender calamari possible, lightly char them over very high heat and remove them from the grill before they overcook.

BRICKYARD CALAMARI SALAD

SERVES: 4
PREP TIME: 25 MINUTES
MARINATING TIME: 30 MINUTES

WAY TO GRILL: DIRECT HIGH HEAT (450° TO 550°F)
GRILLING TIME: ABOUT 4 MINUTES PER BATCH
SPECIAL EQUIPMENT: 2 FOIL-WRAPPED BRICKS

DRESSING
 3 tablespoons fresh lemon juice
 1 teaspoon minced garlic
 ½ teaspoon crushed red pepper flakes
 ½ teaspoon kosher salt
 ¼ teaspoon freshly ground black pepper
 ⅓ cup extra-virgin olive oil

 12 whole, small squid, cleaned (see page 224)
 ¼ teaspoon kosher salt
 ¼ teaspoon freshly ground black pepper
 1½ cups small cherry tomatoes, halved
 ¼ cup ¼-inch-diced red onion
 2 large ripe Haas avocados, cubed
 1½ tablespoons chopped fresh oregano

1. In a medium bowl combine the lemon juice, garlic, red pepper flakes, salt, and pepper. Slowly whisk in the olive oil.

2. Season the calamar with the salt and pepper and place on a sheet pan with 2 tablespoons of the dressing. Toss to coat and let marinate at room temperature for about 30 minutes.

3. Prepare the grill for direct cooking over high heat. Brush the cooking grates clean.

4. Making two rows, place about 4 calamari tubes in a line over **direct high heat** so they can be weighted under the bricks. Place the bricks on top of the tubes, with the smooth side of the foil facing down, and grill, with the lid closed as much as possible, until the tubes easily lift off the cooking grate, about 2 minutes. Wearing insulated barbecue mitts and using tongs, carefully tilt the bricks onto their sides off of the tubes. Turn the tubes over, and set the bricks back in place over the tubes for an additional 2 minutes. Transfer the tubes to a platter. Repeat with the remaining tubes, brushing the cooking grates clean after you remove the first batch. Grill the tentacles beside the bricks for about 4 minutes, turning once

5. Put the tomatoes and onion into the bowl with the remaining dressing and toss to coat. Spoon the tomatoes and diced onion over the calamari tubes and add the avocado. Sprinkle with the oregano.

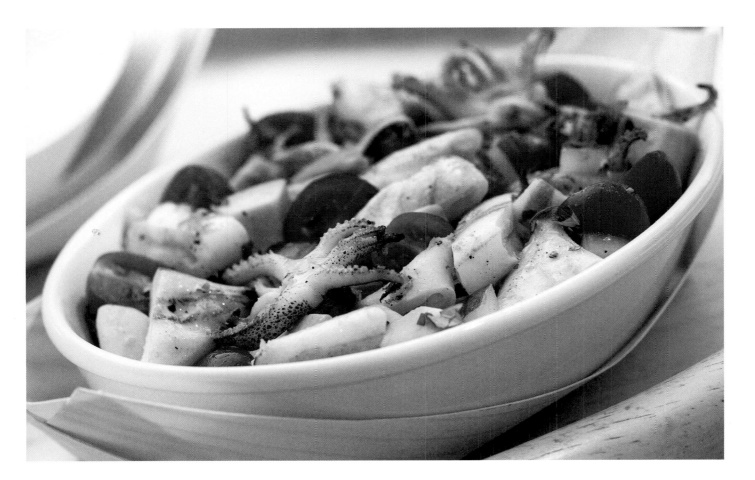

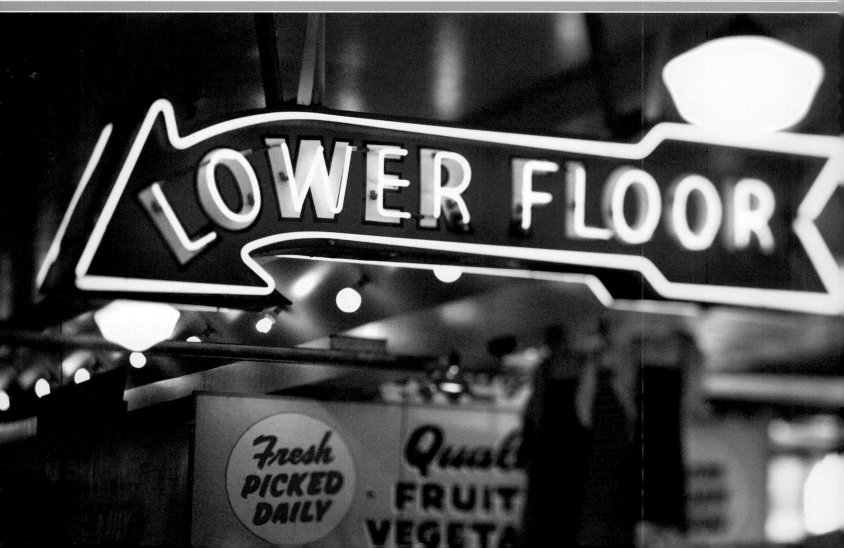

WAY TO GRILL™

VEGETABLES

TECHNIQUES

RECIPES

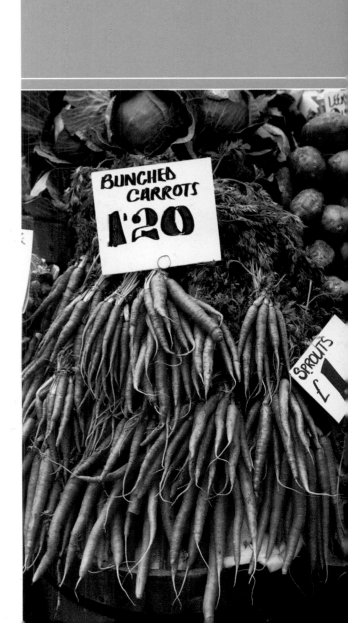

WAY TO MAKE POLENTA

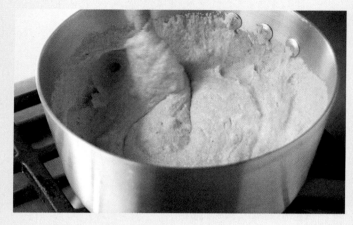

1. As soon as the polenta begins to boil, turn the heat to low and stir with a wooden spoon to prevent the hot mixture from splattering out of the saucepan.

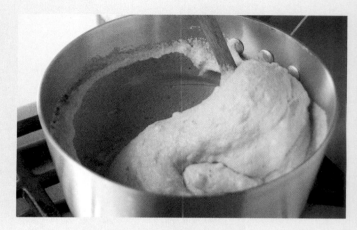

2. Cook over low heat until the polenta is thick and no longer gritty. Continue to stir every few minutes to prevent sticking and scorching on the bottom and sides of the saucepan.

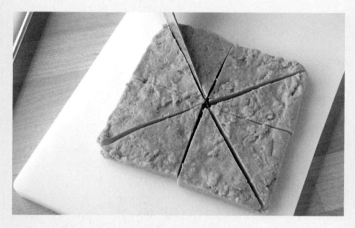

3. Scrape the hot polenta into an oiled pan and smooth it out with the back of a wet spoon or spatula. Allow the mixture to cool and firm up for a couple hours. Then flip it onto a board and cut it into serving pieces.

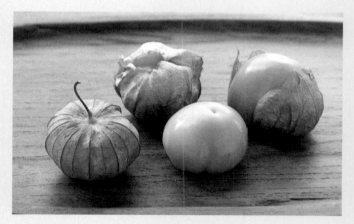

4. Tomatillos provide really nice tangy and herblike flavors to the base of the sauce. You will often find them with papery husks still attached. Peel the husks off and rinse each tomatillo under water to remove the sticky coating.

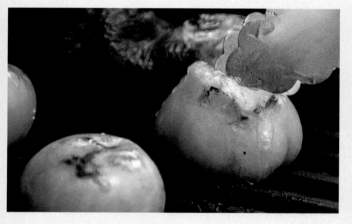

5. Grill the tomatillos over direct medium heat until their skins begin to break, turning occasionally. During this grilling time, their flavors will turn richer, sweeter, and more concentrated.

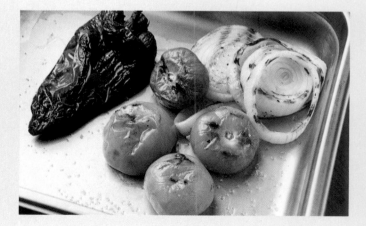

6. Grill the poblano pepper and onion slices at the same time as the tomatillos. Once the pepper has been peeled and seeded, puree the vegetables with some olive oil, fresh cilantro, brown sugar, and salt for a bold vegetarian sauce to serve with grilled polenta.

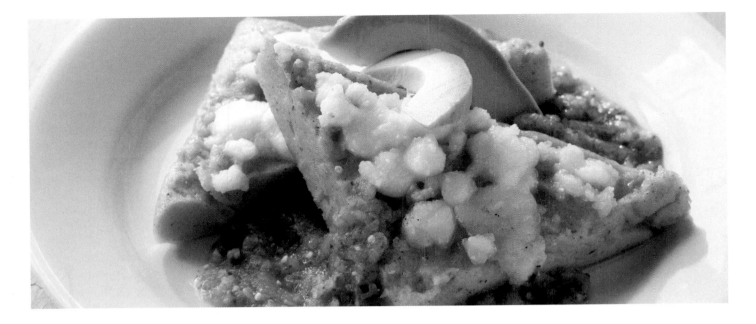

POLENTA WITH QUESO FRESCO AND ROASTED TOMATILLO SAUCE

SERVES: 4
PREP TIME: 40 MINUTES
COOLING TIME: 2 HOURS

WAY TO GRILL: DIRECT AND INDIRECT MEDIUM HEAT
(350° TO 450°F)
GRILLING TIME: 18 TO 22 MINUTES

POLENTA
  2 tablespoons unsalted butter
  ½ cup finely chopped yellow onion
  4 cups milk
  1 cup polenta
  1 teaspoon prepared chili powder
  ¾ teaspoon kosher salt
    Extra-virgin olive oil

SAUCE
  2 slices yellow onion, each about ½ inch thick
  4 tomatillos, about ½ pound total, papery skins
    removed, rinsed
  1 small poblano chile, 3 to 4 inches long
  ¼ cup tightly packed fresh cilantro leaves
  ½ teaspoon brown sugar
  ¼ teaspoon kosher salt

  4 ounces queso fresco cheese, crumbled
  1 ripe Haas avocado

1. In a large saucepan over medium heat, melt the butter. Add the onion and cook until lightly browned, 3 to 5 minutes, stirring occasionally. Add the milk, polenta, chili powder, and salt; whisk to blend. Whisk often until the mixture begins to boil. Turn the heat to very low and stir with a wooden spoon almost constantly to prevent splattering or burning. Cook and stir until the polenta is very thick and no longer gritty to bite, 15 to 20 minutes.

2. Brush the inside of an 8-inch square pan with 1 tablespoon of oil. Scrape the hot polenta into the pan and spread into a smooth, even layer. Let cool at room temperature for 2 hours. Prepare the grill for direct and indirect cooking over medium heat.

3. Brush the onion slices, tomatillos, and chile with olive oil. Brush the cooking grates clean. Grill the vegetables over **direct medium heat**, with the lid closed as much as possible, until the onions are lightly charred, the tomatillos soften and begin to collapse, and the chile is slightly softened and lightly charred, turning as needed. The onions will take 8 to 10 minutes, the tomatillos about 10 minutes, and the chile, 10 to 12 minutes. Remove the vegetables from the grill as they are done. Place the chile in a bowl. Cover with plastic wrap and let steam for 10 to 15 minutes.

4. When the chile is cool enough to handle, pull off and discard the skin, stem, and seeds. Put the vegetables, the cilantro, brown sugar, and salt in a food processor or blender. Whirl until evenly pureed. Add more brown sugar and salt to taste.

5. Invert the pan of polenta onto a cutting board, tapping to release the polenta if necessary. Cut the polenta into 4 to 8 pieces of whatever size and shape you like.

6. Set the pieces of polenta, smooth and oiled side down, over **indirect medium heat**. Carefully pile the crumbed cheese on top of each piece. Grill, with the lid closed, until the polenta is warm and the cheese begins to melt, 8 to 10 minutes, without turning. While the polenta is on the grill, peel and thinly slice the avocado.

7. Transfer the polenta to serving plates. Spoon the tomatillo sauce over the polenta and top with avocado slices.

WAY TO GRILL CORN IN EMBERS

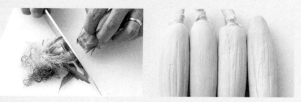

1. Cut off the exposed brownish silk and peel the layers of the husk until you begin to see some kernels showing through the layers. Now the charcoal flavors can penetrate the kernels.

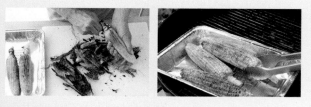

2. Lay the ears of corn on and alongside the embers, turning them as the husks blacken in spots.

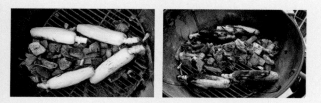

3. Let the ears of corn cool a bit and then peel off the remaining layers of the husk. Finish cooking the corn in a pan of melted lemon-curry butter.

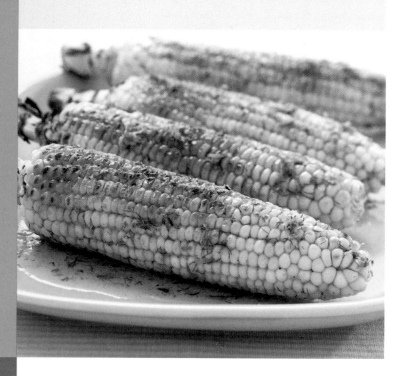

EMBER-ROASTED CORN WITH LEMON-CURRY BUTTER

SERVES: 4
PREP TIME: 10 MINUTES

WAY TO GRILL: DIRECT MEDIUM HEAT (350° TO 450°F)
    FOR CHARCOAL GRILLS ONLY
GRILLING TIME: 20 TO 25 MINUTES

BUTTER
  ¼ cup (½ stick) unsalted butter, softened
  1 tablespoon finely chopped fresh dill
  2 teaspoons finely grated lemon zest
  1 teaspoon curry powder
  ½ teaspoon kosher salt
  ⅛ teaspoon freshly ground black pepper

  4 ears fresh sweet corn, in husks

1. Prepare the charcoal grill as seen on the left. Let the coals burn down to medium heat.

2. In a small bowl mash the butter ingredients with the back of a fork. Mix until the ingredients are evenly distributed.

3. Trim the pointed end of each ear of corn, cutting off and discarding the fine silk sticking out of the husk. Remove and discard a layer or two of the tough outer leaves of each husk. If you can see some kernels through the transparent leaves, that's good.

4. Carefully lay the ears of corn in a single layer on the charcoal grate, on and alongside the coals. Cook the ears of corn there, with the lid closed as much as possible, until the husks are blackened all over and the kernels are tender, 15 to 20 minutes, swapping the positions of the ears and rolling them over a few times for even cooking. If any of the kernels are exposed, keep that side away from direct exposure to the coals. If the outer leaves burn, that's okay.

5. Using long-handled tongs, carefully remove the ears of corn from the grill. Let cool for a few minutes or until you can safely hold them in your hands. Carefully peel off and discard the husk and silk from each ear of corn. Leave the stem ends attached to use as handles.

6. Arrange the corn in a single layer in a pan that will fit on the grill. Add the butter to the pan. When ready to serve, place the pan on the cooking grate and grill over **direct medium heat**, with the lid closed as much as possible, until the butter melts and the ears of corn are warm, about 5 minutes, turning occasionally. If desired, keep the corn warm in the pan over indirect heat while you finish grilling other parts of the meal.

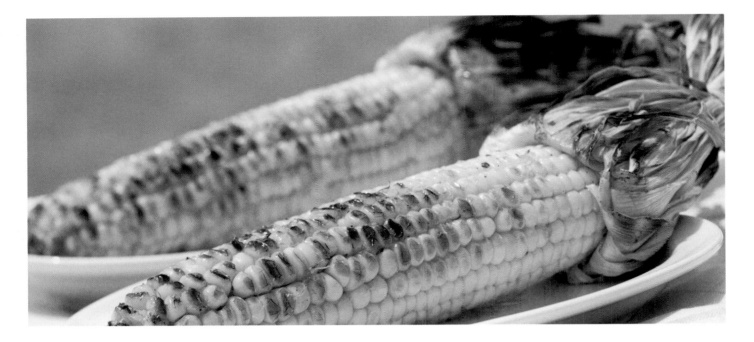

GINGER AND LIME-GLAZED CORN ON THE COB

SERVES: 6
PREP TIME: 15 MINUTES

WAY TO GRILL: DIRECT MEDIUM HEAT (350° TO 450°F)
GRILLING TIME: 10 TO 15 MINUTES

GLAZE
⅓ cup low-sodium chicken broth
4 tablespoons unsalted butter
1 tablespoon granulated sugar
1 teaspoon finely grated lime zest
1 teaspoon kosher salt
1 teaspoon grated fresh ginger

6 ears fresh sweet corn, in husks

1. Prepare the grill for direct cooking over medium heat.

2. In a medium saucepan over medium-high heat, stir the glaze ingredients and bring to a boil. Continue to boil until the glaze slightly thickens, 5 to 7 minutes. Keep the glaze warm.

3. Cut off the top of each ear of corn just above the first row of kernels. Set aside a couple of corn husks to make long strips. Pull the corn husks back, but do not break them off the ears. Remove and discard the corn silk. On each ear, gather the husks together where they narrow toward the ends and use a strip of husk about ½ inch wide to tie the husks together for a handle. Mix and then brush the glaze all over the corn. Brush the cooking grates clean. Grill the corn over **direct medium heat**, with the lid closed as much as possible, letting the husks extend over indirect heat so they do not burn. Cook the corn until it is browned in spots and tender, 10 to 15 minutes, turning several times. Transfer to a platter and baste the kernels with the remaining glaze.

WAY TO PREP CORN ON THE COB

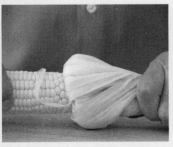
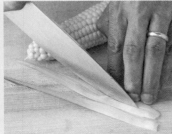
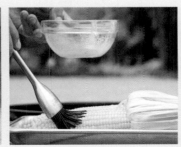
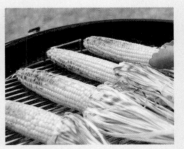

1. Pull the husks back, but leave them attached at the stem end so you have handles. Remove and discard the corn silk.

2. Use a couple of long husks from the outer layers to cut long strips for tying up the handles.

3. Brush the exposed corn kernels with some of the glaze.

4. Grill the corn over direct medium heat, with the handles extending over indirect heat so that they do not burn.

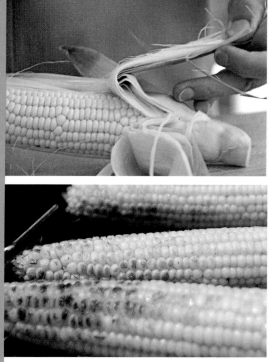

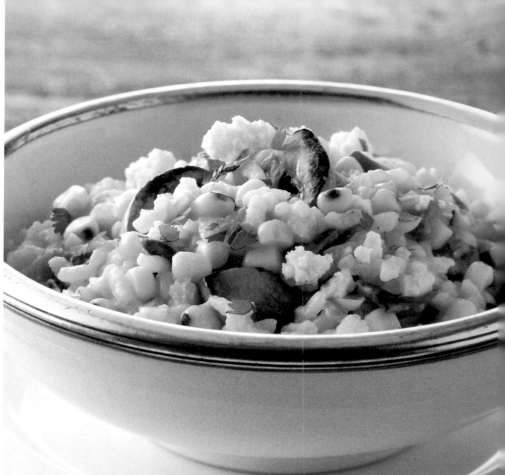

For optimal flavor, fresh corn should be shucked just before grilling. Many of the kernels will turn golden brown and crisp-tender over direct medium heat.

GRILLED CORN AND MUSHROOM RISOTTO

SERVES: 4 TO 6
PREP TIME: 50 MINUTES

WAY TO GRILL: DIRECT MEDIUM HEAT (350° TO 450°F)
GRILLING TIME: 8 TO 10 MINUTES
SPECIAL EQUIPMENT: 12-INCH SKILLET

½ pound button mushrooms, each about 1½ inches wide
1 poblano chile pepper, about 6 inches long
3 ears fresh sweet corn, husked
1 medium yellow onion, cut crosswise into ½-inch slices
   Extra-virgin olive oil
5 cups low-sodium chicken broth
2 tablespoons unsalted butter
1 cup Arborio rice
½ teaspoon kosher salt
1 cup grated chile-jack cheese
½ cup grated cotijia cheese or crumbled feta cheese
¼ cup chopped fresh cilantro leaves

1. Prepare the grill for direct cooking over medium heat.

2. Wipe the mushrooms with a damp cloth or paper towel. Remove and discard the discolored stem ends. Lightly brush the mushrooms, chile, corn, and onion slices with oil.

3. Grill the vegetables over **direct medium heat**, with the lid closed as much as possible, until the mushrooms and onion slices are tender, the chile is blackened and blistered all over, and the corn is browned in spots and tender, 8 to 10 minutes, turning as needed. Remove the vegetables from the grill and let cool. Coarsely chop the mushrooms and cut the corn kernels off the cobs. Scrape off the loosened bits of skin from the chile and discard along with the seeds and stem; finely chop the remaining part of the chile. Roughly chop the onion. In a medium bowl combine the mushrooms, chile, and corn. Set the onion aside. (The vegetables can sit at room temperature for 3 to 4 hours.)

4. In a large saucepan over medium heat, warm the broth until it simmers.

5. In a 12-inch skillet over high heat, melt the butter. Add the onion and rice. Cook until the rice is slightly opaque, 2 to 3 minutes, stirring frequently. Pour in 1 cup of the hot broth and stir the mixture often until the broth is absorbed.

6. Continue to add the hot broth, 1 cup at a time, and cook at a simmer until the broth is absorbed and the rice is tender, 20 to 30 minutes, stirring frequently. When the rice is fully cooked, the mixture should be creamy but not soupy. At this point, add the remaining grilled vegetables and the salt.

7. Remove the risotto from the heat, add the chile-jack cheese, and stir until melted. Spoon risotto into warm, wide bowls, and top with cotijia cheese and cilantro.

VEGETABLES

MARINATED BABY BOK CHOY AND SHIITAKES

SERVES: 4
PREP TIME: 15 MINUTES
MARINATING TIME: 1 TO 2 HOURS

WAY TO GRILL: DIRECT MEDIUM HEAT (350° TO 450°F)
GRILLING TIME: ABOUT 5 MINUTES
SPECIAL EQUIPMENT: PERFORATED GRILL PAN

MARINADE
⅓ cup low-sodium soy sauce
¼ cup dry sherry
1 tablespoon light brown sugar
1 tablespoon dark sesame oil
4 slices peeled fresh ginger, each ⅛ inch thick, crushed
2 garlic cloves, crushed
¼ teaspoon crushed red pepper flakes

4 baby bok choy, larger ones cut in half
20 large shiitake mushrooms

1. In a medium bowl whisk the marinade ingredients until the sugar is dissolved.

2. Plunge the bok choy into a bowl of water and shake to clean off the dirt nestled between the leaves. Wipe the mushrooms clean with a damp cloth or paper towel and then remove and discard the stems.

3. Place the vegetables into a large, resealable plastic bag and pour in the marinade. Press the air out of the bag and seal tightly. Turn the bag to distribute the marinade and let stand at room temperature for 1 to 2 hours, turning occasionally.

4. Prepare the grill for direct cooking over medium heat. Preheat a grill pan over **direct medium heat** for about 10 minutes.

5. Remove the vegetables from the bag and reserve the marinade. When the grill pan is hot, place the bok choy and mushrooms onto the pan, spreading them out in a single layer. Grill over **direct medium heat**, with the lid closed as much as possible, until the bok choy is crisp-tender and the shiitakes are heated through, about 5 minutes, turning once or twice and basting occasionally with the reserved marinade. Serve hot.

WAY TO GRILL BOK CHOY AND SHIITAKE MUSHROOMS

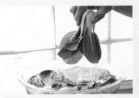
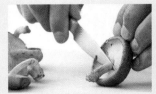

1. Plunge the baby bok choy under water to remove any dirt between the leaves.

2. Remove and discard the tough stems from the mushrooms.

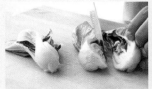
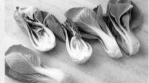

3. Cut the larger bok choy in half, keeping the root ends intact.

4. Leave the smaller bok choy as is.

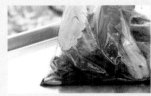
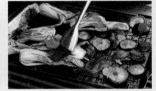
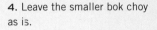

5. Coat the vegetables with the marinade in a large plastic bag.

6. Grill the vegetables on a preheated grill pan, basting occasionally with the marinade.

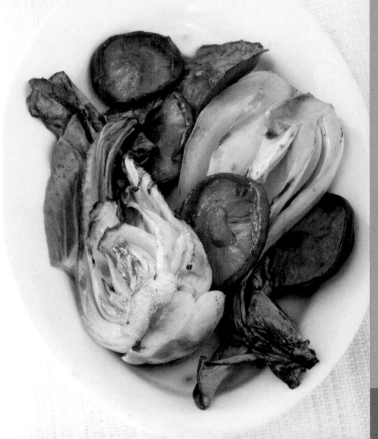

PORTABELLO MUSHROOM SANDWICHES WITH ARUGULA AND BALSAMIC AIOLI

SERVES: 6
PREP TIME: 20 MINUTES
MARINATING TIME: 15 TO 20 MINUTES

WAY TO GRILL: DIRECT MEDIUM HEAT (350° TO 450°F)
GRILLING TIME: 8 TO 12 MINUTES

AIOLI
- ⅓ cup mayonnaise
- 2 tablespoons balsamic vinegar
- 1 teaspoon kosher salt
- ½ teaspoon minced garlic

MARINADE
- ¾ cup extra-virgin olive oil
- ¼ cup red wine vinegar
- 2 tablespoons finely minced shallot
- 1 teaspoon minced garlic
- 1 teaspoon kosher salt
- ½ teaspoon freshly ground black pepper

- 6 large portabello mushrooms, cleaned, stems and black gills removed (see photos below)
  Kosher salt
  Freshly ground black pepper

- 6 Kaiser rolls, cut in half
- 2 ounces arugula, trimmed, rinsed, and dried

1. In a small bowl combine the aioli ingredients. Refrigerate until ready to assemble the sandwiches.

2. In a small bowl whisk the marinade ingredients. Place the mushroom caps, gill sides down, in a large baking pan. Brush the mushroom caps generously with the marinade and turn the caps over. Spoon the rest of the marinade over the gill side. Allow the mushrooms to marinate at room temperature for 15 to 20 minutes.

3. Prepare the grill for direct cooking over medium heat.

4. Remove the mushrooms from the pan and reserve the marinade. Lightly season the mushrooms with salt and pepper. Brush the cooking grates clean. Grill the mushrooms, gill sides down, over **direct medium heat**, with the lid closed as much as possible, until they begin to soften, 4 to 6 minutes. Brush the cap sides of the mushrooms with some of the remaining marinade from the pan. Turn the mushrooms over and grill them until they are tender when pierced with a knife, 4 to 6 minutes.

5. Grill the rolls, cut sides down, over **direct medium heat** until lightly toasted, about 30 seconds.

6. Spread aioli on the toasted buns and top each one with some arugula and a mushroom. Serve warm.

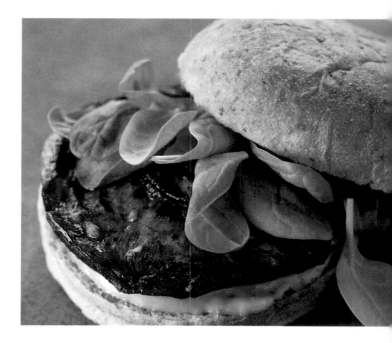

WAY TO GRILL PORTABELLO MUSHROOMS

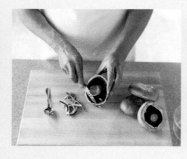

1. Cut away the stems and any curled edges around the rims.

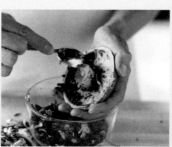

2. With a spoon, gently scrape away the dark gills that might be holding dirt.

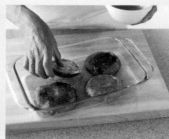

3. Use a vinaigrette to marinate and baste the mushrooms.

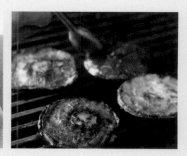

4. Finish grilling the mushrooms with the stem sides facing up so that the juices are held inside the caps.

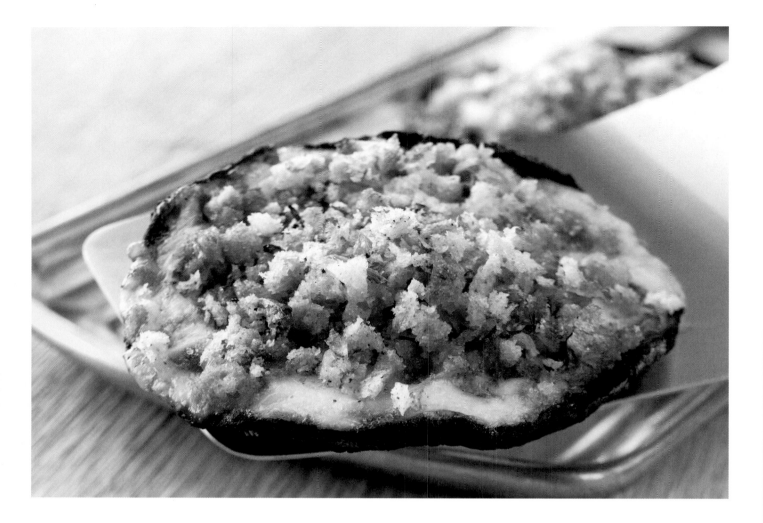

MARINATED PORTABELLO MUSHROOMS WITH ASIAGO

SERVES: 6
PREP TIME: 10 MINUTES
MARINATING TIME: 15 TO 20 MINUTES

WAY TO GRILL: DIRECT MEDIUM HEAT (350° TO 450°F)
GRILLING TIME: 8 TO 12 MINUTES

MARINADE
¼ cup extra-virgin olive oil
3 tablespoons balsamic vinegar
1 tablespoon soy sauce
1 teaspoon chopped fresh rosemary or ½ teaspoon dried
   crushed rosemary
½ teaspoon freshly ground black pepper
¼ teaspoon kosher salt

6 large portabello mushrooms, each 5 to 6 inches
   in diameter
¾ cup fresh bread crumbs
1 tablespoon finely chopped fresh Italian parsley
1½ cups grated Asiago cheese
   Kosher salt
   Freshly ground black pepper

1. In a small bowl whisk the marinade ingredients.

2. Wipe the mushrooms clean with a damp cloth or paper towel. Remove and discard the stems. With a teaspoon, carefully scrape out and discard the black gills from the mushroom caps (see photos on opposite page). Place the mushrooms, cap sides up, on a rimmed plate and brush them with the marinade. Turn the mushrooms over and brush again with the marinade. Let stand for 15 to 20 minutes at room temperature. Prepare the grill for direct cooking over medium heat.

3. In a small bowl combine the bread crumbs with the parsley.

4. Brush the cooking grates clean. Grill the mushrooms, gill sides down, over **direct medium heat**, with the lid closed, until the mushrooms begin to soften, 4 to 6 minutes. Brush the cap sides with some of the remaining marinade from the plate, turn them over, add ¼ cup of cheese on top of each mushroom, close the lid, and cook until tender when pierced with a knife, 4 to 6 minutes. During the last minute of cooking, place the bread crumb mixture evenly on top of each mushroom. Remove from the grill, add salt and pepper to taste, and serve immediately.

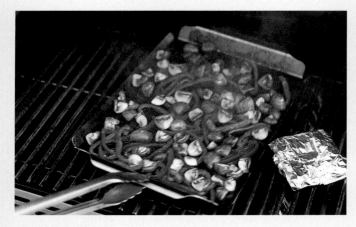

1. A grill pan is a convenient tool for grilling small pizza toppings like chopped mushrooms and bell pepper slices. Roast the garlic in a foil packet.

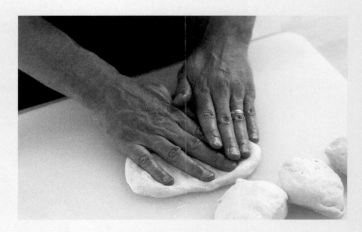

2. To flatten and stretch dough easily, without it springing back, it needs to be at room temperature. If you happen to buy refrigerated dough, let it sit on a counter for a few hours so it will warm up and relax.

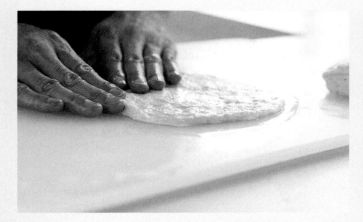

3. A bit of olive oil on your hands and your board will make the dough more pliable. Finish flattening each piece of dough on a sheet of parchment paper.

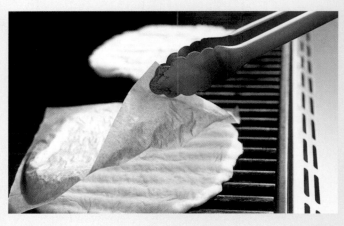

4. The parchment paper will help to hold the shape of the dough as you flip it onto the grill. After a minute or so of grilling, peel off the paper.

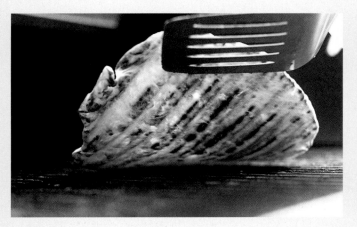

5. The oil will prevent sticking and promote even browning. When the underside is crisp and toasted, transfer the crusts to a work surface, with the grilled sides facing up.

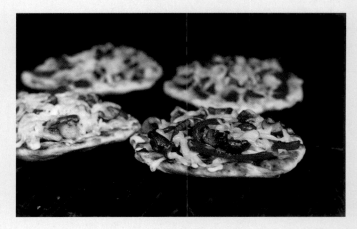

6. Arrange the toppings on the toasted sides and continue to grill the pizzas until the bottoms of the crusts are crisp and the cheese has melted.

PIZZA WITH MUSHROOMS, PEPPERS, GARLIC, AND SMOKED MOZZARELLA

SERVES: 8
PREP TIME: 25 MINUTES
RISING TIME: 1½ TO 2 HOURS

WAY TO GRILL: DIRECT MEDIUM HEAT (350° TO 450°F)
    AND DIRECT MEDIUM-HIGH HEAT (ABOUT 450°F)
GRILLING TIME: 29 TO 46 MINUTES
SPECIAL EQUIPMENT: ELECTRIC STAND MIXER

DOUGH
- 1½ cups warm water (100° to 110°F)
- 1 package rapid-rise active dry yeast
- ½ teaspoon granulated sugar
- 4½ cups all-purpose flour
- 3 tablespoons extra-virgin olive oil
- 2 teaspoons kosher salt

- ¼ cup extra-virgin olive oil
- ½ teaspoon kosher salt
- ¼ teaspoon freshly ground black pepper
- 10 medium garlic cloves, peeled
- 1 large red bell pepper, cut into ¼-inch strips
- ½ pound cremini mushrooms, cleaned, stemmed, and quartered
- 2 cups shredded smoked mozzarella cheese

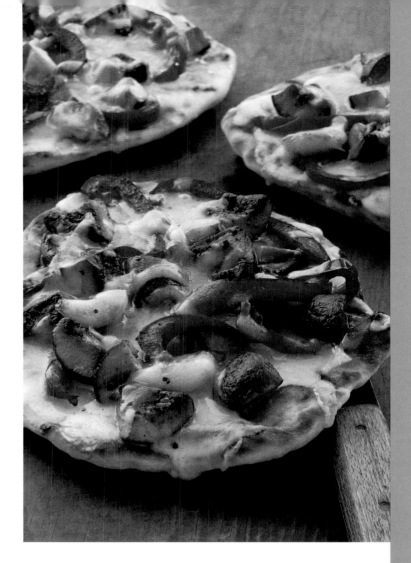

1. In the bowl of an electric stand mixer, combine the water, yeast, and sugar. Stir briefly and let stand for 5 minutes or until the top surface has a thin, frothy layer (this indicates that the yeast is active). Add the flour, oil, and salt. Fit the mixer with the dough hook and mix on low speed for about 1 minute or until the dough begins to come together. Increase the speed to medium. Continue to mix until the dough is slightly sticky, smooth, and elastic, about 10 minutes. Form the dough into a ball and place in a lightly oiled bowl. Turn it over to coat all sides and tightly cover the bowl with plastic wrap. Allow the dough to rise in a warm place until it has doubled in size, 1½ to 2 hours.

2. In a large bowl mix ¼ cup oil with the salt and pepper. Place the garlic cloves in the middle of a small sheet of aluminum foil, about 8 inches square, and pour 1 tablespoon of the oil mixture over the garlic. Fold up the sides to make a sealed packet, leaving a little room for the expansion of steam.

3. Add all the peppers and mushrooms to the bowl with the remaining oil mixture. Toss to coat the vegetables evenly.

4. Prepare the grill for direct cooking over medium-high heat. Preheat a perforated grill pan over **direct medium-high heat** for about 10 minutes. While the pan is preheating, place the packet of garlic over **direct medium-high heat** and cook until the cloves are soft and light brown, 15 to 20 minutes. Remove the packet from the grill. When the grill pan is really hot, using tongs, lift the mushrooms and peppers from the bowl and spread them out in a single layer on the pan. Cook until they are

nicely browned and tender, about 6 minutes, stirring once or twice. Wearing insulated barbecue mitts, remove the pan from the grill and set it down on a heat-proof surface.

5. Cut the dough into 8 equal pieces. Lightly brush eight, 9-inch squares of parchment paper on one side with oil. Using your fingers, flatten each piece of dough on a sheet of parchment paper to create 8 rounds. Each round should be about ⅓ inch thick and 6 to 8 inches in diameter. Lightly brush the tops with oil. Let the rounds sit at room temperature for 5 to 10 minutes.

6. Lower the temperature of the grill to medium heat. Brush the cooking grates clean. Working with 4 rounds at a time, place the dough on the cooking grate with the paper sides facing up. Grill over **direct medium heat**, with the lid closed as much as possible, until the dough is well marked and firm on the underside, 2 to 5 minutes, rotating as needed for even cooking. Peel off and discard the parchment paper. Transfer the crusts to a work surface with the grilled sides facing up. Repeat with the other 4 rounds.

7. Spread the cheese evenly over the crusts and then arrange some garlic, mushrooms, and pepper slices on top. Return the pizzas to the grill and cook over **direct medium heat**, with the lid closed as much as possible, until the cheese is melted and the bottom of the crusts are crisp, 2 to 5 minutes, rotating the pizzas occasionally for even cooking. Transfer to a cutting board and cut into wedges. Serve warm.

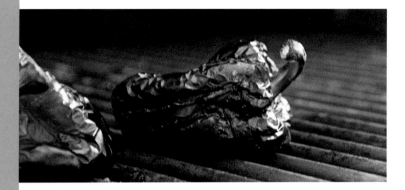

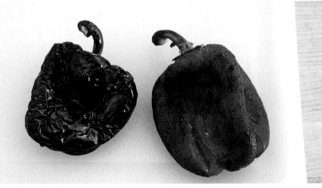

Go ahead and burn them. Roasting chile peppers is one technique where it is okay to burn the food...to a degree. Charring the peppers until black (see above, left) helps to loosen the skin so you can peel it away and enjoy the sweet flesh below (see above, right).

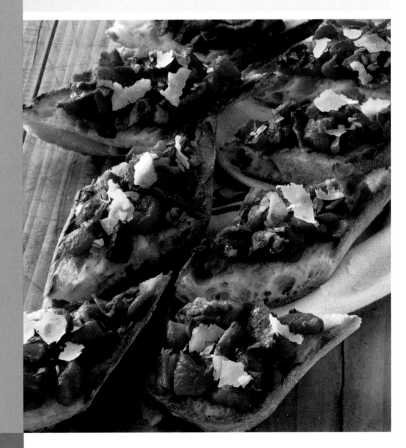

ROASTED PEPPER AND BACON BRUSCHETTA

SERVES: 6 AS AN APPETIZER (MAKES 18 PIECES)
PREP TIME: 15 MINUTES

WAY TO GRILL: DIRECT MEDIUM HEAT (350° TO 450°F)
GRILLING TIME: 13 TO 17 MINUTES

- 3 medium red bell peppers
- 6 strips bacon, cooked and finely chopped
- 2 tablespoons extra-virgin olive oil, divided
- 1 tablespoon red wine vinegar
  Kosher salt
- 1 loaf Italian or French bread, cut in half lengthwise
- ⅓ cup freshly grated Parmigiano-Reggiano cheese
- ¼ cup finely chopped fresh basil

1. Prepare the grill for direct cooking over medium heat. Brush the cooking grates clean. Grill the peppers over **direct medium heat**, with the lid closed as much as possible, until blackened and blistered all over, 12 to 15 minutes, turning every 3 to 5 minutes. Place the peppers in a bowl and cover with plastic wrap. Let stand for 10 to 15 minutes. Remove the peppers from the bowl and peel away and discard the charred skins. Cut off and discard the tops and seeds, and then finely chop the peppers. Transfer the chopped peppers to a medium bowl and toss with the bacon, 2 teaspoons of the oil, and the vinegar. Season to taste with salt.

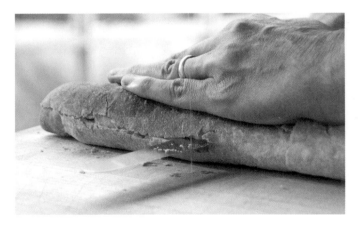

2. Lightly brush or spray the cut sides of the bread with the remaining 4 teaspoons of oil and grill over **direct medium heat** until toasted, 1 to 2 minutes. Remove from the grill and cut the bread on the diagonal into 2-inch-wide pieces.

3. Just before serving, add the cheese to the bell pepper mixture. Spoon the mixture on the toasted pieces of bread. Sprinkle the basil on top and serve at room temperature.

WAY TO GRILL ONIONS

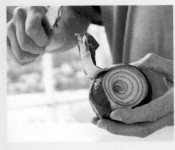 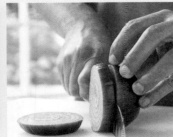 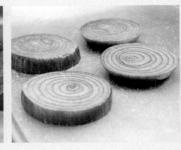 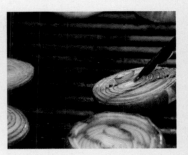

1. Cut off the root and stem ends from each onion. Peel off the papery skin.

2. Cut each onion crosswise into ½-inch slices.

3. The layers will hold together best if they are evenly sliced.

4. When turning the slices, hold the layers closest to the center with tongs.

ROASTED PEPPERS, GRILLED ONIONS, AND FETA CHEESE SALAD

SERVES: 6
PREP TIME: 15 MINUTES

WAY TO GRILL: DIRECT MEDIUM HEAT (350° TO 450°F)
GRILLING TIME: 12 TO 15 MINUTES

VINAIGRETTE
- ¼ cup extra-virgin olive oil
- 2 tablespoons red wine vinegar
- ½ tablespoon finely minced garlic
- ½ teaspoon kosher salt
- ¼ teaspoon freshly ground black pepper

- 2 medium red onions, cut crosswise into ½-inch slices
  Extra-virgin olive oil
- 2 large red bell peppers
- 6 cups arugula, rinsed and dried
- ½ cup toasted walnuts, coarsely chopped
- 1 cup feta cheese, crumbled

1. Prepare the grill for direct cooking over medium heat.

2. In a small bowl whisk the vinaigrette ingredients until emulsified.

3. Lightly brush the onion slices with oil. Brush the cooking grates clean. Grill the onions and bell peppers over ***direct medium heat***, with the lid closed as much as possible, until the onions are tender and the skins of the peppers are evenly charred and blistered, turning occasionally. The onions will take 8 to 12 minutes and the peppers, 12 to 15 minutes. Remove the veggies from the grill. Place the peppers in a medium bowl, cover with plastic wrap, and let them steam for 10 to 15 minutes. When the peppers are cool enough to handle, remove and discard the charred skins, stems, and seeds and cut them into strips about ½ inch wide.

4. Place the peppers and onions in a bowl. Add 2 tablespoons of the vinaigrette and toss to coat.

5. In a salad bowl toss the arugula with the remaining dressing. Top with the onions and peppers and then add the walnuts and feta cheese. Serve right away.

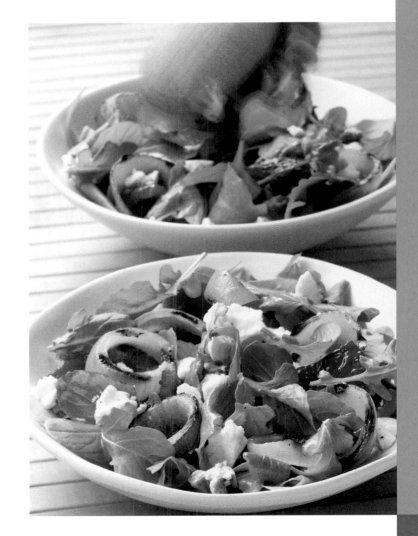

GRILL-ROASTED TOMATO SOUP
WITH PARMESAN CROUTONS

SERVES: 4
PREP TIME: 30 MINUTES

WAY TO GRILL: DIRECT LOW HEAT (250° TO 350°F)
GRILLING TIME: 8 TO 10 MINUTES
SPECIAL EQUIPMENT: PERFORATED GRILL PAN

2	pounds plum tomatoes, firm but ripe
1	red onion, quartered through the stem and peeled
10	medium garlic cloves, peeled
¼	cup lightly packed fresh thyme sprigs
¼	cup extra-virgin olive oil
4	cups low-sodium chicken broth
1	teaspoon granulated sugar
1	teaspoon kosher salt
½	teaspoon freshly ground black pepper
2	tablespoons unsalted butter, softened
8	slices baguette, each about ¼ inch thick
½	cup grated Parmigiano-Reggiano cheese, divided
2	tablespoons roughly chopped fresh basil

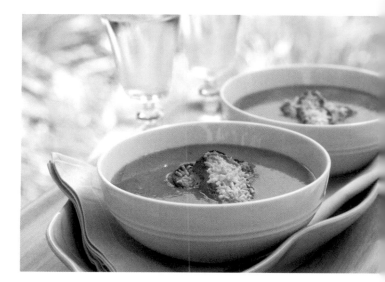

1. Prepare the grill for direct cooking over low heat. Preheat a grill pan over **direct low heat** for about 10 minutes.

2. In a medium bowl combine the tomatoes, onion, garlic, thyme, and oil and toss to coat. Using tongs arrange all the vegetables and herbs on the grill pan and cook over **direct low heat**, with the lid closed as much as possible, until the tomato skins wrinkle and start to brown, 20 to 25 minutes, turning occasionally. Transfer the tomatoes to a large saucepan. Continue to cook the onions, garlic, and thyme until the onions and garlic are lightly charred on all sides, 5 to 10 minutes. Add the onions and garlic to the saucepan. Discard the thyme.

3. Add the chicken broth to the saucepan. Bring to a boil, reduce the heat, and simmer until the tomatoes collapse

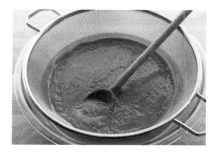

completely, 8 to 10 minutes. Transfer the soup to a blender and puree until very smooth. Pour the soup through a mesh strainer to remove all the tomato seeds and skin. Season with the sugar, salt, and pepper.

4. If the grill has an infrared burner above the warming rack, preheat the burner on **high**, with the grill lid open. Butter one side of each slice of bread. Top each buttered side with about 1 teaspoon of cheese. Using tongs position the bread slices on the warming rack (toward the back) just in front of the burner. Cook, with the lid open, until the cheese melts and browns, about 2 minutes. Watch carefully so the cheese doesn't burn. Remove the croutons from the warming rack. If your grill does not have an infrared burner, toast the croutons under a broiler.

5. Just before serving, reheat the soup, if necessary, and add the basil. Ladle the soup into bowls and float the croutons on top. Garnish with any remaining cheese. Serve warm.

WAY TO GRILL-ROAST TOMATOES

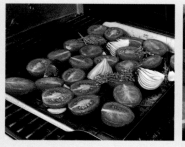

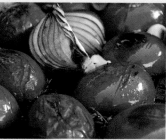

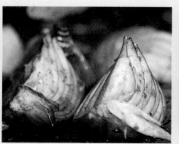

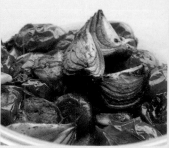

1. Coat the tomatoes and other vegetables with oil and spread them out on a preheated grill pan.

2. Cook over direct low heat until the tomato skins wrinkle and brown.

3. Turn the vegetables occasionally for even caramelization.

4. Don't be afraid of deep, dark colors on the vegetables. That's where the flavor is.

VEGETABLES

242

PANZANELLA SKEWERS
WITH SHERRY VINAIGRETTE

SERVES: 4
PREP TIME: 15 MINUTES

WAY TO GRILL: DIRECT MEDIUM HEAT (350° TO 450°F)
GRILLING TIME: ABOUT 4 MINUTES
SPECIAL EQUIPMENT: 4 BAMBOO SKEWERS,
    SOAKED IN WATER FOR AT LEAST 30 MINUTES

VINAIGRETTE
  2 tablespoons sherry vinegar
  1 teaspoon Dijon mustard
  ½ teaspoon finely chopped garlic
  6 tablespoons extra-virgin olive oil
  ¼ teaspoon kosher salt
  ¼ teaspoon freshly ground black pepper

  1 small loaf focaccia or Italian bread, cut into
     1-inch cubes
  1 pint cherry tomatoes, firm but ripe
  4 cups baby arugula
  ⅓ cup fresh basil leaves, coarsely chopped
  2 tablespoons freshly grated Parmigiano-Reggiano cheese

1. Prepare the grill for direct cooking over medium heat.

2. In a small bowl whisk the vinegar, mustard, and garlic. Slowly drizzle and whisk in the oil until it is emulsified. Season with the salt and pepper.

3. In a large bowl combine the bread cubes and tomatoes with 2 tablespoons of the vinaigrette and toss to coat. Thread the bread cubes and tomatoes alternately on the skewers.

4. Brush the cooking grates clean. Grill the skewers over **direct medium heat**, with the lid open, until the tomato skins brown and the bread is lightly toasted, about 4 minutes, turning every minute (if the bread starts to burn, move the skewer over indirect heat for the remaining time).

5. In a large bowl toss the arugula and basil with 2 tablespoons of vinaigrette. Brush the skewers with the remaining vinaigrette. To serve, divide the salad greens evenly onto serving plates and top with a panzanella skewer. Sprinkle with the cheese.

WAY TO PREP VINAIGRETTE

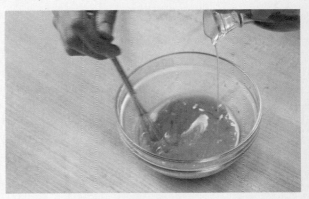

1. Whisk the vinegar, mustard, and garlic first. The mustard will help to emulsify the oil.

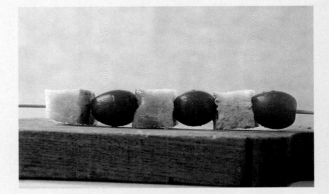

2. Add the extra-virgin olive oil slowly, whisking all the time for a smooth dressing.

WAY TO PREP SKEWERS

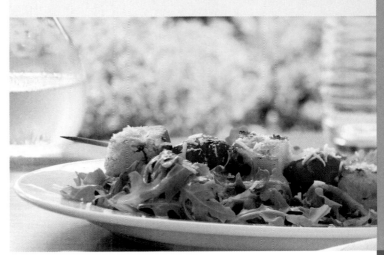

Cut the bread cubes just a little bigger than the tomatoes so that the cubes will toast nicely before the tomatoes collapse.

WAY TO GRILL ARTICHOKE HEARTS

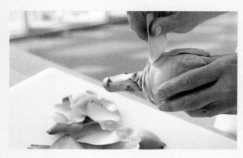
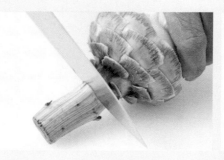
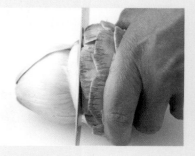

1. Bend back the dark outer leaves of each artichoke, breaking them just above the base. Stop when you see the pale green and yellowish leaves exposed.

2. Trim the stem of each artichoke, leaving ¾ inch or so attached.

3. With a sharp knife remove the pale green and yellowish leaves above the base of each artichoke.

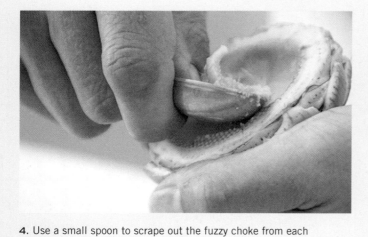
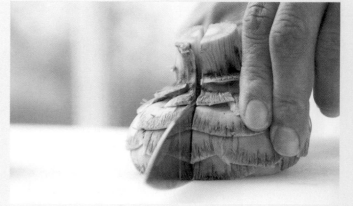

4. Use a small spoon to scrape out the fuzzy choke from each artichoke heart.

5. Cut each artichoke heart in half lengthwise through its stem.

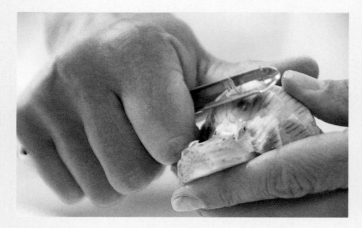
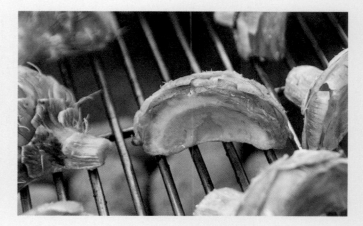

6. Using a vegetable peeler or paring knife, trim most of the rough edges from the artichoke hearts and trim off a thin layer of the stem to expose the softer interior.

7. After blanching the artichoke hearts in boiling water to make them tender, brush them with oil, season them with salt, and grill them over direct medium heat until warm and lightly charred on all sides.

ARTICHOKE HEARTS WITH SMOKED TOMATO AND ROASTED GARLIC AIOLI

SERVES: 4 TO 6
PREP TIME: 35 MINUTES

WAY TO GRILL: INDIRECT AND DIRECT MEDIUM HEAT
 (350° TO 450°F)
GRILLING TIME: 24 TO 26 MINUTES

 3 plum tomatoes, about 4 ounces each, halved, cored, seeds removed
  Extra-virgin olive oil
 3 large garlic cloves
 2 handfuls oak or hickory wood chips, soaked in water for at least 30 minutes
 ¾ cup mayonnaise
 1½ teaspoons balsamic vinegar
 1 teaspoon kosher salt, divided
 ¼ teaspoon freshly ground black pepper

 6 large artichokes, 10 to 12 ounces each
  Juice of 1 lemon

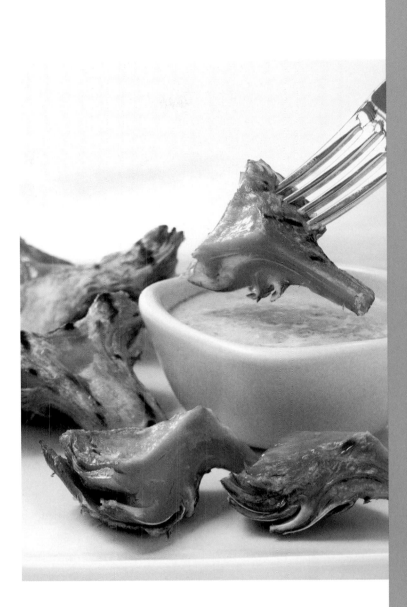

1. Prepare the grill for indirect and direct cooking over medium heat.

2. Lightly brush the tomatoes with oil. Cut a sheet of aluminum foil about 8 by 12 inches. Put the garlic cloves in the center of the foil. Drizzle ½ teaspoon of oil over the garlic cloves and fold up all four sides to make a packet.

3. Drain and add the wood chips directly onto burning coals or to the smoker box of a gas grill, following manufacturer's instructions. Brush the cooking grates clean. As soon as the wood begins to smoke, place the tomatoes and the packet of garlic over **indirect medium heat**. Cook until the tomatoes are lightly smoked and browned in spots, and the garlic is browned along the edges, about 20 minutes.

4. In the bowl of a food processor, puree the tomatoes and garlic until they are smooth. Add the mayonnaise, vinegar, ½ teaspoon of the salt, and the pepper. Pour the sauce into individual serving bowls. (Cover and refrigerate if you are not planning to serve the sauce within the next hour. Let stand at room temperature for about 30 minutes before serving.)

5. Bring a large pot of salted water to a boil.

6. Prepare the artichokes by snapping off the dark outer leaves until you expose the yellowish leaves with pale green tips. Lay each artichoke on its side. With a sharp knife cut off the remaining leaves just above the base. Using a small teaspoon, scoop out the fuzzy choke. Cut the base of each artichoke in half lengthwise, through the stem, and then trim the stem, leaving about ¾ inch attached. Using a small, sharp knife or

vegetable peeler, trim and smooth the rough and greenish areas around the base. Trim about 1⁄16 inch all the way around the stem to expose the tender part of the stem. After each artichoke heart is trimmed, place it into a large bowl mixed with lemon juice.

7. Cook the artichokes in the boiling salted water until you can pierce them easily with a knife, 10 to 12 minutes, being careful not to overcook them. Drain the artichokes in a colander and place them in a large bowl. While still warm, add 2 tablespoons of oil and the remaining ½ teaspoon of salt. Toss gently to coat the artichokes. (The artichokes may be made up to this point and refrigerated for up to 4 hours. Bring to room temperature before grilling.)

8. Lift the artichoke hearts from the bowl letting any excess oil drip back into the bowl. Grill the artichokes over **direct medium heat**, with the lid closed as much as possible, until warm and lightly charred, 4 to 6 minutes, turning them once or twice. Serve warm or at room temperature with the sauce.

WAY TO GRILL ASPARAGUS

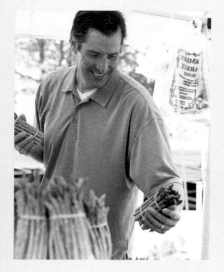

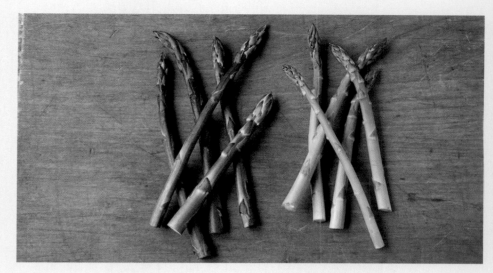

1. During springtime, the peak season for asparagus, look for firm spears with smooth skins and tightly closed heads.

2. Spears of medium thickness do better on the grill than pencil-thin spears. They are less likely to fall through the cooking grate and they usually have fuller flavors. Both purple and green spears will be green when they are cooked.

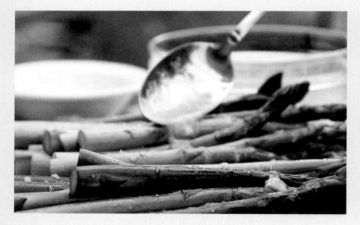

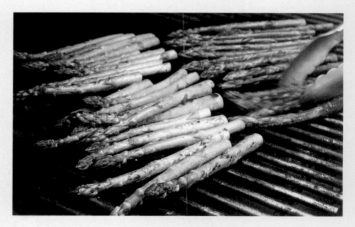

3. Coat raw, trimmed asparagus spears with a vinaigrette. The dressing will add flavor and promote even browning on the grill; however, the spears should not be dripping wet when you lay them on the grill. That would cause flare-ups.

4. So that you don't lose spears through the cooking grate, align them so that they run perpendicular to the bars. Roll the spears over every few minutes with tongs to cook them evenly.

WAY TO GRILL PROSCIUTTO

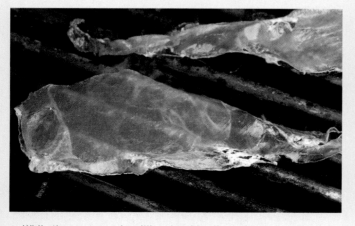

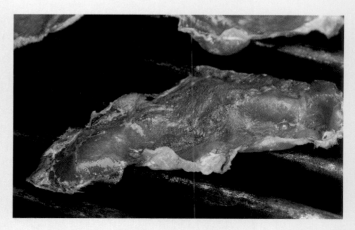

1. While the asparagus is grilling, lay thin slices of prosciutto over direct heat and grill them until crispy, turning once or twice.

2. It will take only a minute or two for most of the prosciutto fat to melt, making the meat golden brown and delicious. Let the slices cool and then break them into bits and pieces for garnish.

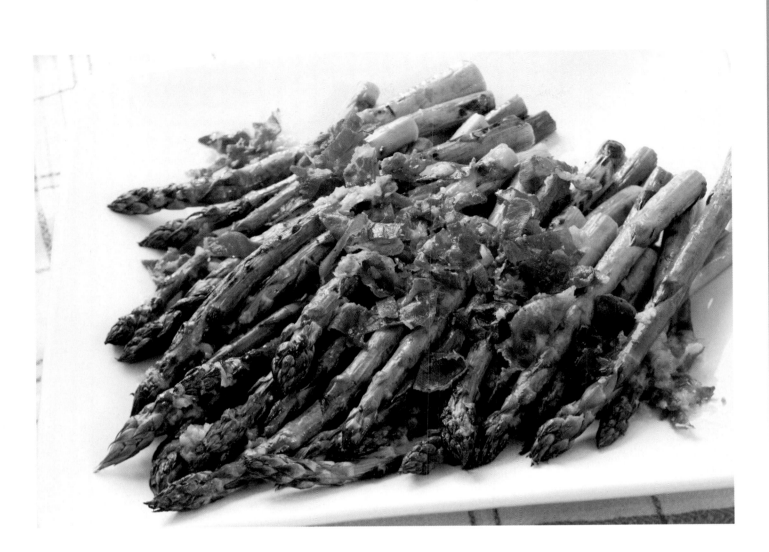

ASPARAGUS AND PROSCIUTTO WITH LEMON VINAIGRETTE

SERVES: 4
PREP TIME: 20 MINUTES

WAY TO GRILL: DIRECT MEDIUM HEAT (350° TO 450°F)
GRILL TIME: 6 TO 8 MINUTES

VINAIGRETTE
- 2 tablespoons apple cider vinegar
- 1 tablespoon finely diced shallot
- 2 teaspoons finely grated lemon zest
- 1 teaspoon Dijon mustard
- ¼ cup extra-virgin olive oil
- ¼ teaspoon kosher salt
- ¼ teaspoon freshly ground black pepper

- 1½ pounds asparagus
- ½ teaspoon kosher salt
- 4 thin slices prosciutto, about 2 ounces total

1. Prepare the grill for direct cooking over medium heat.

2. In a small bowl whisk the vinegar, shallot, lemon zest, and mustard. Slowly drizzle and whisk in the oil until it is emulsified. Season with the salt and pepper.

3. Remove and discard the tough bottom of each asparagus spear by grasping each end and bending it gently until it snaps at its natural point of tenderness, usually two-thirds of the way down the spear. If desired, use a vegetable peeler to peel off the outer skin from the bottom half of each spear. Spread the asparagus on a large plate. Drizzle with a few tablespoons of the vinaigrette and season evenly with the salt.

4. Brush the cooking grates clean. Grill the asparagus and the prosciutto over *direct medium heat*, with the lid closed as much as possible, until the asparagus is tender and the prosciutto is crisp, turning once or twice. The asparagus will take 6 to 8 minutes and the prosciutto will take 1 to 2 minutes.

5. Arrange the asparagus on a platter, spoon on the vinaigrette, and crumble the crispy prosciutto on top.

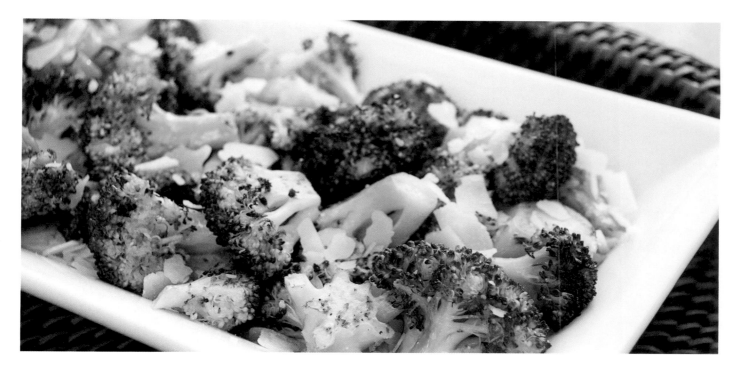

LEMON BROCCOLI

SERVES: 4
PREP TIME: 10 MINUTES

WAY TO GRILL: DIRECT MEDIUM HEAT (350° TO 450°F)
GRILLING TIME: 4 TO 6 MINUTES
SPECIAL EQUIPMENT: PERFORATED GRILL PAN

2½ teaspoons kosher salt, divided
1 pound broccoli florets, about 6 cups
2 tablespoons extra-virgin olive oil
1 tablespoon finely grated lemon zest
⅓ cup grated Parmigiano-Reggiano cheese

1. Fill a large saucepan with water to within a few inches of the top. Add 2 teaspoons of the salt to the water and bring to a boil over high heat. Add the broccoli to the boiling water and cook until bright green and crisp-tender, 3 to 5 minutes. Remove from the saucepan and plunge into an ice bath to rapidly cool them. Then remove the broccoli from the ice bath and drain.

2. Prepare the grill for direct cooking over medium heat. Brush the cooking grates clean. Preheat a grill pan over **direct medium heat** for about 10 minutes.

3. In a large bowl mix the broccoli, oil, lemon zest, and the remaining ½ teaspoon salt.

4. Spread the broccoli on the grill pan in a single layer. Grill over **direct medium heat**, with the lid closed as much as possible, until the broccoli is warm and just begins to brown, 4 to 6 minutes, turning occasionally.

5. Remove from the grill and garnish with the cheese. Serve warm.

WAY TO GRILL BROCCOLI

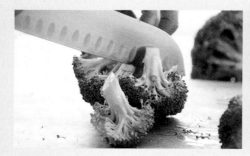

1. Cut broccoli florets into evenly sized pieces before blanching them.

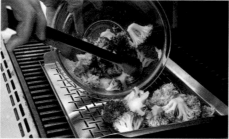

2. For quick browning, preheat the grill pan before laying out the florets.

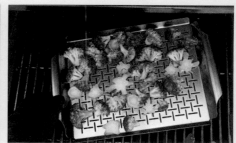

3. Turn the florets occasionally with tongs or shake the grill pan with an insulated barbecue mitt.

GREEN BEANS WITH LEMON OIL

SERVES: 4
PREP TIME: 20 MINUTES
COOLING TIME: 30 MINUTES TO 1 HOUR

WAY TO GRILL: DIRECT MEDIUM HEAT (350° TO 450°F)
GRILLING TIME: 5 TO 7 MINUTES
SPECIAL EQUIPMENT: PERFORATED GRILL PAN

LEMON OIL
   1   lemon
   ¼   cup extra-virgin olive oil
   2   large garlic cloves, thinly sliced
   ¼   teaspoon crushed red pepper flakes

   1   pound fresh, skinny green beans
   2   tablets (500 mg each) vitamin C
       Kosher salt

1. Using a vegetable peeler remove wide strips of yellow zest from the lemon. Put them in a small saucepan with the oil, garlic, and red pepper flakes. Cook over low heat until the oil simmers. Let simmer for about 2 minutes, and then remove the saucepan from the heat. Let the oil cool and steep for 30 minutes to 1 hour.

2. Remove and discard the stem ends from the green beans. Pile the beans into a large bowl.

3. Remove and discard the lemon zest and garlic from the oil. Using the sharp blade and the side of a knife, chop and crush the vitamin C tablets into a powder. Add the powder and ½ teaspoon salt to the oil. Mix well.

4. Prepare the grill for direct cooking over medium heat. Preheat the grill pan over *direct medium heat* for about 10 minutes.

5. Pour the oil mixture over the green beans. Toss the green beans over and over again to make sure they are well coated.

6. Using tongs lift the green beans from the bowl and shake off any excess oil, letting it fall back into the bowl. Spread the green beans on the grill pan in a single layer. Grill over *direct medium heat*, with the lid closed as much as possible, until browned in spots and crisp-tender, 5 to 7 minutes, turning occasionally.

7. Remove the green beans from the pan. Season to taste with salt and freshly squeezed lemon juice. Serve warm.

WAY TO GRILL GREEN BEANS

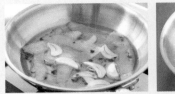
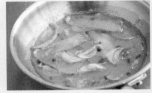

1. To infuse olive oil with more flavor, heat it with strips of lemon zest, garlic, and crushed red pepper flakes.

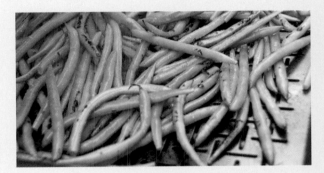

2. Crushed vitamin C (an antioxidant) in the oil will help to keep the beans bright green as they cook.

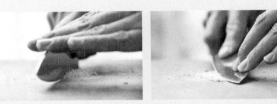

3. Spread the beans on a preheated grill pan so they cook quickly in direct contact with the pan.

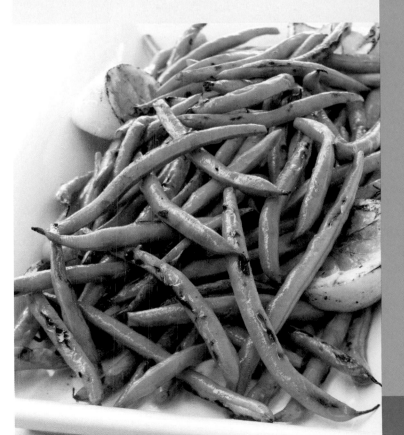

WAY TO GRILL CARROTS

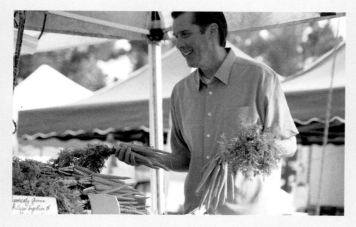

1. I once considered carrots too crunchy to grill. Then I realized that I should just boil them first to make them tender. Now they are one of my favorite side dishes, especially when I find young carrots with their stems still attached. They are so sweet and fabulous.

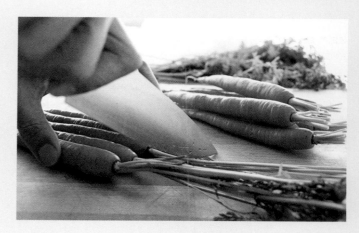

2. Trim off the stems and leaves an inch or so above the end of each carrot. Then peel the carrots and blanch them in boiling salted water until they are barely tender.

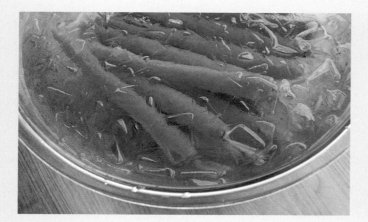

3. Stop the cooking by plunging the carrots in a bowl of ice water. At this point, you could drain the carrots and set them aside for several hours before grilling them.

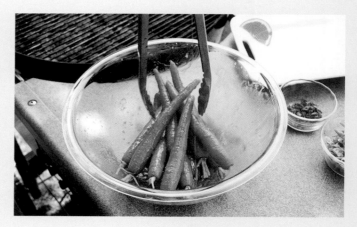

4. When you are ready to grill, coat the carrots in a bowl with melted butter, honey, orange zest, and a little balsamic vinegar.

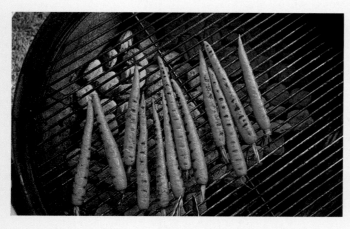

5. Arrange the carrots more or less perpendicular to the bars of the cooking grate so that you don't lose any. Grill them over direct medium heat until they develop handsome grill stripes.

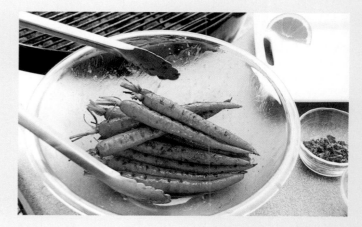

6. Finally, return the carrots to the bowl with the glaze and coat them again for extra flavor.

VEGETABLES

ORANGE-GLAZED CARROTS

SERVES: 4 TO 6
PREP TIME: 8 TO 10 MINUTES

WAY TO GRILL: DIRECT MEDIUM HEAT (350° TO 450°F)
GRILLING TIME: 4 TO 6 MINUTES

2¼ teaspoons kosher salt, divided
12 medium carrots, each 6 to 8 inches long and about 1 inch wide at the stem, peeled and trimmed
3 tablespoons unsalted butter, melted
2 tablespoons honey or maple syrup
2 teaspoons finely grated orange zest
2 teaspoons balsamic vinegar
2 tablespoons finely chopped fresh Italian parsley

1. Fill a large saucepan with water to within a few inches of the top. Add 2 teaspoons of the salt to the water and bring to a boil over high heat. Add the carrots to the boiling water and cook until tender but still crisp, 4 to 6 minutes. Remove from the saucepan and plunge into an ice bath to cool them rapidly. Then remove the carrots from the ice bath and drain.

2. Prepare the grill for direct cooking over medium heat.

3. In a large bowl combine the melted butter, honey, orange zest, vinegar, and the remaining ¼ teaspoon of salt. Add the carrots to the bowl and toss to coat them evenly.

4. Brush the cooking grates clean. Remove the carrots from the bowl and let the excess butter mixture drip back into the bowl. Set the bowl aside. Grill the carrots over **direct medium heat**, with the lid closed as much as possible, until lightly caramelized, 4 to 6 minutes, turning occasionally. Place the carrots back into bowl with the remaining butter mixture. Toss to coat thoroughly. Garnish with the parsley and serve warm.

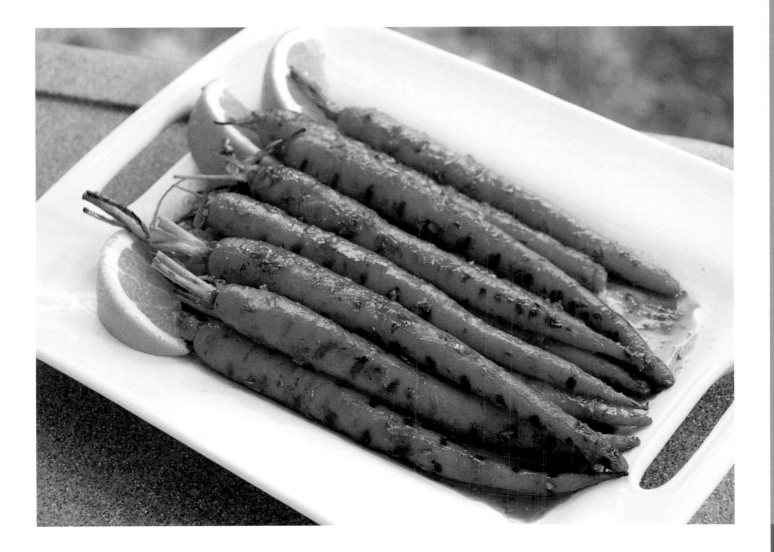

WAY TO GRILL TOFU

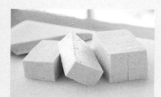 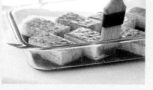

1. "Steaks" of tofu can be a delicious alternative to meat. Buy extra-firm tofu so that it holds together well on the grill.

2. To give tofu some added flavor, coat the steaks in a marinade based on lemon juice, fresh ginger, and soy sauce.

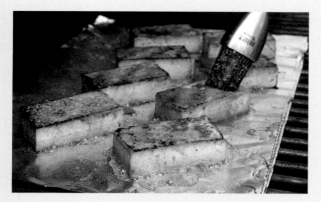

3. Grilling tofu steaks on sheets of aluminum foil avoids any risk of sticking. The heat conducted through the foil browns the surfaces nicely.

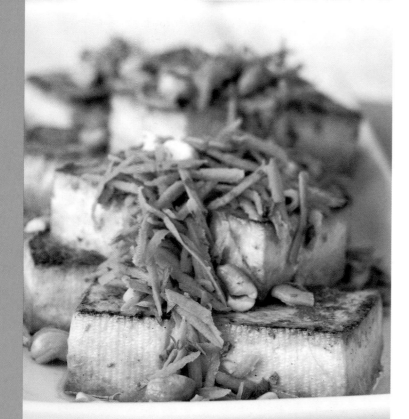

LEMON-GINGER TOFU STEAKS WITH CARROT AND CASHEW SALAD

SERVES: 4
PREP TIME: 20 MINUTES
MARINATING TIME: 3 TO 4 HOURS

WAY TO GRILL: DIRECT HIGH HEAT (450° TO 550°F)
GRILLING TIME: 6 TO 8 MINUTES

MARINADE
- ¼ cup fresh lemon juice
- ¼ cup canola oil
- ¼ cup soy sauce
- 2 tablespoons freshly grated ginger
- 2 tablespoons light brown sugar
- 1 teaspoon chile-garlic sauce, such as Sriracha

- 2 packages (14 ounces each) extra-firm tofu (not silken-style)

SALAD
- 2 cups coarsely grated carrot
- ½ cup roughly chopped cashews
- ⅓ cup minced scallions, white and light green parts
- ⅓ cup finely chopped fresh cilantro or Italian parsley
- 2 teaspoons fresh lemon juice
- 1 teaspoon dark sesame oil
- 1 teaspoon soy sauce

1. In a medium bowl whisk the marinade ingredients. Remove the blocks of tofu from their containers, leaving the liquid behind. Cut each block lengthwise into 4 slices, each about 1 inch thick. Arrange the slices in a single layer on a rimmed platter or in a baking dish.

2. Pour the marinade over the tofu slices and brush the marinade on all sides. Cover with plastic wrap and refrigerate for 3 to 4 hours, turning the slices over once or twice.

3. In a large bowl combine the salad ingredients and mix well. Set aside at room temperature.

4. Prepare the grill for direct cooking over high heat. Brush the cooking grates clean. Lay a large sheet of aluminum foil, about 12 by 16 inches, directly on the cooking grate. Lift the tofu slices from the platter and arrange them in a single layer on the foil, reserving the marinade for glazing. Grill the tofu over **direct high heat**, with the lid closed as much as possible, until both sides are nicely caramelized and the slices are warm, 6 to 8 minutes, turning once and brushing occasionally with some of the reserved marinade. Using a spatula, transfer the slices of tofu to serving plates. Stack the salad on top. Serve warm or at room temperature.

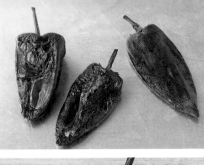

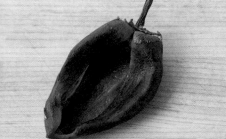

When roasting, peeling, and opening the chiles, be careful that you maintain enough structure in the chiles that they can hold the cheese filling.

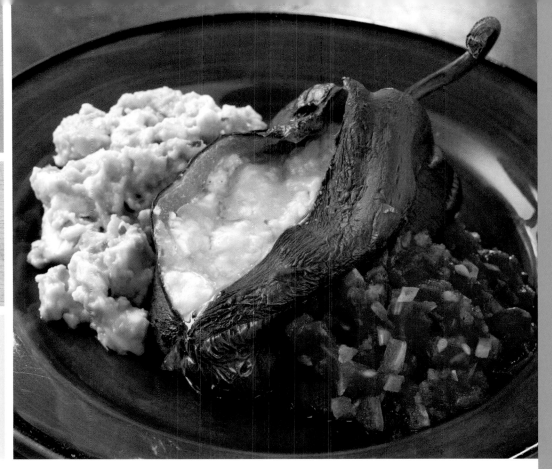

CHILES RELLENOS WITH TOMATO SALSA AND GUACAMOLE

SERVES: 6
PREP TIME: 30 MINUTES

WAY TO GRILL: DIRECT AND INDIRECT MEDIUM HEAT
(350° TO 450°F)
GRILLING TIME: 22 TO 31 MINUTES

SALSA
- 3 medium tomatoes, firm but ripe, halved and cored
- 1 small white onion, cut crosswise into ½-inch slices
  Extra-virgin olive oil
- 2 tablespoons finely chopped fresh cilantro leaves
- 1 tablespoon fresh lime juice
- 1 teaspoon minced serrano or jalapeño chile pepper
- 1 teaspoon kosher salt

GUACAMOLE
- 3 large ripe Haas avocados
- ¼ cup finely chopped red onion
- 2 tablespoons fresh lime juice
- 1 teaspoon kosher salt

- 6 large poblano chile peppers
- 1 cup grated Monterey Jack cheese
- 1 cup grated cheddar cheese
- ½ cup crumbled fresh goat cheese

1. Prepare the grill for direct and indirect cooking over medium heat. Brush the cooking grates clean.

2. Lightly brush or spray the tomatoes and onion slices with oil. Grill over *direct medium heat*, with the lid closed as much as possible, until lightly charred all over, 6 to 8 minutes. turning once. Remove from the grill, finely chop, and transfer to a medium bowl. Stir in the remaining salsa ingredients.

3. In a medium bowl using a fork, coarsely mash the avocados. Stir in the onion and lime juice and season with the salt. Cover with plastic wrap, placing the wrap directly on the surface of the guacamole to prevent it from browning, and refrigerate until about 1 hour before serving.

4. Grill the chiles over *direct medium heat*, with the lid open, until the skins are blackened and blistered all over, 10 to 15 minutes, turning occasionally. (The goal is to char the skins quickly so that you can peel them without the chiles collapsing. You will need chiles with enough structure, even when roasted, to hold the filling.) Place the chiles in a large bowl, cover with plastic wrap, and let them steam for about 10 minutes. Gently peel and discard the skin from the chiles. Leaving the stems intact, carefully cut a slit down one side of each chile and remove and discard the seeds and veins.

5. In a medium bowl combine the cheeses and mix together with a fork. Carefully stuff the mixture into the chile cavities. Brush the chiles with olive oil.

6. Grill the stuffed chiles, seam sides up, over *indirect medium heat*, with the lid closed, until the cheese melts, 6 to 8 minutes. Gently remove them from the grill with a spatula. Serve warm with the salsa and guacamole.

WAY TO ROAST GARLIC

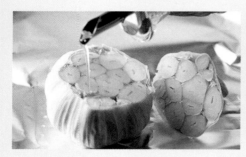

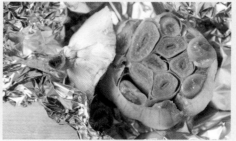

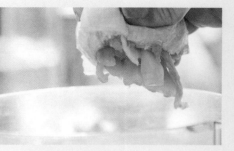

1. Cut off the top of a head of garlic to expose the cloves, and drizzle some oil on the cloves.

2. Wrap the head in foil and grill it over indirect heat until the cloves are soft and beginning to brown.

3. Let cool and then squeeze out the soft, mellow-tasting garlic cloves

WAY TO PREP EGGPLANT

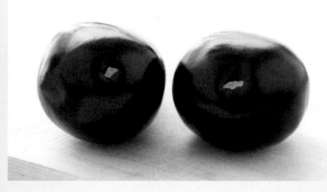

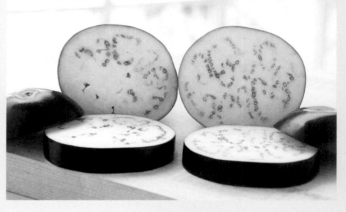

1. Globe eggplants should be quite firm, with glossy, unblemished skins. Look for cylindrical shapes that feel heavy for their size.

2. A male eggplant (left) will often have fewer seecs than a female eggplant (right), making the pulp of the male sweeter and less bitter.

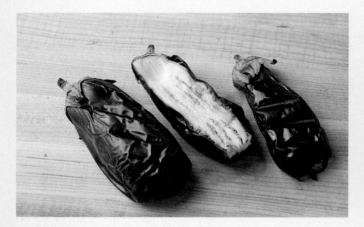

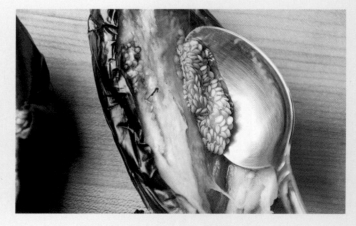

3. Prick the whole eggplants several times with a fork and grill them over direct high heat until the skins are charred and beginning to collapse.

4. Cut the cooled eggplants in half lengthwise and scoop out the pulp for the dip, but remove and discard any clumps of seeds that could turn the dip bitter.

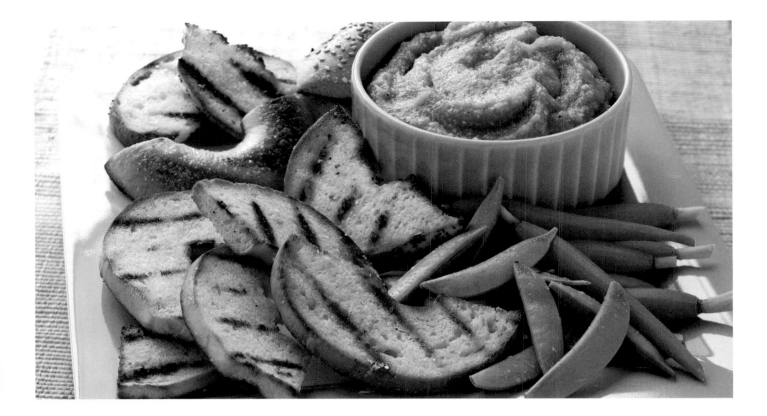

ROASTED EGGPLANT DIP

SERVES: 8 TO 10 AS AN APPETIZER
PREP TIME: 10 MINUTES

WAY TO GRILL: INDIRECT AND DIRECT HIGH HEAT
   (450° TO 550°F), DIRECT MEDIUM HEAT (350° TO 450°F)
GRILLING TIME: 42 TO 52 MINUTES

- 1 head garlic
- 1 teaspoon extra-virgin olive oil
- 2 medium globe eggplants, about 1 pound total
- 1 tablespoon fresh lemon juice
- 1 teaspoon fresh oregano leaves
- ½ teaspoon kosher salt
- ½ teaspoon freshly ground black pepper

BAGEL CHIPS
- 2 bagels
- 2 tablespoons extra-virgin olive oil
- ¼ teaspoon kosher salt

1. Prepare the grill for indirect and direct cooking over high heat.

2. Remove the loose, papery outer skin from the head of garlic and cut off the top to expose the cloves. Place the garlic on a large square of aluminum foil and drizzle the oil over the top of the cloves. Fold up the sides to make a sealed packet, leaving a little room for the expansion of steam. Brush the cooking grates clean. Grill over **indirect high heat**, with the lid closed, until the cloves are soft, 40 to 50 minutes.

3. Prick the eggplants several times with a fork. Grill over **direct high heat**, with the lid closed as much as possible, until the skins are charred and they begin to collapse, 15 to 20 minutes, turning occasionally. A knife should slide in and cut of the flesh without resistance.

4. Once the garlic and eggplants are cool enough to handle, squeeze out the garlic cloves into the large bowl of a food processor fitted with a metal blade. Cut the eggplants in half lengthwise and, using a large spoon, scrape away the flesh from the skin. Discard the skin and any large seed pockets. Add the flesh of the eggplants to the food processor bowl and pulse to create a thick paste. Add the lemon juice and oregano and process until the mixture is smooth. Season with the salt and pepper. Decrease the temperature of the grill to medium heat.

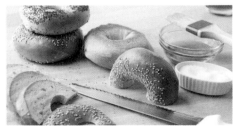

5. Slice the bagels in half so you have two half-moons. Slice the bagel halves lengthwise into ¼-inch-thick slices.

6. Lightly brush the bagel slices with the oil. Sprinkle with salt and grill over **direct medium heat** until the chips begin to brown and get crispy, about 2 minutes, turning once.

7. Serve the dip warm with bagel chips and fresh vegetables.

WAY TO GRILL SANDWICHES

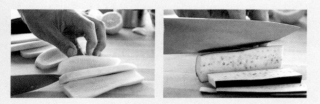

1. Cut the squashes and eggplants lengthwise and evenly into ⅓-inch slices and grill them over direct medium heat before assembling the sandwiches.

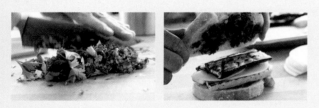

2. Coarsely chop the fresh herbs, garlic, and sun-dried tomatoes. Distribute the spread on the inside of each bread slice.

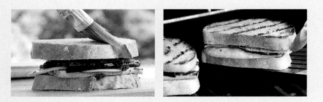

3. Brush the outside of each slice of bread with oil and grill the sandwiches until toasted on each side.

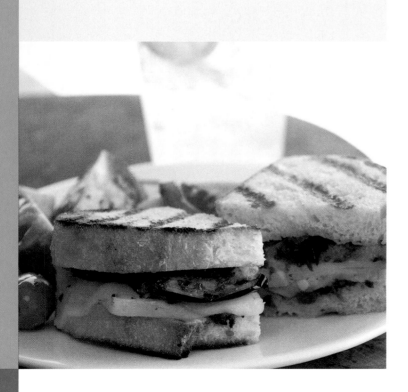

VEGETABLE SANDWICHES WITH SUN-DRIED TOMATO SPREAD

SERVES: 4
PREP TIME: 20 MINUTES

WAY TO GRILL: DIRECT MEDIUM HEAT (350° TO 450°F)
GRILLING TIME: 10 TO 14 MINUTES

SPREAD
- 1 cup lightly packed fresh basil
- 1 cup lightly packed fresh Italian parsley
- 1 medium garlic clove
- ¼ cup finely chopped oil-packed sun-dried tomatoes
- 2 tablespoons oil from the jar of oil-packed sun-dried tomatoes
- 1 teaspoon finely grated lemon zest
- 1 teaspoon fresh lemon juice
- ¼ teaspoon kosher salt

- 2 Japanese eggplants, about 1 pound total, trimmed and cut lengthwise into ⅓-inch slices
- 1–2 yellow squashes, about 8 ounces total, trimmed and cut lengthwise into ⅓-inch slices
  Extra-virgin olive oil
- ½ teaspoon kosher salt
- ¼ teaspoon freshly ground black pepper
- 8 slices country-style sourdough bread, each about ½ inch thick
- 4 slices provolone cheese, cut to fit the bread

1. Prepare the grill for direct cooking over medium heat.

2. Finely chop the basil and parsley with the garlic. Place the herb mixture in a small bowl. Add the remaining spread ingredients and mix well to form a paste.

3. Lightly brush both sides of the eggplant and squash slices with oil. Season with the salt and pepper. Grill the vegetable slices over **direct medium heat**, with the lid closed as much as possible, until nicely marked on both sides, 8 to 10 minutes, turning once or twice. The squash will cook a little faster than the eggplant. Transfer the vegetables from the grill to a platter as they are done.

4. Distribute the spread on the inside of each bread slice. Arrange the cheese and grilled vegetables in layers on half of the bread slices, making sure the cheese is in the center. Place the top slice of bread on and gently press with your hand to keep the sandwich together. Lightly brush the outsides of the bread with oil.

5. Grill over **direct medium heat**, with the lid open, until the bread is toasted and the cheese has melted, 2 to 4 minutes, turning once. Serve warm.

HONEY AND CURRY-GLAZED SQUASH

SERVES: 4 TO 6
PREP TIME: 15 MINUTES

WAY TO GRILL: INDIRECT MEDIUM HEAT (350° TO 450°F)
GRILLING TIME: 1 HOUR TO 1 HOUR AND 10 MINUTES

 5–6 pounds winter squashes, such as acorn and butternut
 ¼ cup extra-virgin olive oil
   Kosher salt
   Freshly ground black pepper

GLAZE
 4 tablespoons (½ stick) unsalted butter
 ¼ cup honey
 1 tablespoon cider vinegar
 2 teaspoons mild curry powder
 ¼ teaspoon ground chipotle chile powder

1. Prepare the grill for indirect cooking over medium heat.

2. Wash the squashes under cold water. Using a heavy, sharp knife, cut the ends off of each squash and then cut each squash into 4 or 6 pieces. Using a tablespoon, scoop out and discard the seeds and pulp. Place the squash pieces on a sheet pan and brush the flesh with the oil. Season to taste with salt and pepper.

3. Brush the cooking grates clean. Grill the squash pieces, skin sides down, over *indirect medium heat*, with the lid closed, for about 30 minutes.

4. In a small saucepan over medium heat, combine the glaze ingredients and cook until the butter is melted and the glaze is smooth, about 2 minutes, stirring often. Remove from the heat.

5. After the first 30 minutes of cooking, return the squash pieces to the sheet pan. Close the grill's lid to maintain the heat inside. Brush the flesh with the glaze, return the squash to the grill, and continue to roast over *indirect medium heat*, with the lid closed as much as possible, until soft and tender, 30 to 40 minutes, glazing every 15 to 20 minutes. Season with more salt, if desired. Drizzle with the remaining glaze and serve warm.

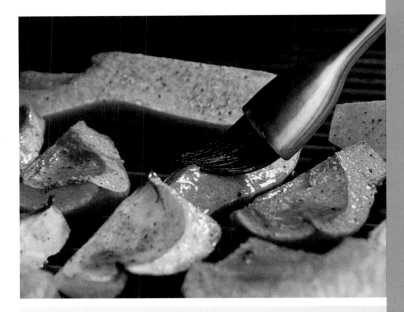

Grill the squash pieces over indirect medium heat for about 30 minutes before glazing them. Applying a sweet glaze too early could cause burning. During the final 30 to 40 minutes of cooking, glaze the squash every 15 to 20 minutes, but close the lid as quickly as possible to maintain the right heat.

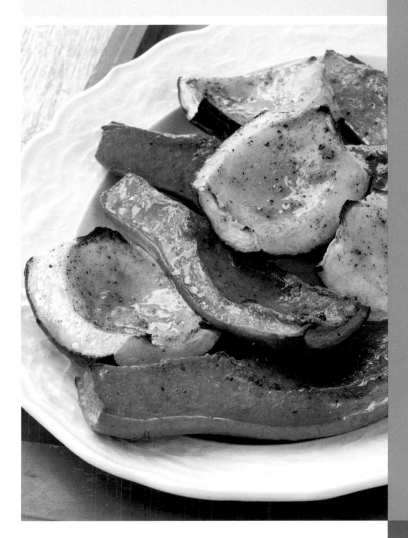

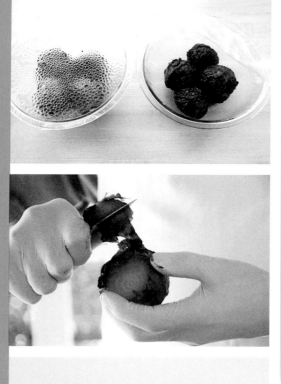

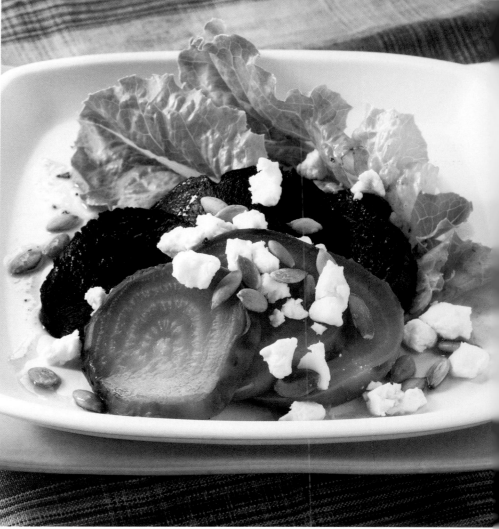

After roasting red and golden beets over indirect heat, put them in separate bowls so their colors won't run together, and cover the bowls with plastic wrap to loosen their skins with steam. Wear rubber gloves to avoid staining your hands when peeling the beets with a paring knife.

GRILL-ROASTED BEET SALAD WITH PEPITAS AND FETA

SERVES: 4
PREP TIME: 30 TO 40 MINUTES

WAY TO GRILL: INDIRECT MEDIUM HEAT (350° TO 450°F)
GRILLING TIME: 1 TO 1½ HOURS

    4   golden or red beets (or a combination of both), about 2 pounds total
       Extra-virgin olive oil

DRESSING
    2   tablespoons red wine vinegar
    1   teaspoon Dijon mustard
    1   teaspoon honey
    1   teaspoon ground cumin
   ¼   teaspoon crushed red pepper flakes
   ½   cup extra-virgin olive oil
   ½   teaspoon kosher salt
   ¼   teaspoon freshly ground black pepper

    3   cups baby romaine leaves, whole or torn into pieces
   ¼   cup pepitas (shelled pumpkin seeds), toasted
    1   cup crumbled feta or goat cheese

1. Prepare the grill for indirect cooking over medium heat. Brush the cooking grates clean.

2. Trim off the leafy tops and root ends from the beets and scrub them under cold water. Lightly brush them with oil. Grill the beets over *indirect medium heat*, with the lid closed as much as possible, until they are tender with pierced with the tip of a knife, 1 to 1½ hours, depending on size, turning occasionally. Remove from the grill and place the red beets and golden beets in separate bowls. Cover the bowls with plastic wrap and allow to stand at room temperature until cool enough to handle. With a sharp paring knife, cut off the ends and remove the skins. Cut the beets crosswise into ¼- to ½-inch slices and keep the slices in their separate bowls (to keep the red beets from dying the golden beets red).

3. In a medium bowl or in a blender, whisk or pulse the vinegar, mustard, honey, cumin, and red pepper flakes. Slowly drizzle in the oil while whisking until the dressing has emulsified. Season with the salt and pepper.

4. Divide the romaine and beet slices between 4 salad plates and drizzle with some dressing. Garnish each plate with pepitas and cheese. Serve warm.

FENNEL AND FONTINA

SERVES: 4 TO 6
PREP TIME: 10 MINUTES

WAY TO GRILL: DIRECT MEDIUM-LOW HEAT (ABOUT 350°F)
GRILLING TIME: 23 TO 28 MINUTES

- 3 medium fennel bulbs
- 3 tablespoons extra-virgin olive oil
- 1 tablespoon fresh lemon juice
- ½ teaspoon kosher salt
- ⅛ teaspoon freshly ground black pepper
- ½ cup (4 ounces) shredded Italian fontina cheese

1. Prepare the grill for direct cooking over medium-low heat.

2. If the fennel stalks have the fronds attached, trim off the fronds and chop enough to make 2 tablespoons. Cut off the thick stalks above the bulbs and save the stalks for another use. Cut each fennel bulb into quarters and then remove the thick triangular-shaped core. Cut the fennel vertically into ¼-inch-thick slices.

3. Pile the fennel off to one side of a sheet of heavy-duty aluminum foil, about 12 by 24 inches, leaving enough foil to completely cover and envelope the fennel. Pour the oil and lemon juice over the fennel. Season with the salt and pepper. Fold the foil over the fennel and seal the packet tightly so that no liquid can escape.

4. Grill the packet over **direct medium-low heat**, with the lid closed, until the fennel is barely tender, 20 to 25 minutes. Carefully open the packet with tongs and sprinkle the cheese over the fennel. Grill, with the foil packet open, until the cheese melts slightly, 2 to 3 minutes. Carefully remove the packet from the grill and garnish with chopped fennel fronds. Serve warm.

WAY TO GRILL FENNEL

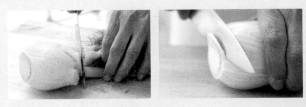

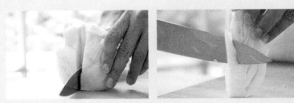

1. Cut off the thick stalks and the root end from each bulb, but reserve some of the fronds for garnish.

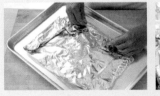

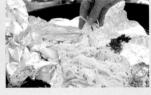

2. Cut each bulb lengthwise into quarters and cut away nearly all the tough core.

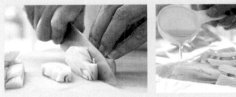

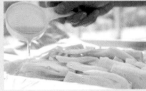

3. Thinly slice the fennel, arrange the slices on a large sheet of foil, and coat them with good olive oil.

4. Grill the fennel in a sealed packet until barely tender. Open the foil packet and finish cooking the fennel with shredded fontina cheese.

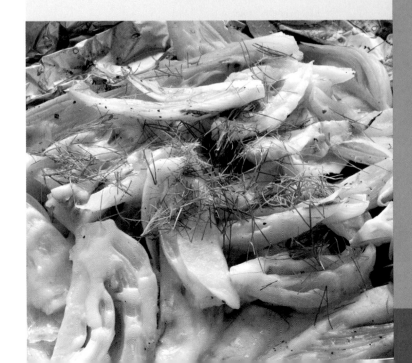

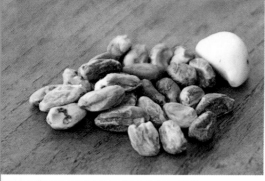

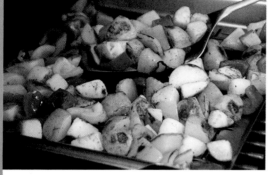

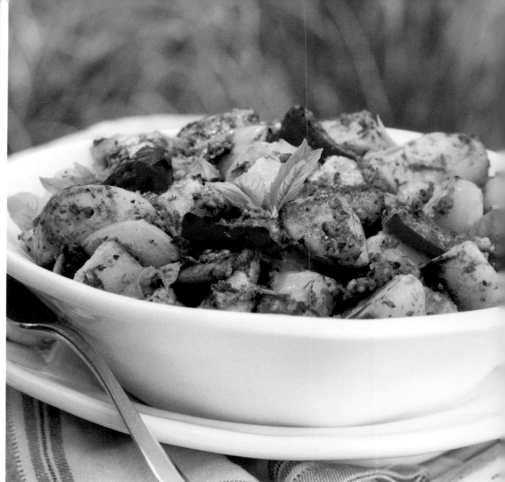

Shelled pistachios and garlic are at the heart of a nontraditional but delicious pesto for coating grill-roasted potatoes.

YELLOW POTATO SALAD WITH PISTACHIO PESTO

SERVES: 4 TO 6
PREP TIME: 20 MINUTES

WAY TO GRILL: DIRECT MEDIUM HEAT (350° TO 450°F)
GRILLING TIME: 10 TO 15 MINUTES
SPECIAL EQUIPMENT: PERFORATED GRILL PAN

PESTO
   1 garlic clove
   1 cup tightly packed fresh basil leaves
  ¼ cup shelled unsalted pistachios
  ⅓ cup mayonnaise
  2 teaspoons white wine vinegar
  ½ teaspoon kosher salt
  ¼ teaspoon freshly ground black pepper

  8 medium yellow potatoes, each 2 to 3 inches in diameter, about 2 pounds total, scrubbed (do not peel)
     Kosher salt
  2 large red or yellow (or 1 of each) bell peppers
  2 tablespoons extra-virgin olive oil
     Freshly ground black pepper
  2 tablespoons torn fresh basil, optional

1. In the bowl of a food processor mince the garlic. Add the basil and pistachios and pulse until they are finely chopped. Transfer the mixture to a large bowl and mix with the remaining pesto ingredients.

2. Cut each potato into eighths and put them into a large saucepan. Cover by at least 1 inch with water. Add 2 teaspoons of salt to the water and bring to a boil over high heat. Reduce the heat to a simmer and cook until the potatoes are barely tender, 5 to 10 minutes. Meanwhile cut each bell pepper in half lengthwise. Remove and discard the stem, seeds, and large white veins. Cut each pepper into 1- to 1½-inch pieces.

3. When the potatoes are barely tender, drain them in a colander and return them to the dry saucepan. Add the bell pepper pieces. Add the oil and ½ teaspoon of salt. Toss to coat the vegetables evenly.

4. Prepare the grill for direct cooking over medium heat. Preheat the grill pan over ***direct medium heat*** for about 10 minutes. When the pan is hot, spoon the potatoes and peppers onto the pan, spreading them out in a single layer. Grill over ***direct medium heat***, with the lid closed as much as possible, until the potatoes are seared with golden brown marks on all sides and they are quite tender, 10 to 15 minutes, turning occasionally. Transfer the vegetables to the bowl with the pesto. Gently toss to coat the vegetables completely. Allow to cool for at least 5 minutes. Season to taste with salt and pepper. Garnish with basil, if desired. Serve warm or at room temperature.

COCONUT-GLAZED SWEET POTATOES

SERVES: 4 TO 6
PREP TIME: 15 MINUTES

WAY TO GRILL: DIRECT MEDIUM HEAT (350° TO 450°F)
    FOR CHARCOAL GRILLS ONLY
GRILLING TIME: ABOUT 1 HOUR
SPECIAL EQUIPMENT: 12-INCH CAST-IRON SKILLET

  4 medium sweet potatoes

GLAZE
  1 can (13½ ounces) coconut milk
    Finely grated zest and juice of 1 lime
  2 tablespoons brown sugar
  1 tablespoon unsalted butter
  1 jalapeño chile pepper, minced
  ½ teaspoon kosher salt

  ¼ cup shredded coconut

1. Wash and dry the potatoes and then wrap them individually in sheets of aluminum foil.

2. Prepare a bull's-eye fire for medium heat (see below). When the coals are ready, place the sweet potatoes directly on the charcoal grate resting on the edge of the charcoal. Close the lid and cook until the potatoes are soft, 45 to 55 minutes, turning them occasionally. To check for doneness, squeeze the potatoes with a pair of tongs.

3. Remove the potatoes from the grill and let them cool for about 15 minutes before unwrapping them. Slit the skins with a knife and peel off and discard the skin. Cut the flesh into ½-inch cubes. Set aside while you make the glaze.

4. Place a 12-inch cast-iron skillet over **direct medium heat**

(you can also do this step on your stove top). Combine the glaze ingredients in the skillet and bring the mixture to a simmer, stirring occasionally. Let the mixture reduce until half the volume remains, 5 to 8 minutes, stirring occasionally. The glaze will be slightly thick. Remove the skillet from the heat and add the sweet potato cubes, gently stirring to coat with the glaze, being careful not to mash them.

5. In a small skillet over high heat, toast and brown the coconut, about 2 minutes.

6. Place the potatoes in a serving bowl and sprinkle the toasted coconut over the top. Serve warm.

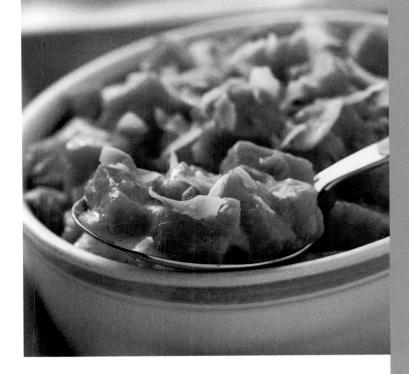

WAY TO GRILL SWEET POTATOES

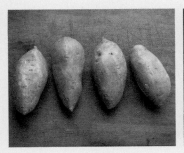

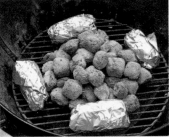

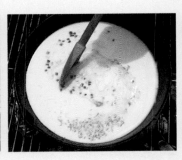

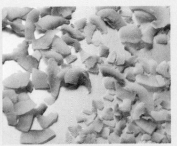

1. Choose cylindrical sweet potatoes of similar size and thickness so that they cook evenly.

2. Wrap them in foil and lay them against the coals, turning them occasionally.

3. Moisten and flavor the potatoes with a thick glaze based on coconut milk and brown sugar.

4. Garnish with shredded coconut that has been toasted in a skillet.

WAY TO MAKE FLAT BREAD

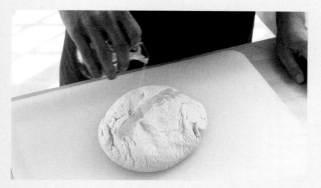

1. To make sticky dough easier to handle, add a little oil to the dough and the cutting board.

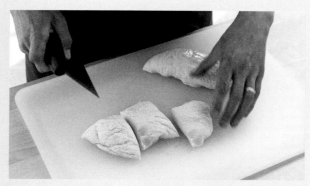

2. Use a "bench scraper" (shown here) or a large knife to cut the dough into equal portions.

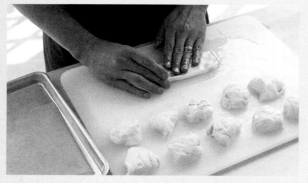

3. Make 12 individual balls and use your hands to press and stretch each one into whatever shape you like, as long as they are about ⅓ inch thick.

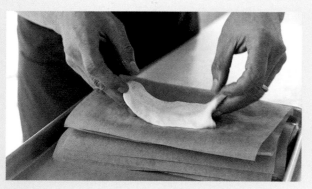

4. Stack the flattened pieces of dough between sheets of parchment paper. Make sure every piece of dough has a coating of oil on each side to prevent them from sticking on the grill.

GRILLED FLAT BREAD WITH THREE TOPPINGS

SERVES: 4
PREP TIME: 15 MINUTES
RISING TIME: 1½ TO 2 HOURS

WAY TO GRILL: DIRECT MEDIUM HEAT (350° TO 450°F)
GRILLING TIME: ABOUT 6 MINUTES FOR EACH BATCH
SPECIAL EQUIPMENT: ELECTRIC STAND MIXER

DOUGH
- 1½ cups warm water (100° to 110°F)
- 1 package rapid-rise active dry yeast
- ½ teaspoon granulated sugar
- 4½ cups all-purpose flour
- 3 tablespoons extra-virgin olive oil
- 2 teaspoons kosher salt

1. In the bowl of an electric stand mixer, combine the water, yeast, and sugar. Stir briefly and let stand for 5 minutes or until the top surface has a thin, frothy layer (this indicates that the yeast is active). Add the flour, oil, and salt. Fit the mixer with the dough hook and mix on low speed for about 1 minute or until the dough begins to come together. Increase the speed to medium. Continue to mix until the dough is slightly sticky, smooth, and elastic, about 10 minutes. Form the dough into a ball and place in a lightly oiled bowl. Turn it over to coat all sides and tightly cover the bowl with plastic wrap. Allow the dough to rise in a warm place until it has doubled in size, 1½ to 2 hours.

2. Prepare the grill for direct cooking over medium heat.

3. Turn the dough out onto a lightly oiled surface and cut it into 12 equal portions, 2 to 3 ounces each. Using your fingers and the palms of your hands (oil them, too), stretch the dough to a length of about 8 inches. The first stretch will probably shrink back, but continue to pull and stretch using gentle pressure until you achieve the proper length. As needed, add more oil to the surface to keep the dough moist and pliable. Stack the pieces of dough between sheets of parchment paper.

4. Brush the cooking grates clean. Carefully lay the pieces of dough, a few at a time, over ***direct medium heat***. Within 1 to 2 minutes the undersides of the dough should crisp, darken, and harden, and the tops will puff slightly. Turn them over and continue to cook until both sides are dark brown, about 6 minutes total, turning every minute. If desired, keep warm over indirect heat. Serve warm or at room temperature with the topping(s) of your choice.

WHITE BEAN PUREE WITH ROASTED GARLIC
MAKES: 1½ TO 2 CUPS
PREP TIME: 10 MINUTES

WAY TO GRILL: INDIRECT MEDIUM HEAT (350° TO 450°F)
GRILLING TIME: 45 MINUTES TO 1 HOUR

- 1 small head garlic
- 2 tablespoons plus 1 teaspoon extra-virgin olive oil, divided
- 1 can (15 ounces) cannellini or navy beans, rinsed and drained
- 1 teaspoon finely grated lemon zest
- 2 tablespoons fresh lemon juice
- 1 teaspoon kosher salt
- ¼ teaspoon freshly ground black pepper
- ¼ cup loosely packed fresh Italian parsley leaves
- 2–3 small fresh sage leaves

1. Prepare the grill for indirect cooking over medium heat.

2. Remove the loose, papery outer skin from a head of garlic and cut off the top to expose the cloves. Place the garlic on a large square of aluminum foil and drizzle 1 teaspoon of the oil over the top of the cloves. Fold up the sides to make a sealed packet, leaving a little room for the expansion of steam. Grill over **indirect medium heat**, with the lid closed, until the cloves are soft, 45 minutes to 1 hour.

3. In the bowl of a food processor, squeeze out the garlic cloves, being careful not to add any of the papery skin, and then add and puree the beans, the remaining 2 tablespoons of oil, the lemon zest, lemon juice, salt, and pepper. Add the parsley and sage and process to give the puree a consistency that resembles the texture of hummus. If necessary, add additional oil to create a smoother consistency.

TOMATO TAPENADE
MAKES: 1 CUP
PREP TIME: 10 MINUTES

- ½ cup pitted kalamata olives, drained
- ½ cup oil-packed, sun-dried tomatoes, drained
- 1 small garlic clove or several roasted garlic cloves
- 3–4 tablespoons extra-virgin olive oil
- ¼ cup loosely packed fresh basil leaves
- 2 tablespoons capers, drained
- 2 teaspoons balsamic vinegar
- ¼ teaspoon freshly ground black pepper

1. In the bowl of a food processor, pulse the olives, tomatoes, and garlic several times to coarsely chop them. Add in 3 tablespoons of the oil and the rest of the ingredients. Continue to puree until the mixture is well combined. Add the remaining tablespoon of oil if the tapenade seems too chunky.

BLUE CHEESE-WALNUT SPREAD
MAKES: 1 CUP
PREP TIME: 10 MINUTES

- 4 ounces crumbled blue cheese, such as Maytag, Roquefort, or Danish
- ¼ cup (½ stick) unsalted butter, softened
- ½ cup walnuts, lightly toasted and coarsely chopped
- ¼ cup minced shallot
- 1 tablespoon fresh lemon juice
- ¼ teaspoon freshly ground black pepper
  Finely chopped fresh Italian parsley

1. Using a fork or an electric stand mixer fitted with the paddle attachment on low speed, mix the blue cheese and butter to form a semi-smooth spread. It's okay if there are some chunks of blue cheese. Fold in the remaining ingredients, including parsley to taste.

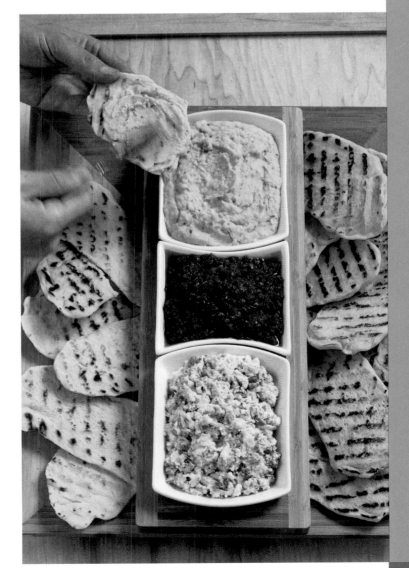

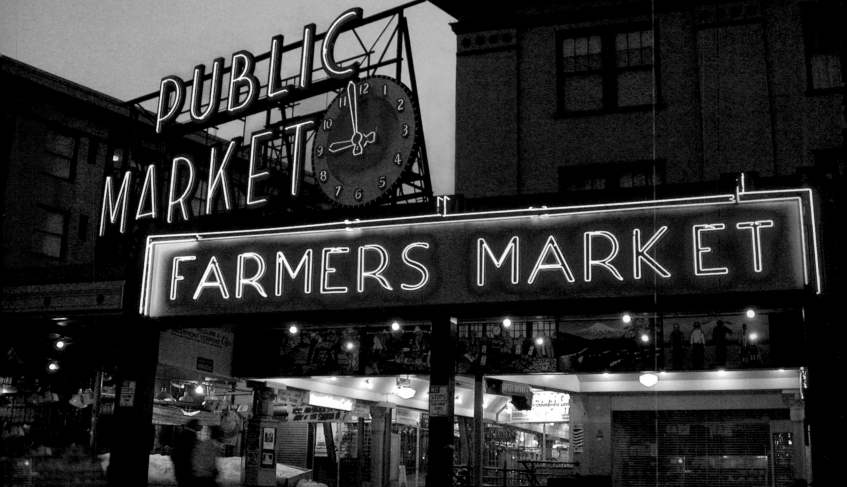

WAY TO GRILL™
FRUIT

TECHNIQUES

RECIPES

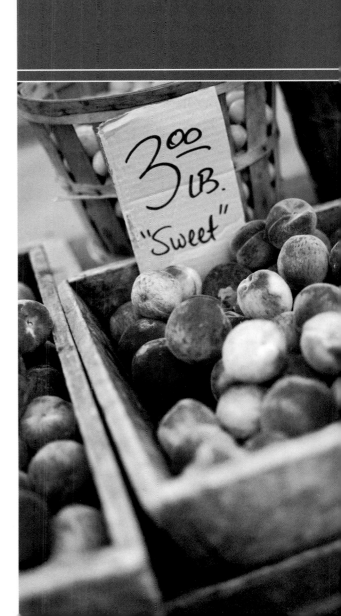

WAY TO GRILL PINEAPPLE UPSIDE-DOWN CAKE

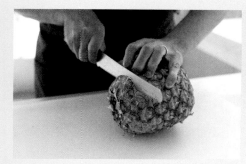

1. Trim about an inch from both the top and bottom of a ripe pineapple.

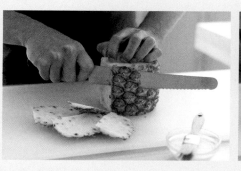

2. Stand the pineapple upright and rotate it as you cut off the tough skin.

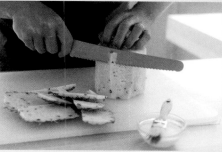

3. Go back around the pineapple to trim off the dark "eyes."

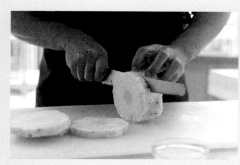

4. Cut the pineapple crosswise into ½-inch slices.

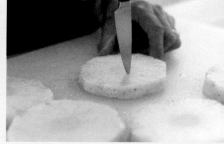

5. Use a paring knife to cut around the core of each slice (on both sides) and remove it.

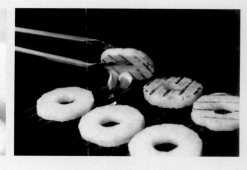

6. Brush the slices with butter and grill them over direct medium heat.

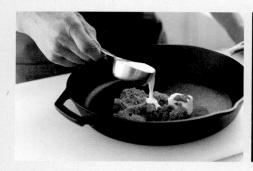

7. In a 12-inch cast-iron skillet, combine brown sugar, cream, and cinnamon.

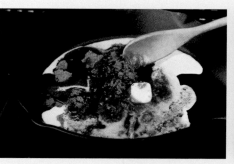

8. Melt the brown sugar mixture over direct medium heat.

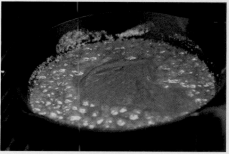

9. When the mixture bubbles around the outer edge, remove the skillet from the heat.

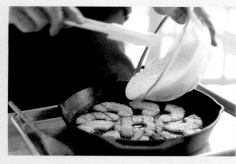

10. Very carefully arrange cut pineapple slices in the hot mixture and pour the batter on top.

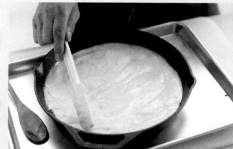

11. Spread the batter evenly to all edges of the skillet.

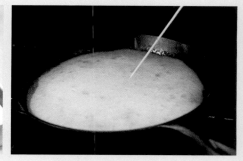

12. Cook over indirect heat until a skewer comes out clean. Then invert the cake onto a large platter.

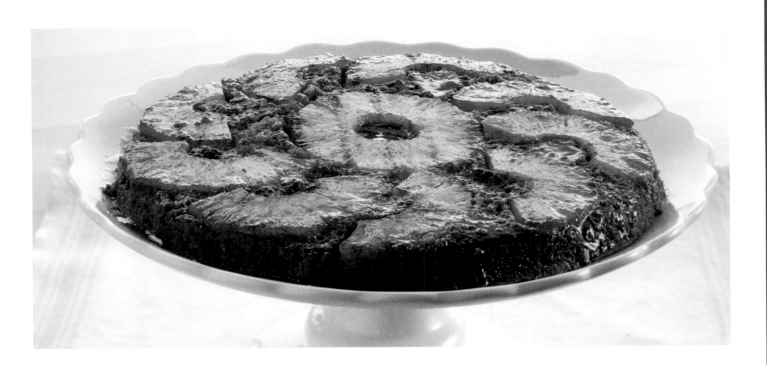

PINEAPPLE UPSIDE-DOWN CAKE

SERVES: 6 TO 8
PREP TIME: 30 MINUTES

WAY TO GRILL: DIRECT AND INDIRECT MEDIUM HEAT (350°
    TO 450°F) **FOR GAS GRILLS ONLY**
GRILLING TIME: 46 TO 58 MINUTES
SPECIAL EQUIPMENT: 12-INCH CAST-IRON SKILLET

TOPPING

  6 rings fresh (not canned) pineapple, each ½ inch thick,
     peeled and cored
  2 tablespoons unsalted butter, melted
  ½ cup dark brown sugar, packed
  ¼ cup heavy cream
  ½ teaspoon ground cinnamon

BATTER

  1 cup all-purpose flour
  1 teaspoon baking powder
  ½ teaspoon kosher salt
  ¼ teaspoon baking soda
  ⅔ cup buttermilk
  2 large eggs
  1 teaspoon vanilla extract
  ¼ pound (1 stick) unsalted butter, softened
  ¾ cup granulated sugar

1. Prepare the grill for direct and indirect cooking over medium
heat. Brush the cooking grates clean.

2. Brush the pineapple rings with the melted butter. Grill them
over **direct medium heat**, with the lid open, until nicely marked,
4 to 6 minutes, turning once. Remove from the grill and let cool.
Leave one pineapple ring whole and cut the others into halves.

3. In a 12-inch cast-iron skillet over **direct medium heat**,
combine the brown sugar, cream, cinnamon, and any melted
butter remaining from brushing the pineapple slices. Cook until
the sugar has melted and the liquid starts to bubble around the
outer edge, about 2 minutes. Remove the skillet from the heat
and place on a sheet pan. Place the whole pineapple ring in
the center of the skillet, and then arrange the pineapple halves
around it. Set aside.

4. In a large bowl mix the flour, baking powder, salt, and baking
soda. In a small bowl whisk the buttermilk, eggs, and vanilla.

5. In a large bowl, using an electric mixer, cream the butter
and sugar on medium-high speed until light and fluffy, 2 to
4 minutes. With the mixer on low, add the buttermilk mixture
and then gradually add the flour mixture. Blend until smooth,
scraping down the sides as necessary. Using a rubber spatula,
spread the batter evenly over the pineapple slices in the skillet.

6. Bake the cake over **indirect medium heat**, keeping the
temperature of the grill as close to 350°F as possible, with the
lid closed, until the top is golden brown and a skewer inserted
into the center comes out clean, 40 to 50 minutes. Wearing
insulated barbecue mitts, remove the cake from the grill and let
cool at room temperature for about 10 minutes.

7. Before removing the cake from the skillet, run a paring knife
around the edge to loosen it. Place a serving platter, large
enough to hold the cake, over the top of the skillet. Wearing
insulated barbecue mitts, carefully invert the skillet and platter
at the same time, and then slowly remove the skillet. Replace
any pineapple that has stuck to the bottom of the skillet. Let the
cake cool briefly before slicing into wedges and serving. The cake
is best served warm or at room temperature the day it is made.

WAY TO MAKE CRÈME FRAICHE

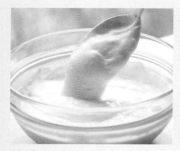

1. After 8 hours at room temperature, a bit of buttermilk turns heavy cream into thick crème fraiche.

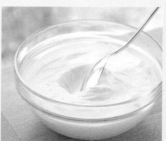

2. After 24 hours, the same crème fraiche is even thicker and more delicious.

WAY TO GRILL APPLES

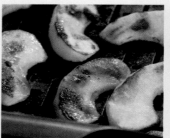

1. Apple slices coated with butter quickly turn brown and tender on the grill.

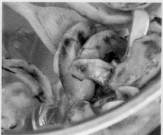

2. Toss them with caramel sauce before assembling the dessert.

APPLE CARAMEL ON PUFF PASTRY

SERVES: 4
PREP TIME: 20 MINUTES

WAY TO GRILL: DIRECT MEDIUM HEAT (350° TO 450°F)
GRILLING TIME: 8 TO 10 MINUTES
SPECIAL EQUIPMENT: PERFORATED GRILL PAN

    1 sheet frozen puff pastry, about 9 inches square, thawed

SAUCE
  ½ cup light brown sugar
  ¼ cup heavy cream
  ¼ cup (½ stick) unsalted butter

  4 Granny Smith apples, peeled and cored, cut into
     ½-inch-thick wedges
  ¼ cup (½ stick) unsalted butter, melted
     Coarse sea salt, optional
  ¼ cup crème fraiche (recipe follows) or whipped cream

1. Using a 4-inch biscuit cutter, cut 4 rounds from the pastry sheet. Using a fork, prick each pastry round about 12 times to prevent the dough from rising too much in the oven. Following package directions, bake the pastry rounds on a baking sheet until golden brown. Transfer to a wire rack to cool.

2. In a small saucepan over medium heat, combine the sauce ingredients, stirring constantly until the sugar is dissolved and the butter is melted, 4 to 5 minutes. Remove from the heat and set aside.

3. In a large bowl toss the apple slices with the melted butter to coat well.

4. Prepare the grill for direct cooking over medium heat. Preheat a perforated grill pan over **direct medium heat** for about 10 minutes. Add the apple slices to the pan and grill them, with the lid closed as much as possible, until they are well browned and tender, 8 to 10 minutes, turning once or twice.

Transfer the apple slices to a bowl. Reheat the sauce over low heat, if necessary, and spoon some of the sauce over the apple slices, gently tossing to coat.

5. To assemble, place each pastry round on a dessert plate. Arrange the apple slices on top of the pastry rounds. Spoon the remaining sauce over the apples, allowing it to run down onto the plates. Sprinkle with a little coarse sea salt, if desired. Finish with a dollop of crème fraiche or whipped cream.

CRÈME FRAICHE
MAKES: 1⅛ CUPS
PREP TIME: 2 MINUTES
STANDING TIME: 8 TO 24 HOURS

  1 cup heavy cream
  2 tablespoons buttermilk

1. In a small bowl combine the cream and buttermilk. Cover and let stand at room temperature for 8 to 24 hours. It can be kept in the refrigerator for up to 10 days.

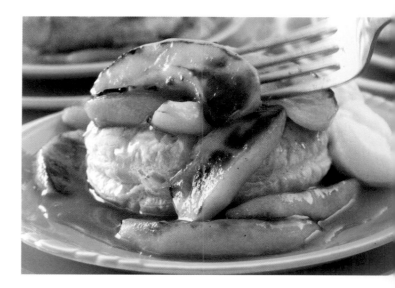

GINGERBREAD
WITH GRILLED APRICOTS

SERVES: 12
PREP TIME: 30 MINUTES

WAY TO GRILL: INDIRECT AND DIRECT MEDIUM HEAT
   (350° TO 450°F) **FOR GAS GRILLS ONLY**
GRILLING TIME: 39 TO 41 MINUTES
SPECIAL EQUIPMENT: 9- OR 10-INCH CAST-IRON SKILLET

1½ cups all-purpose flour
  1 teaspoon ground ginger
  ¾ teaspoon ground cinnamon
  ¾ teaspoon baking soda
  ¾ teaspoon kosher salt
  ½ cup (1 stick) unsalted butter, softened,
       plus more for the pan
  ½ cup granulated sugar
  1 large egg, at room temperature
  ½ cup unsulphured light molasses
  ½ cup hot water
  3 tablespoons chopped crystallized ginger

 12 apricots, firm but ripe, cut in half lengthwise and pitted
  3 tablespoons unsalted butter, melted
  3 tablespoons granulated sugar
  1 tablespoon dark rum, optional

 12 scoops vanilla ice cream

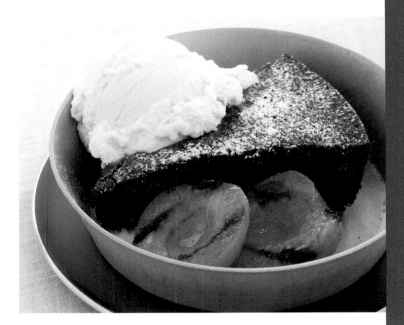

1. In a small bowl combine the flour, ginger, cinnamon, soda, and salt. In a medium bowl, using an electric mixer, beat ½ cup butter and the sugar on high speed until the mixture is light and fluffy, about 3 minutes. Beat in the egg and then the molasses. With the mixer on low speed, gradually add in the flour mixture, scraping down the sides of the bowl with a rubber spatula. Add the water and mix until smooth. Stir in the ginger. Lightly butter the inside of a 9- or 10-inch cast-iron skillet. Evenly spread the batter in the skillet.

2. Prepare the grill for indirect cooking over medium heat. Brush the cooking grates clean.

3. Grill the gingerbread over **indirect medium heat**, with the lid closed, until a toothpick inserted in the center comes out clean, about 35 minutes. Keep the grill's temperature as close to 350°F as possible. Wearing insulated barbecue mitts, carefully remove the skillet from the grill.

4. In a large bowl gently toss the apricots with the melted butter, sugar, and rum. Lift the apricots from the butter mixture, letting the excess butter fall back into the bowl. Grill the apricots, cut sides down, over **direct medium heat**, with the lid closed as much as possible, until heated through, 4 to 6 minutes, turning and brushing with the butter mixture once. Cooking times will vary depending on the ripeness of the apricots.

5. Cut the gingerbread into wedges and serve warm with the apricots. Spoon any remaining butter mixture over the top and serve with ice cream.

WAY TO GRILL GINGERBREAD AND APRICOTS

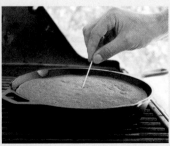

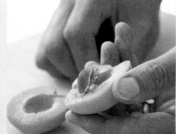

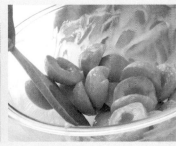

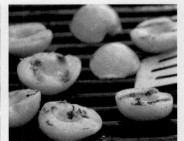

1. Cook gingerbread over indirect medium heat until a toothpick comes out clean.

2. Cut each apricot in half and remove the pits.

3. Toss the apricots in a bowl with sugar and melted butter.

4. Grill the apricots, cut sides down first, over direct medium heat.

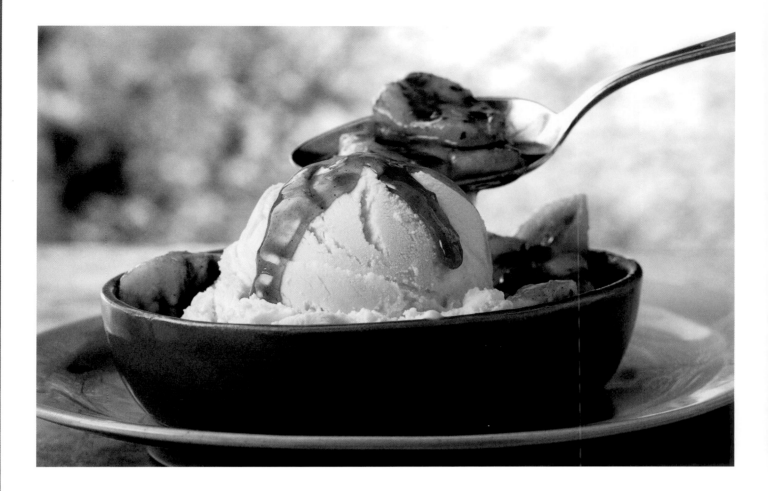

BANANAS FOSTER

SERVES: 6 TO 8
PREP TIME: 10 MINUTES

WAY TO GRILL: DIRECT MEDIUM HEAT (350° TO 450°F)
GRILLING TIME: 2 TO 3 MINUTES

  4 medium bananas, firm but ripe
  2 tablespoons unsalted butter, melted

SAUCE
  ½ cup (1 stick) unsalted butter
  ½ cup firmly packed dark brown sugar
  ¼ teaspoon ground cinnamon
  ⅛ teaspoon ground nutmeg
  ½ cup dark rum
  ¼ cup banana liqueur

    Vanilla ice cream

1. Prepare the grill for direct cooking over medium heat.

2. Cut each banana in half lengthwise and leave the skins attached (they will help the bananas hold their shape on the grill). Brush the cut sides with the melted butter.

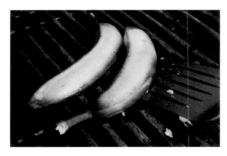

Grill banana halves in their skins to hold the fruit together. Peel and cut the fruit before adding it to the rum sauce.

3. Brush the cooking grates clean. Grill the bananas over **direct medium heat**, with the lid open, until warmed and well marked but not too soft, 2 to 3 minutes, without turning. Remove from the grill. Peel the banana halves, cut them into quarters, and set aside.

4. In a large skillet over medium-high heat, melt the ½ cup of butter. Add the brown sugar, cinnamon, and nutmeg, and cook, stirring constantly, until it bubbles, about 2 minutes. Stir in the rum and banana liqueur. Allow the liquid to warm for a few seconds and then carefully ignite the rum with a long match or multipurpose lighter. Let the flames die down. Add the banana pieces and cook over medium heat for 2 to 3 minutes or until the bananas curl slightly. Spoon the banana mixture over ice cream and serve immediately.

FRUIT

GRILLED BANANA S'MORES

SERVES: 8
PREP TIME: 15 MINUTES

WAY TO GRILL: INDIRECT AND DIRECT MEDIUM HEAT
   (ABOUT 400°F)
GRILLING TIME: 15 TO 21 MINUTES
SPECIAL EQUIPMENT: 8X8-INCH BAKING PAN
   SUITABLE FOR THE GRILL

CRUST
   1   cup graham cracker crumbs
   4   tablespoons unsalted butter, melted
   1   egg yolk

   1   tablespoon unsalted butter, melted
   1   teaspoon brown sugar
   2   medium bananas, firm but ripe
   4   cups mini marshmallows
   ½   cup semisweet chocolate chips

1. Prepare the grill for indirect and direct cooking over medium heat.

2. In a large bowl combine the crust ingredients and mix well. Firmly and evenly press the mixture into the bottom of an 8x8-inch baking pan. Grill the crust over *indirect medium heat*, with the lid closed as much as possible, until firm, 6 to 8 minutes. Remove the crust from the grill and set aside to cool for about 10 minutes. This will allow the crust to set.

3. In a small bowl combine the butter and brown sugar. Cut each banana in half lengthwise and leave the skins attached (they will help the bananas hold their shape on the grill). Liberally brush the cut sides of the bananas with the butter mixture.

4. Grill the bananas, cut sides down, over *direct medium heat*, with the lid open, until they start to soften, 2 to 4 minutes, without turning. Let cool briefly and then score the bananas into ½-inch-thick slices, cutting through just to the peel.

5. Fill the pan with 2 cups of the marshmallows, making sure they cover the bottom of the crust evenly. Next, scoop out and distribute the slices of grilled banana, followed by the remaining 2 cups of marshmallows.

6. Grill the pie over *indirect medium heat*, with the lid closed, keeping the temperature of the grill as close to 400°F as possible, until the marshmallows have puffed up and start to brown, 5 to 7 minutes. At this point carefully sprinkle the chocolate chips over the top and continue cooking until the chips appear glossy and melted, about 2 minutes. Remove the pie from the grill and let cool for 5 minutes. Spoon into small serving bowls and serve warm.

WAY TO GRILL BANANA S'MORES

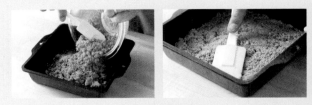

1. Pour the graham cracker mixture into a pan and press it into place with a spatula.

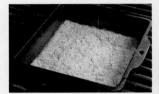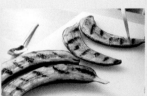

2. Cook the crust until firm. Grill the buttered bananas in their skins so they hold their shapes.

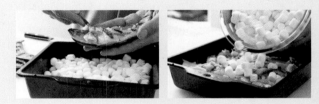

3. Cut the bananas into bite-sized pieces and layer them in the pan between the marshmallows.

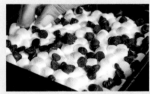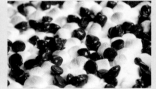

4. During the last couple minutes, sprinkle chocolate chips on top so that they melt into the sweet gooey marshmallows.

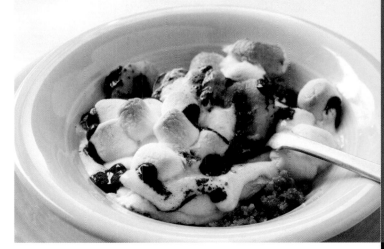

WAY TO PREP PANNA COTTA

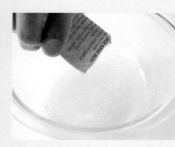

1. Sprinkle gelatin over cold water to soften it.

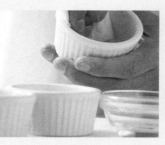

2. Oil the ramekins to help the panna cotta slide out later.

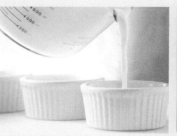

3. Fill the ramekins and chill the panna cotta for at least 8 hours.

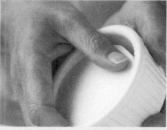

4. Very gently separate the chilled dessert from each ramekin with your thumb.

LEMON-BUTTERMILK PANNA COTTA WITH GRILLED FIGS

SERVES: 6
PREP TIME: 20 MINUTES
CHILLING TIME: AT LEAST 8 HOURS

WAY TO GRILL: DIRECT MEDIUM HEAT (350° TO 450°F)
GRILLING TIME: 4 MINUTES
SPECIAL EQUIPMENT: SIX 6-OUNCE RAMEKINS OR
   CUSTARD CUPS

PANNA COTTA
2½   teaspoons (1 envelope) gelatin
 ¼   cup cold water
  1   cup heavy cream
 ½   cup granulated sugar
  2   cups low-fat buttermilk, well shaken
 ½   teaspoon vanilla extract
  1   tablespoon finely grated lemon zest

     Vegetable oil

  9   ripe figs, about 1¼ ounces each, stems removed,
      cut in half lengthwise
  1   tablespoon honey
  1   bunch fresh mint, optional

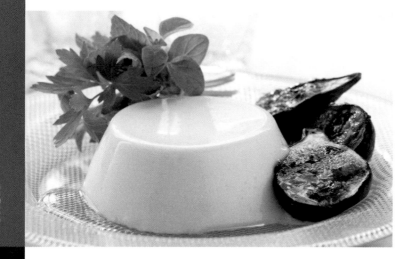

1. In a small cup sprinkle the gelatin over the water and let stand until the gelatin softens, about 5 minutes.

2. In a medium saucepan over medium-low heat, bring the cream and sugar to a simmer, stirring to dissolve the sugar. Once the mixture is simmering, remove from the heat and add the softened gelatin; stir constantly until the gelatin is completely dissolved, about 2 minutes. Stir in the buttermilk and vanilla. Strain the mixture through a wire sieve into a large glass measuring cup or pitcher, and then stir in the lemon zest.

3. Using a paper towel, completely oil the insides of 6 ramekins. Pour equal amounts of the mixture, about ⅔ of a cup, into each ramekin. Place the ramekins on a sheet pan and loosely cover with plastic wrap. Refrigerate until the panna cottas are chilled and set, at least 8 hours, or up to 1 day.

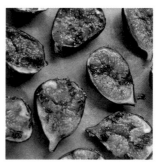

4. Prepare the grill for direct cooking over medium heat. Lightly brush the cuts sides of the figs with oil. Brush the cooking grates clean. Grill the figs over **direct medium heat**, with the lid closed as much as possible, until well marked and heated through, about 4 minutes, turning once after 3 minutes.

5. To remove the panna cotta from the ramekin, one at a time, use your thumb to gently press each pudding around its circumference to pull it away from the sides of the ramekin. You may need to go around a couple of times before it totally releases. This works better than running a knife around the inside of each pudding, which could cut into the pudding. Place a dessert plate on top of the ramekin, and invert the plate. Shake firmly, and let the pudding fall onto the plate.

6. For each serving, stand 3 warm fig halves opposite the panna cotta and drizzle a little honey on the plate. Serve with fresh mint, if desired.

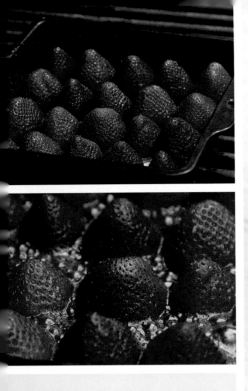

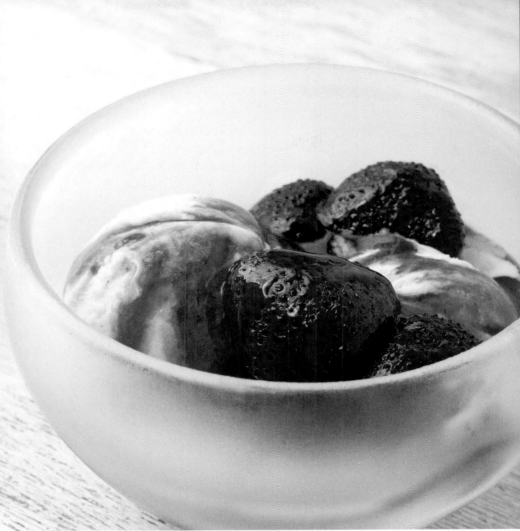

Arrange ripe strawberries snugly in a pan and cook them over direct heat so that their juices bubble and thicken with butter, sugar, vanilla, and orange liqueur.

FIRE-ROASTED STRAWBERRIES

SERVES: 6 TO 8
PREP TIME: 10 MINUTES

WAY TO GRILL: DIRECT HIGH HEAT (450° TO 550°F)
    FOR GAS GRILLS ONLY
GRILLING TIME: 8 TO 12 MINUTES
SPECIAL EQUIPMENT: 8X8-INCH BAKING PAN
    SUITABLE FOR THE GRILL

- 2 pints (20 to 24) fresh, large strawberries, washed and blotted dry
- 4 tablespoons granulated sugar
- ½ teaspoon vanilla extract
- 4 tablespoons orange-flavored liqueur, or 2 tablespoons water and 1 tablespoon lemon juice
- 1 tablespoon unsalted butter, softened
  Vanilla ice cream

1. Hull and trim the stem end of the strawberries so that they are flat. In a medium bowl combine the berries, sugar, vanilla, and liqueur, and toss to coat.

2. Use the soft butter to generously coat the bottom and sides of an 8x8-inch ovenproof pan or disposable aluminum pan. The pan should be just large enough to hold the berries in a single layer with their sides almost touching (this allows the berries to gently support one another as they begin to soften). Prepare the grill for direct cooking over high heat.

3. Remove the berries from the bowl and line them up so that they fit snuggly, pointing up, in the prepared pan. Pour the contents from the bowl over the berries and cook over **direct high heat**, with the lid closed, until they're bubbling and beginning to slump, 8 to 12 minutes. Cooking times will vary depending on the variety, size, and ripeness of the strawberries. Watch closely to catch them before they collapse.

4. Spoon the pan juices over the berries to moisten them, let cool for 5 minutes, and then carefully cut them into quarters or leave whole. Ladle berries over ice cream.

    ■■■

The woodsy smoke of charcoal doesn't belong in fruit desserts like this one. Grill them over gas instead.

    ■■■

WAY TO MAKE SHORTCAKES

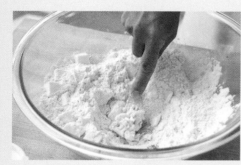

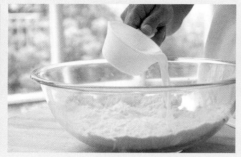

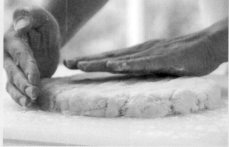

1. Using the back of a fork, mix the butter with the dry ingredients to create a crumbly mixture. Leave some pea-sized clumps of butter for flaky biscuits.

2. Add the half-and-half and gently stir the mixture just until it comes together, but don't toughen the dough by overworking it.

3. Turn the dough onto a lightly floured surface and pat it to a thickness of about ¾ inch.

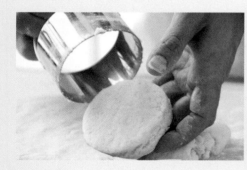

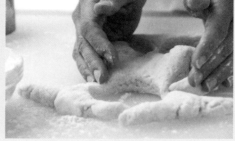

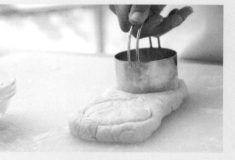

4. Use a floured biscuit cutter to make smooth rounds.

5. Gently gather the scraps into another single strip of dough.

6. Cut a couple more rounds from the strip.

WAY TO GRILL PEACHES

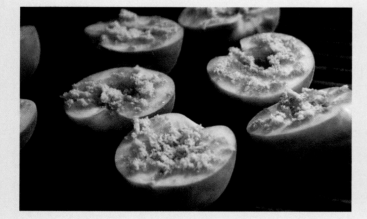

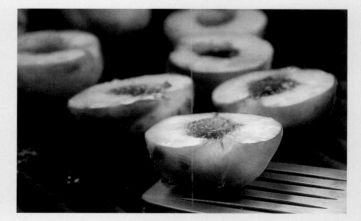

1. Fill the centers of the peach halves with brown sugar, and grill until the sugar melts and the peaches are tender.

2. Remove the peaches with a spatula. Peel and discard the charred skins, chop the peaches, and serve them with split biscuits and whipped cream.

PEACH SHORTCAKES

SERVES: 8
PREP TIME: 20 MINUTES

WAY TO GRILL: DIRECT MEDIUM HEAT (350° TO 450°F)
   FOR GAS GRILLS ONLY
BAKING AND GRILLING TIME: 23 TO 30 MINUTES

- 2 cups all-purpose flour, plus more for dusting
- 5 tablespoons granulated sugar
- 1 tablespoon baking powder
- ½ teaspoons kosher salt
- ½ cup (1 stick) unsalted butter, cold, cut into small pieces
- ½ cup half-and-half, cold
- 1 tablespoon unsalted butter, melted

- 1 cup heavy cream
- 1 teaspoon pure vanilla extract
- 2 tablespoons powdered sugar
- 4 large freestone peaches, firm but ripe, cut in half lengthwise, pits removed
- ¼ cup light brown sugar
- 8 fresh mint sprigs, optional

1. Preheat oven to 400°F.

2. In a large bowl combine the flour, granulated sugar, baking powder, and salt, and blend well. Add the butter and mix with a fork or a pastry blender just until the mixture resembles coarse bread crumbs. Add the half-and-half and gently stir it in (the mixture will be crumbly). Then use your hands to mix the dough quickly and gently in the bowl just until it comes together. Turn the dough out onto a lightly floured work surface. Lightly dust your hands with flour and gently pat out the dough to about ¾ inch thick. Dip a round biscuit cutter, 2½ to 3 inches in diameter, in flour and cut out rounds of dough. Gather scraps of dough and pat out, using a light touch so you don't overwork the dough; cut to make a total of 8 shortcakes. Place the shortcakes about 2 inches apart on a baking sheet lined with parchment paper. Brush the tops with the melted butter. Bake the shortcakes for 15 to 20 minutes. Set aside to cool.

3. In a large bowl combine the cream, vanilla, and powdered sugar and whip just to stiff peaks; do not over beat. Cover and refrigerate until serving.

4. Prepare the grill for direct cooking over medium heat. Brush the cooking grates clean. Sprinkle the cut sides of the peach halves with the brown sugar. Grill the peach halves, cut sides up, over **direct medium heat**, with the lid closed, until the sugar melts and the peaches are soft, 8 to 10 minutes. Carefully remove from the grill and pour the melted brown sugar from the peaches into a medium bowl.

5. Pull the charred skin off the peaches and discard. Cut the peaches into bite-sized pieces and add them to the bowl with the melted brown sugar. Gently toss to coat. Split each shortcake horizontally and top each bottom half with equal portions of the peaches and whipped cream. Add the shortcake tops and garnish with mint sprigs, if desired.

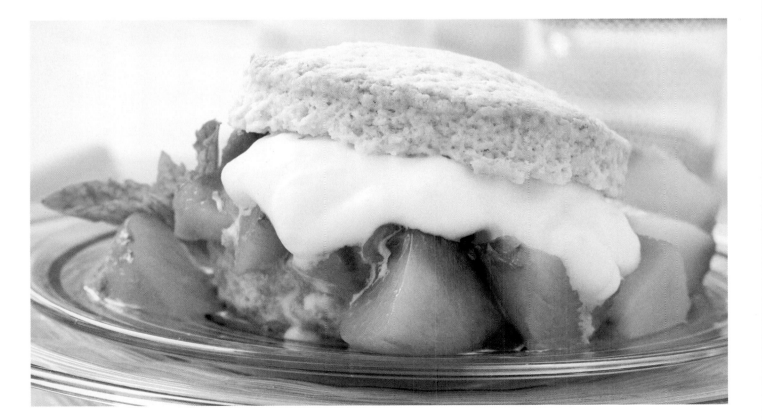

PEAR AND PROSCIUTTO SALAD WITH CHAMPAGNE VINAIGRETTE

SERVES: 4
PREP TIME: 20 MINUTES

WAY TO GRILL: DIRECT MEDIUM HEAT (350° TO 450°F)
GRILLING TIME: 4 TO 6 MINUTES

VINAIGRETTE
- ¼ cup champagne or white wine vinegar
- 2 tablespoons minced shallot
- 1 teaspoon Dijon mustard
- ½ teaspoon granulated sugar
- ¼ teaspoon kosher salt
- ¼ teaspoon freshly ground black pepper
- ¼ cup extra-virgin olive oil
- 2 tablespoons toasted hazelnut oil or olive oil

- 8 paper-thin slices prosciutto
- 2 Bartlett pears, firm but ripe, quartered and cored
- 8 cups lightly packed arugula or mesclun greens
- 2 ounces manchego or Parmigiano-Reggiano cheese
- ¾ cup skinned hazelnuts, toasted and coarsely chopped
  Kosher salt
  Freshly ground black pepper

1. In a small bowl whisk the vinegar, shallot, mustard, sugar, salt, and pepper. Gradually drizzle in both oils, whisking constantly, until emulsified. Taste, and if the vinaigrette is too acidic, add 1 tablespoon or so of water.

2. Prepare the grill for direct cooking over medium heat. Brush the cooking grates clean.

3. Wrap a slice of prosciutto around each pear wedge, pressing the loose ends of the prosciutto down so the meat stays together. Lightly brush the outside of the wrapped pears with some vinaigrette and grill them over **direct medium heat**, with the grill lid open, until the prosciutto is slightly crispy and golden brown and the pears are warm, 4 to 6 minutes, turning as needed.

4. Whisk the vinaigrette again to emulsify the ingredients. In a large bowl, toss the arugula with enough vinaigrette to lightly coat the leaves (you may not need all the vinaigrette) and divide among 4 salad plates. Top each salad with 2 warm pear wedges and drizzle with some additional vinaigrette. Using a vegetable peeler, shave wide ribbons of cheese over each salad, and then sprinkle with the hazelnuts. Season to taste with salt and pepper. Serve immediately.

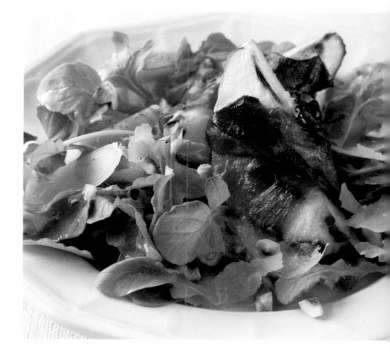

WAY TO PREP PEAR AND PROSCIUTTO

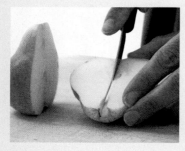

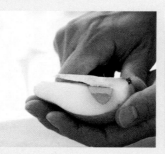

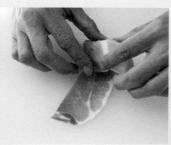

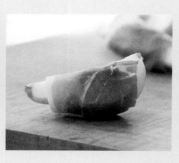

1. Quarter each pear lengthwise.

2. Trim away the core and seeds.

3. Cut the prosciutto into strips for wrapping the quarters.

4. Overlap and press each strip of prosciutto on itself so that it stays in place on the grill.

WAY TO WRAP BRIE IN GRAPE LEAVES

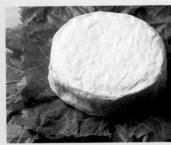

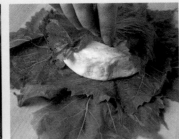

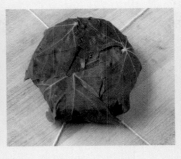

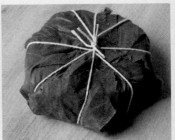

1. Overlap rinsed and dried grape leaves, vein-side up, and place the cheese in the center.

2. Pull the edges over the cheese, overlapping them on top.

3. Create an X with two long pieces of butcher's twine and put the cheese bundle on top.

4. Wrap the twine around the cheese bundle a couple times, knotting in the center each time.

GRAPE LEAF-WRAPPED BRIE WITH GRAPE SALSA

SERVES: 4 TO 6 AS AN APPETIZER
PREP TIME: 15 MINUTES

WAY TO GRILL: DIRECT MEDIUM HEAT (350° TO 450°F)
GRILLING TIME: 4 TO 5 MINUTES
SPECIAL EQUIPMENT: BUTCHER'S TWINE

SALSA
1 tablespoon balsamic vinegar
½ teaspoon granulated sugar
1 cup coarsely chopped seedless red and/or purple grapes
1 tablespoon chopped fresh mint

6 large grape leaves
1 wheel triple-cream Brie cheese, about 8 ounces
1 baguette, about 8 ounces, cut diagonally into ½-inch slices
1 tablespoon grapeseed oil or olive oil

1. In a small sauté pan over medium heat, combine the vinegar and sugar. Add the grapes and cook to soften them, about 2 minutes, stirring occasionally. Transfer to a small bowl and cover to keep warm. Add the mint just before serving.

2. Prepare the grill for direct cooking over medium heat.

3. Unroll and rinse the grape leaves. Spread out the leaves on a work surface and pat dry with paper towels. Cut off and discard the tough stems. Overlap 4 grape leaves, vein-side up, into an 11- or 12-inch circle. Put another leaf in the center, and then put the cheese on top. Cover the cheese with another grape leaf. Wrap the leaves around the cheese, overlapping them to prevent the cheese from ultimately leaking out. Knot together two 3-foot pieces of butcher's twine in the middle. Lay on a work surface in the shape of an X. Set the cheese bundle on top. Bring the twine to the top and tie snugly. Wrap the twine around the cheese 1 or 2 more times like spokes on a wheel, knotting

snugly in the center each time. Tuck in any loose leaf edges. Trim the ends of the twine.

4. Lightly brush the cheese bundle and bread slices all over with oil. Brush the cooking grates clean. Grill the cheese over **direct medium heat**, with the lid closed as much as possible, until each side is soft when gently pressed, 3 to 4 minutes, turning once. Carefully remove the cheese and let rest for about 2 minutes. After you remove the cheese, grill the bread slices over **direct medium heat** until they are lightly toasted on one side only, about 1 minute. By grilling only one side of the bread it ensures a nice sturdy base for the melted cheese and salsa.

5. Arrange the cheese and grilled bread on a serving plate or tray. Cut the twine and discard it. Pull the grape leaves open to reveal the cheese inside. Be sure to do this just before serving as the cheese begins to ooze out as soon as you remove the grape leaves. Top the cheese with some of the grape salsa or serve it alongside in a bowl. Use spoons to scoop up cheese and salsa, and place on slices of grilled bread.

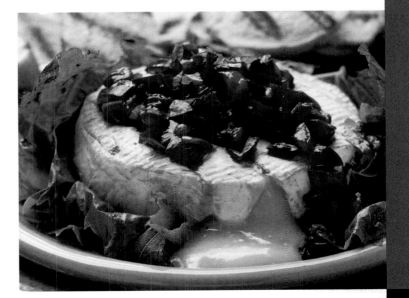

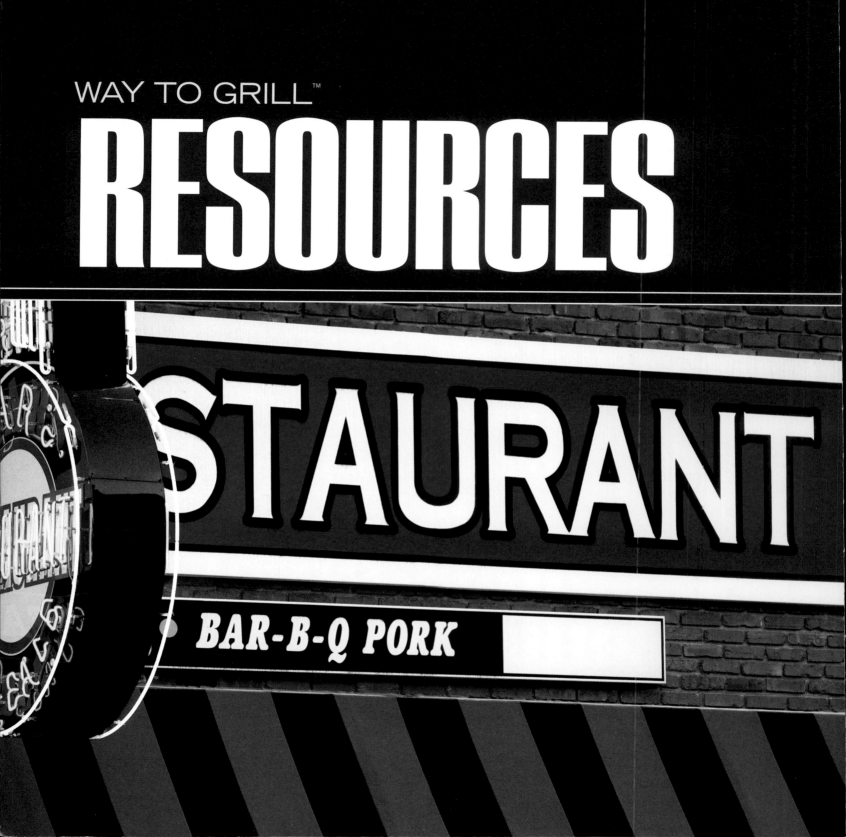

WAY TO GRILL™

RESOURCES

GRILLING GUIDES AND TIPS

RECIPES

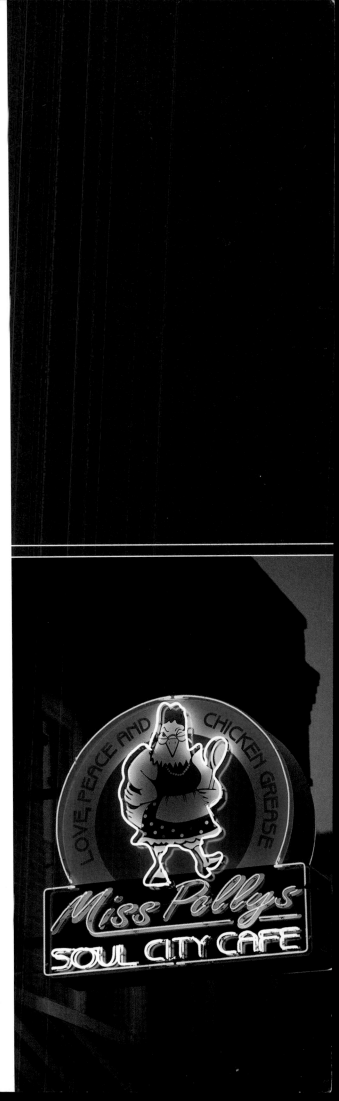

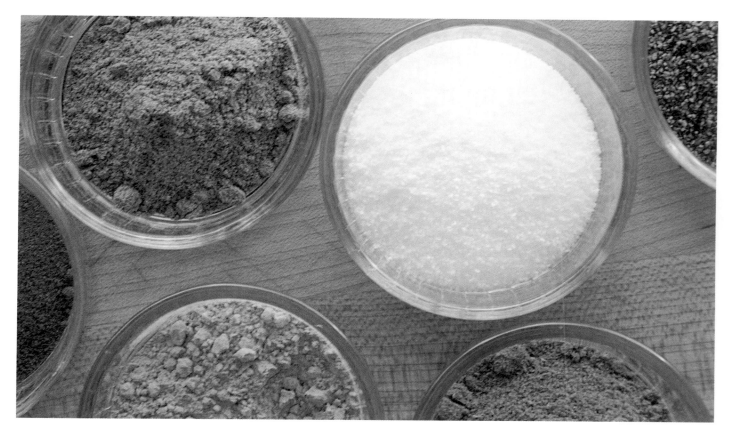

RUBS

A rub is a mixture of spices, herbs, and other seasonings (often including sugar) that can quickly give a boost of flavors to foods before grilling. The following pages provide some mighty good examples, along with recommendations for which foods they complement, but dare to be different. One of the steps toward developing your own style at the grill is to concoct a signature rub recipe or two. Only you will know exactly what ingredients are blended in your special jar of "magic dust."

A word about freshness: Ground spices lose their aromas in a matter of months (8 to 10 months maximum). If you have been holding onto a little jar of coriander for years, waiting to blend the world's finest version of curry powder, forget about it. Dump the old, tired coriander and buy some freshly ground. Better yet, buy whole coriander seeds and grind them yourself. Whatever you do, store your spices and spice rubs in airtight containers away from light and heat, to give them a long, aromatic life.

HOW LONG?

If you leave a rub on for a long time, the seasonings intermix with the juices in the meat and produce more pronounced flavors, as well as a crust. This is good to a point, but a rub with a lot of salt and sugar will draw moisture out of the meat over time, making the meat tastier, yes, but also drier. So how long should you use a rub? Here are some guidelines.

1 TO 15 MINUTES	Small foods, such as shellfish, cubed meat for kabobs, and vegetables
15 TO 30 MINUTES	Thin cuts of boneless meat, such as chicken breasts, fish fillets, pork tenderloin, chops, and steaks
30 TO 90 MINUTES	Thicker cuts of boneless or bone-in meat, such as leg of lamb, whole chickens, and beef roasts
2 TO 8 HOURS	Big or tough cuts of meat, such as racks of ribs, whole hams, pork shoulders, and turkeys

CLASSIC BARBECUE SPICE RUB

MAKES: ABOUT ¼ CUP

- 4 teaspoons kosher salt
- 2 teaspoons pure chile powder
- 2 teaspoons light brown sugar
- 2 teaspoons granulated garlic
- 2 teaspoons paprika
- 1 teaspoon celery seed
- 1 teaspoon ground cumin
- ½ teaspoon freshly ground black pepper

CHICKEN AND SEAFOOD RUB

MAKES: ABOUT ¼ CUP

- 4 teaspoons granulated onion
- 4 teaspoons granulated garlic
- 1 tablespoon kosher salt
- 2 teaspoons prepared chili powder
- 2 teaspoons freshly ground black pepper

CRACKED PEPPER RUB

MAKES: ABOUT 1½ TABLESPOONS

- 1 teaspoon whole black peppercorns
- 1 teaspoon mustard seed
- 1 teaspoon paprika
- ½ teaspoon granulated garlic
- ½ teaspoon kosher salt
- ½ teaspoon light brown sugar
- ⅛ teaspoon ground cayenne pepper

Using a spice mill or mortar and pestle, crush the black peppercorns and mustard seed. Transfer to a small bowl and combine with the remaining ingredients.

CAJUN RUB

MAKES: ABOUT 3 TABLESPOONS

- 2 teaspoons finely chopped fresh thyme
- 1½ teaspoons kosher salt
- 1 teaspoon granulated garlic
- 1 teaspoon granulated onion
- 1 teaspoon paprika
- 1 teaspoon light brown sugar
- ¾ teaspoon freshly ground black pepper
- ¼ teaspoon ground cayenne pepper

PORK RUB

MAKES: ABOUT ⅓ CUP

- 2 teaspoons pure chile powder
- 2 teaspoons freshly ground black pepper
- 2 teaspoons kosher salt
- 2 teaspoons ground cumin
- 2 teaspoons dried oregano
- 1 teaspoon granulated garlic

BEEF RUB

MAKES: ¼ CUP

- 4 teaspoons kosher salt
- 1 tablespoon pure chile powder
- 1 tablespoon granulated onion
- 1½ teaspoons granulated garlic
- 1 teaspoon paprika
- 1 teaspoon dried marjoram
- ½ teaspoon ground cumin
- ½ teaspoon freshly ground black pepper
- ¼ teaspoon ground cinnamon

FENNEL RUB

MAKES: ¼ CUP

- 3 teaspoons ground fennel seed
- 3 teaspoons kosher salt
- 3 teaspoons pure chile powder
- 1½ teaspoons celery seed
- 1½ teaspoons freshly ground black pepper

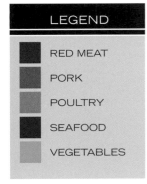

LEGEND

RED MEAT
PORK
POULTRY
SEAFOOD
VEGETABLES

WAY MORE RUBS

SOUTHWEST RUB

MAKES: ABOUT ¼ CUP

2 teaspoons pure chile powder
2 teaspoons granulated garlic
2 teaspoons paprika
2 teaspoons kosher salt
1 teaspoon ground coriander
1 teaspoon ground cumin
1 teaspoon freshly ground black pepper

CARIBBEAN RUB

MAKES: ABOUT ¼ CUP

1 tablespoon light brown sugar
1 tablespoon granulated garlic
1 tablespoon dried thyme
2¼ teaspoons kosher salt
¾ teaspoon freshly ground black pepper
¾ teaspoon ground allspice

TARRAGON RUB

MAKES: ABOUT ¼ CUP

1½ tablespoons dried tarragon
2½ teaspoons kosher salt
2 teaspoons freshly ground black pepper
1½ teaspoons dried thyme
1 teaspoon rubbed dried sage, packed

MAGIC RUB

MAKES: 2 TABLESPOONS

1 teaspoon dry mustard
1 teaspoon granulated onion
1 teaspoon paprika
1 teaspoon kosher salt
½ teaspoon granulated garlic
½ teaspoon ground coriander
½ teaspoon ground cumin
½ teaspoon freshly ground black pepper

ESPRESSO-CHILE RUB

MAKES: ABOUT ¼ CUP

2 tablespoons dark-roast coffee or espresso beans
2 teaspoons cumin seed, toasted
1 tablespoon ground ancho chile pepper
1 teaspoon sweet paprika
1 teaspoon kosher salt
1 teaspoon freshly ground black pepper

In a spice mill pulse the coffee beans and cumin seed until finely ground. Transfer to a small bowl, add the remaining ingredients, and stir to combine.

ASIAN RUB

MAKES: ABOUT ¼ CUP

2 tablespoons paprika
2 teaspoons kosher salt
2 teaspoons ground coriander
2 teaspoons Chinese five-spice powder
1 teaspoon ground ginger
½ teaspoon ground allspice
½ teaspoon ground cayenne pepper

LEGEND	
■	RED MEAT
■	PORK
■	POULTRY
■	SEAFOOD
■	VEGETABLES

BABY BACK RIBS RUB

MAKES: ½ CUP

2 tablespoons kosher salt
2 tablespoons paprika
4 teaspoons granulated garlic
4 teaspoons pure chile powder
2 teaspoons dry mustard
2 teaspoons freshly ground black pepper

BAJA FISH RUB

MAKES: 4 TEASPOONS

1 teaspoon pure chile powder
1 teaspoon ground cumin
1 teaspoon kosher salt
½ teaspoon ground cayenne pepper
½ teaspoon ground cinnamon

MEXICAN RUB

MAKES: ABOUT ¼ CUP

1 tablespoon ground cumin
1 tablespoon packed brown sugar
2 teaspoons kosher salt
1 teaspoon pasilla or pure chile powder
1 teaspoon ground coriander
1 teaspoon dried oregano

NEW WORLD RUB

MAKES: ABOUT 2 TABLESPOONS

1 teaspoon granulated garlic
1 teaspoon granulated onion
1 teaspoon paprika
½ teaspoon cumin
½ teaspoon dried lemongrass
½ teaspoon dried basil
½ teaspoon dried thyme
½ teaspoon kosher salt
¼ teaspoon freshly ground black pepper
⅛ teaspoon ground cayenne pepper

BARBECUE CHICKEN RUB

MAKES: ABOUT 3 TABLESPOONS

1 tablespoon smoked paprika
2 teaspoons dry mustard
1 teaspoon kosher salt
½ teaspoon granulated garlic
½ teaspoon granulated onion
¼ teaspoon ground chipotle chile

LEMON-PAPRIKA RUB

MAKES: ABOUT 2 TABLESPOONS

2 teaspoons smoked paprika
2 teaspoons kosher salt
Finely grated zest of 1 lemon
½ teaspoon granulated garlic
½ teaspoon freshly ground black pepper

ALL-PURPOSE RUB

MAKES: ABOUT 2 TABLESPOONS

1 teaspoon pure chile powder
1 teaspoon granulated garlic
1 teaspoon paprika
1 teaspoon kosher salt
½ teaspoon ground coriander
½ teaspoon ground cumin
½ teaspoon freshly ground black pepper

PULLED PORK RUB

MAKES: ABOUT ¼ CUP

2 tablespoons pure chile powder
2 tablespoons kosher salt
4 teaspoons granulated garlic
2 teaspoons freshly ground black pepper
1 teaspoon dry mustard

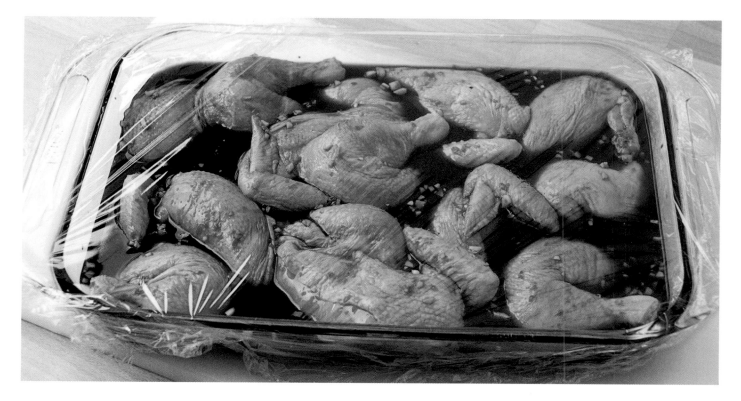

MARINADES

Marinades work more slowly than rubs, but they can seep in a little deeper. Typically, a marinade is made with some acidic liquid, some oil, and some combination of herbs and spices. These ingredients can "fill in the gaps" when a particular meat, fish, or vegetable (yes, vegetable) lacks enough taste or richness. They can also give food characteristics that reflect regional/ethnic cooking styles.

If indeed your marinade includes some acidic liquid, be sure to use a non-reactive container. This is a dish or bowl made of glass, plastic, stainless steel, or ceramic. A container made of aluminum, or some other metals, will react with acids and add a metallic flavor to food.

HOW LONG?

The right times vary depending on the strength of the marinade and the food you are marinating. If your marinade includes intense ingredients such as soy sauce, liquor, or hot chiles and spices, don't overdo it. A fish fillet should still taste like fish, not a burning-hot, salt-soaked piece of protein. Also, if an acidic marinade is left too long on meat or fish, it can make the surface mushy or dry. Here are some general guidelines to get you going.

15 to 30 MINUTES	Small foods, such as shellfish, fish fillets, cubed meat for kabobs, and tender vegetables
1 to 3 HOURS	Thin cuts of boneless meat, such as chicken breasts, pork tenderloin, chops, and steaks, as well as sturdy vegetables
2 to 6 HOURS	Thicker cuts of boneless or bone-in meat, such as leg of lamb, whole chickens, and beef roasts
6 to 12 HOURS	Big or tough cuts of meat, such as racks of ribs, whole hams, pork shoulders, and turkeys

BEER MARINADE

MAKES: ABOUT 1¼ CUPS

1 cup dark Mexican beer
2 tablespoons dark sesame oil
1 tablespoon finely chopped garlic
1 teaspoon dried oregano
1 teaspoon kosher salt
½ teaspoon freshly ground black pepper
¼ teaspoon ground cayenne pepper

JERK MARINADE

MAKES: ABOUT 1 CUP

½ cup roughly chopped yellow onion
1 jalapeño chile pepper, roughly chopped
3 tablespoons white wine vinegar
2 tablespoons soy sauce
2 tablespoons canola oil
½ teaspoon ground allspice
¼ teaspoon granulated garlic
¼ teaspoon ground cinnamon
¼ teaspoon kosher salt
¼ teaspoon freshly ground black pepper
⅛ teaspoon ground nutmeg

PACIFIC RIM MARINADE

MAKES: ABOUT 2 CUPS

1 small yellow onion, roughly chopped
(about 1 cup)
⅓ cup soy sauce
¼ cup fresh lemon juice
¼ cup vegetable oil
2 tablespoons dark brown sugar
2 tablespoons minced garlic
½ teaspoon ground allspice

LEGEND

RED MEAT

PORK

POULTRY

SEAFOOD

VEGETABLES

MOJO MARINADE

MAKES: ABOUT ¾ CUP

¼ cup fresh orange juice
3 tablespoons fresh lime juice
3 tablespoons extra-virgin olive oil
2 tablespoons finely chopped fresh cilantro
1 tablespoon finely chopped jalapeño chile pepper,
including seeds
1 tablespoon minced garlic
¾ teaspoon ground cumin
½ teaspoon kosher salt

LEMON-SAGE MARINADE

MAKES: ABOUT 1 CUP

1 tablespoon finely grated lemon zest
¼ cup fresh lemon juice
¼ cup extra-virgin olive oil
3 tablespoons finely chopped fresh sage
2 tablespoons minced shallot
2 tablespoons whole-grain mustard
1 tablespoon finely chopped garlic
1 tablespoon freshly cracked black peppercorns

TERIYAKI MARINADE

MAKES: ABOUT 2¼ CUPS

1 cup pineapple juice
½ cup low-sodium soy sauce
½ cup finely chopped yellow onion
1 tablespoon dark sesame oil
1 tablespoon grated fresh ginger
1 tablespoon minced garlic
1 tablespoon dark brown sugar
1 tablespoon fresh lemon juice

GREEK MARINADE

MAKES: ABOUT ½ CUP

¼ cup plus 2 tablespoons extra-virgin olive oil
3 tablespoons red wine vinegar
½ teaspoon minced garlic
½ teaspoon kosher salt
½ teaspoon dried oregano
¼ teaspoon crushed red chile flakes

WAY MORE MARINADES

MEDITERRANEAN MARINADE

MAKES: ABOUT ¼ CUP

- 2 tablespoons extra-virgin olive oil
- 2 teaspoons paprika
- 1 teaspoon ground coriander
- 1 teaspoon ground cumin
- 1 teaspoon granulated garlic
- 1 teaspoon kosher salt
- ¼ teaspoon freshly ground black pepper

SOUTHWEST MARINADE

MAKES: ABOUT 1 CUP

- ½ cup fresh orange juice
- 3 tablespoons extra-virgin olive oil
- 2 tablespoons red wine vinegar
- 1 tablespoon minced garlic
- 2 teaspoons pure chile powder
- 1½ teaspoons dried oregano
- 1 teaspoon kosher salt
- ½ teaspoon freshly ground black pepper
- ½ teaspoon ground cinnamon

TEQUILA MARINADE

MAKES: ABOUT 1¾ CUPS

- 1 cup fresh orange juice
- ½ cup tequila
- 2 tablespoons fresh lime juice
- 2 tablespoons light brown sugar
- 2 teaspoons ground cumin
- 1 jalapeño chile pepper, cut into ⅛-inch slices

BOURBON MARINADE

MAKES: ABOUT 1 CUP

- ½ cup bourbon
- ¼ cup ketchup
- 2 tablespoons extra-virgin olive oil
- 2 tablespoons soy sauce
- 1 tablespoon white wine vinegar
- 2 teaspoons minced garlic
- ½ teaspoon hot sauce, or to taste
- ½ teaspoon freshly ground black pepper

HONEY-MUSTARD MARINADE

MAKES: ABOUT 1 CUP

- ½ cup Dijon mustard
- ¼ cup honey
- 2 tablespoons extra-virgin olive oil
- 2 teaspoons curry powder
- 1 teaspoon freshly grated lemon zest
- ½ teaspoon granulated garlic
- ½ teaspoon kosher salt
- ¼ teaspoon ground cayenne pepper
- ¼ teaspoon freshly ground black pepper

TARRAGON-CITRUS MARINADE

MAKES: ABOUT 1 CUP

- ¼ cup extra-virgin olive oil
- ¼ cup roughly chopped fresh tarragon
  Zest and juice of 1 orange
  Zest and juice of 1 lemon
- 2 tablespoons sherry vinegar
- 2 teaspoons kosher salt
- 1 teaspoon minced garlic
- 1 teaspoon grated ginger
- ½ teaspoon prepared chili powder
- ½ teaspoon freshly ground black pepper

LEGEND
■ RED MEAT
■ PORK
■ POULTRY
■ SEAFOOD
■ VEGETABLES

MONGOLIAN MARINADE

MAKES: ABOUT 1¼ CUPS

½ cup hoisin sauce
2 tablespoons oyster sauce
2 tablespoons soy sauce
2 tablespoons dry sherry
2 tablespoons rice vinegar
2 tablespoons canola oil
1 tablespoon honey
1 tablespoon minced ginger
1 tablespoon minced garlic
½ teaspoon crushed red pepper flakes (optional)

SPICY CAYENNE MARINADE

MAKES: ABOUT ½ CUP

¼ cup extra-virgin olive oil
2 tablespoons fresh lemon juice
1 tablespoon minced garlic
2 teaspoons dried oregano
2 teaspoons paprika
1½ teaspoons kosher salt
1 teaspoon celery seed
1 teaspoon ground cayenne pepper

CUBAN MARINADE

MAKES: ABOUT 2 CUPS

½ cup fresh orange juice
½ cup fresh lemonade
½ cup finely chopped yellow onion
¼ cup extra-virgin olive oil
2 tablespoons minced garlic
2 tablespoons dried oregano
2 tablespoons fresh lime juice

CHINESE HOISIN MARINADE

MAKES: ABOUT ¾ CUP

½ cup hoisin sauce
2 tablespoons red wine vinegar
1 tablespoon canola oil
2 teaspoons minced garlic
1 teaspoon grated fresh ginger
1 teaspoon hot sauce, or to taste
1 teaspoon dark sesame oil

TANDOORI MARINADE

MAKES: ABOUT 1¼ CUPS

1 cup plain yogurt
1 tablespoon grated fresh ginger
1 tablespoon paprika
1 tablespoon vegetable oil
2 teaspoons minced garlic
2 teaspoons kosher salt
1½ teaspoons ground cumin
1 teaspoon ground turmeric
½ teaspoon ground cayenne pepper

BARCELONA MARINADE

MAKES: ABOUT ¾ CUP

5 scallions, cut into 1-inch pieces
1 cup lightly packed fresh basil leaves
3 large garlic cloves
2 serrano chile peppers, roughly chopped
¼ cup extra-virgin olive oil
2 tablespoons sherry vinegar
1 teaspoon kosher salt
½ teaspoon freshly ground black pepper

In a food processor or blender, process the ingredients to a smooth paste, 1 to 2 minutes.

CILANTRO PESTO MARINADE

MAKES: ABOUT 1 CUP

2 tablespoons coarsely chopped walnuts
2 medium garlic cloves
1½ cups loosely packed fresh cilantro leaves and tender stems
½ cup loosely packed fresh Italian parsley leaves and tender stems
½ teaspoon kosher salt
¼ teaspoon freshly ground black pepper
¼ cup extra-virgin olive oil

In a food processor finely chop the walnuts and garlic. Scrape down the sides of the bowl. Add the cilantro, parsley, salt, and pepper and process until finely chopped. With the motor running, slowly add the oil to create a smooth puree.

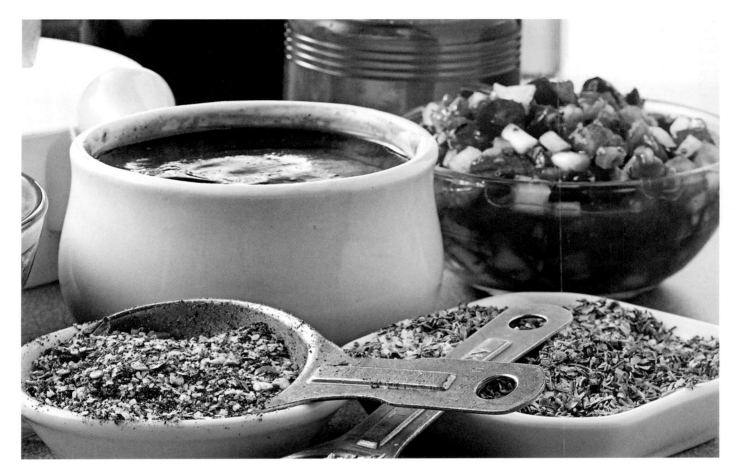

SAUCES

Sauces open up a world of flavors for grillers. They offer us almost limitless ways for distinguishing our food and making it more interesting. Once you have learned some of the fundamentals about balancing flavors and some of the techniques for holding sauces together, you are ready to develop your own. I've included several styles of sauces on the following pages, some of them featuring a grilled ingredient or two for greater depth. Find the sauces that suit you and the kind of food you like to grill. Return to them a couple times so that you understand how and why they work. Then start pushing the parameters. A little more of this. A little less of that. Maybe a few more minutes simmering over the fire. Sauces are playgrounds for discovery. Learn the basics and build from there.

PASILLA BARBECUE SAUCE

MAKES: ABOUT 2 CUPS

2 tablespoons extra-virgin olive oil
6 medium garlic cloves, peeled
⅓ cup finely chopped red onion
2 dried pasilla chile peppers, stemmed, seeded, and cut into strips
1 cup diced canned tomatoes with juice
1 cup amber Mexican beer
1 tablespoon cider vinegar
1 teaspoon kosher salt
½ teaspoon dried oregano
¼ teaspoon freshly ground black pepper

In a small, heavy-bottomed saucepan over medium heat, warm the oil and cook the garlic until lightly browned, 4 to 5 minutes, turning occasionally. Add the onion and chiles. Cook for about 3 minutes, stirring occasionally. Add the remaining ingredients, bring to a boil, then simmer for 15 minutes. Remove the saucepan from the heat and let the mixture stand for 15 minutes to soften the chiles and blend the flavors. Puree in a blender.

CLASSIC RED BARBECUE SAUCE

MAKES: ABOUT 1½ CUPS

- ¾ cup apple juice
- ½ cup ketchup
- 3 tablespoons cider vinegar
- 2 teaspoons soy sauce
- 1 teaspoon Worcestershire sauce
- 1 teaspoon molasses
- ½ teaspoon pure chile powder
- ½ teaspoon granulated garlic
- ¼ teaspoon freshly ground black pepper

In a small saucepan mix the ingredients. Simmer for a few minutes over medium heat, and then remove the saucepan from the heat.

RED CHILE BARBECUE SAUCE

MAKES: ABOUT 2 CUPS

- 4 dried pasilla chile peppers, about ¾ ounce total
- 2 tablespoons canola oil
- ½ cup ketchup
- 3 tablespoons soy sauce
- 2 tablespoons balsamic vinegar
- 3 medium garlic cloves, crushed
- 1 teaspoon ground cumin
- ½ teaspoon dried oregano
- ¼ teaspoon kosher salt
- ¼ teaspoon freshly ground black pepper

Remove the stems and cut the chiles crosswise into sections about 2 inches long. Remove most of the seeds. In a medium skillet over high heat, warm the oil. Add the chiles and toast them until they puff up and begin to turn color, 2 to 3 minutes, turning once. Transfer the chiles and oil to a small bowl. Cover with 1 cup of hot water and soak the chiles for 30 minutes. Pour the chiles, along with the oil and water, into a blender or food processor. Add the remaining ingredients and process until very smooth.

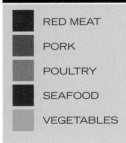

LEGEND	
	RED MEAT
	PORK
	POULTRY
	SEAFOOD
	VEGETABLES

SASSY BARBECUE SAUCE

MAKES: ABOUT 1 CUP

- ½ cup water
- ½ cup ketchup
- 2 tablespoons molasses
- 1 tablespoon white wine vinegar
- 1 tablespoon Dijon mustard
- 1 tablespoon light brown sugar
- 2 teaspoons Worcestershire sauce
- ½ teaspoon kosher salt
- ¼ teaspoon hot sauce, or to taste
- ¼ teaspoon granulated garlic
- ¼ teaspoon freshly ground black pepper

In a small, heavy-bottomed saucepan whisk the ingredients. Bring to boil over medium heat, then reduce the heat and simmer for 10 minutes, stirring occasionally.

ANCHO BARBECUE SAUCE

MAKES: ABOUT 1 CUP

- ⅓ cup slivered almonds
- 2 medium dried ancho chile peppers, about ½ ounce total
- 6 tablespoons fresh orange juice
- ⅓ cup roughly chopped roasted red bell peppers from a jar
- 3 tablespoons ketchup
- 2 tablespoons extra-virgin olive oil
- 1 tablespoon red wine vinegar
- ½ teaspoon granulated garlic
- ¼ teaspoon kosher salt
- ¼ teaspoon freshly ground black pepper

In a medium skillet over medium heat, toast the almonds until golden brown, 3 to 5 minutes, stirring occasionally. Transfer the almonds to a food processor. Remove the stems from the chiles, make a slit down the side of each one with scissors, and remove the veins and seeds. Flatten the chiles and place them in the skillet over medium heat. With a spatula hold the chiles flat for 5 seconds, turn over and repeat for another 5 seconds. Transfer the chiles to a medium bowl and soak in hot water for 15 minutes. Remove the chiles, squeeze out the excess water, and then roughly chop (you should have about ¼ cup). Place the chiles and the remaining ingredients in the food processor with the almonds. Process to create a coarse puree.

WAY MORE SAUCES

CREAMY HORSERADISH SAUCE

MAKES: ABOUT 1 CUP

¾ cup sour cream
2 tablespoons prepared horseradish
2 tablespoons finely chopped fresh Italian parsley
2 teaspoons Dijon mustard
2 teaspoons Worcestershire sauce
½ teaspoon kosher salt
¼ teaspoon freshly ground black pepper

In a medium bowl thoroughly mix the ingredients. Cover and refrigerate until about 30 minutes before serving.

CHIMICHURRI SAUCE

MAKES: ABOUT 1½ CUPS

4 large garlic cloves
1 cup loosely packed fresh Italian parsley leaves
1 cup loosely packed fresh cilantro leaves
½ cup loosely packed fresh basil leaves
¾ cup extra-virgin olive oil
¼ cup rice vinegar
1 teaspoon kosher salt
½ teaspoon freshly ground black pepper
½ teaspoon hot sauce, or to taste

In a food processor with the motor running, mince the garlic. Add the parsley, cilantro, and basil. Pulse to finely chop the herbs. With the motor running, slowly add the oil in a thin stream, and then add the remaining ingredients.

ROMESCO SAUCE

MAKES: ABOUT ¾ CUP

2 medium red bell peppers
1 medium garlic clove
¼ cup whole almonds, toasted
½ cup loosely packed fresh Italian parsley leaves
2 teaspoons sherry wine vinegar
½ teaspoon kosher salt
⅛ teaspoon ground cayenne pepper
¼ cup extra-virgin olive oil

Grill the bell peppers over **direct medium heat** (350° to 450°F), with the lid closed as much as possible, until they are blackened and blistered all over, 12 to 15 minutes, turning occasionally. Place the peppers in a small bowl and cover with plastic wrap. Set aside for about 10 minutes, then remove and discard the skins, stems, and seeds. In a food processor, finely chop the garlic. Add the almonds and process until finely chopped. Add the peppers, parsley, vinegar, salt, and cayenne. Process to create a coarse paste. With the motor running, slowly add the oil and process until you have a fairly smooth sauce.

GARLIC AND RED PEPPER SAUCE

MAKES ABOUT ⅔ CUP

1 large red bell pepper
⅓ cup sour cream
¼ cup mayonnaise
1 tablespoon finely chopped fresh basil
2 teaspoons minced garlic
2 teaspoons balsamic vinegar
¼ teaspoon salt

Grill the bell pepper over **direct medium heat** (350° to 450°F), with the lid closed as much as possible, until the skin is blackened and blistered all over, 12 to 15 minutes, turning occasionally. Place the pepper in a small bowl and cover with plastic wrap to trap the steam. Set aside for at least 10 minutes, then remove the pepper from the bowl and peel away the charred skin. Cut off the top, remove the seeds, and roughly chop the pepper. Place in a food processor along with the remaining ingredients. Process until smooth. Cover and refrigerate until about 20 minutes before serving.

COOL GREEN CHILE SAUCE

MAKES: ABOUT 1½ CUPS

- 3 long Anaheim chile peppers
- 3 scallions, root ends discarded, all the rest roughly chopped
- ¼ cup lightly packed fresh cilantro leaves and tender stems
- 1 small garlic clove
- ½ cup sour cream
- ½ cup mayonnaise
  Finely grated zest and juice of 1 lime
- ¼ teaspoon kosher salt

Grill the chile peppers over **direct high heat** (450° to 550°F), with the lid open, until they are blackened and blistered in spots all over, 3 to 5 minutes, turning occasionally. Remove the chiles from the grill. When cool enough to handle, remove and discard the stem ends. Using a sharp knife, scrape off and discard nearly all the blackened skins. Roughly chop the remaining parts of the chiles and drop them into a food processor or blender. Add the scallions, cilantro, and garlic. Process to make a coarse paste, scraping down the sides once or twice. Add the remaining ingredients and process for a minute or two to create a smooth sauce. If it seems too thick, add a little water. Adjust the seasonings. Cover and refrigerate until about 30 minutes before serving.

TOMATILLO SALSA

MAKES: ABOUT 2 CUPS

- 1 medium yellow onion, cut into ½-inch slices
  Extra-virgin olive oil
- 10 medium tomatillos, husked and rinsed, about ½ pound total
- 1 small jalapeño chile pepper, stem removed
- ¼ cup lightly packed fresh cilantro leaves and tender stems
- 1 medium garlic clove
- ½ teaspoon dark brown sugar
- ½ teaspoon kosher salt

Lightly brush the onion slices on both sides with oil. Brush the cooking grate clean. Grill the onion slices, tomatillos, and jalapeño over **direct high heat** (450° to 550°F), with the lid closed as much as possible, until lightly charred, 6 to 8 minutes, turning once or twice and swapping their positions as needed for even cooking. Be sure the tomatillos are completely soft as you remove them from the grill. Combine the onion slices, tomatillos, and jalapeño in a food processor, along with the remaining ingredients. Process until fairly smooth. Taste and adjust the seasonings.

RÉMOULADE

MAKES ABOUT ¾ CUP

- ½ cup mayonnaise
- 1 tablespoon capers, drained and minced
- 1 tablespoon sweet pickle relish
- 1 tablespoon finely chopped fresh tarragon
- 2 teaspoons minced shallot
- 1 teaspoon tarragon vinegar
- 1 teaspoon minced garlic
- ½ teaspoon Dijon mustard
- ¼ teaspoon paprika
- ⅛ teaspoon kosher salt

In a medium bowl whisk the ingredients. If not using right away, cover and refrigerate for as long as 24 hours.

BALINESE PEANUT SAUCE

MAKES: ABOUT 1¼ CUP

- ½ cup smooth peanut butter
- ½ cup stirred coconut milk
- 2 tablespoons fresh lime juice
- 2 teaspoons garlic-chile sauce, such as Sriracha
- 2 teaspoons fish sauce

In a small saucepan combine the ingredients. Set the saucepan over very low heat and cook until the sauce is smooth, 3 to 5 minutes, whisking occasionally, but do not let the sauce simmer. If the sauce seems too thick, whisk in 1 to 2 tablespoons of water.

TOMATO SALSA

MAKES: ABOUT 2 CUPS

- 1½ cups finely diced ripe tomatoes
- ½ cup finely diced white onion, rinsed in a sieve under cold water
- 2 tablespoons finely chopped fresh cilantro
- 1 tablespoon extra-virgin olive oil
- 2 teaspoons fresh lime juice
- 1 teaspoon minced jalapeño chile pepper (with seeds)
- ¼ teaspoon dried oregano
- ¼ teaspoon kosher salt
- ¼ teaspoon freshly ground black pepper

In a medium bowl mix the ingredients. Allow the salsa to stand at room temperature for about 1 hour. Drain in a sieve just before serving.

RED MEAT

WHAT YOU NEED TO KNOW

TASTE AND TENDERNESS ARE TRADE-OFFS

When you pay more for steak, usually you are paying for tenderness. That's why a filet mignon is more expensive than a flank steak, even though the flank steak has more flavor. The pricey and tender steaks, like the porterhouse, the T-bone, the filet mignon, and the New York strip, come from the loin area of a cow, which gets very little exercise while the cow lumbers around. Other steaks, like the flank and the top sirloin, come from parts of the cow that get more of a workout.

FEED MATTERS

It's natural for cows to eat grass. But feeding them grass their whole lives is expensive. It requires moving the animals from pasture to pasture as the seasons change. It's cheaper to herd them in one place and feed them a grain-based diet, which fattens them up faster than grass, too, and makes them more tender. Grass-fed cattle are usually leaner and free of the added hormones and antibiotics that grain-fed animals often receive, but the meat is a little tougher and stronger in flavor.

GRADES ARE HELPFUL, BUT YOU MAKE THE FINAL CALL

The USDA uses meat grades, at the request of the producer, to reflect the age and marbling of beef. Most of the steaks you'll find in supermarkets are graded Choice or Select. I recommend staying away from Select steaks, as they are just too dry for grilling. And not all Choice steaks are necessarily great. Be selective and choose the ones with a coarse marbling of milky white fat. The flesh should be a rich pink or light cherry color. If you see any with a deep red or brown color, it could mean those steaks came from older, tougher animals. And the surface should be moist, but not wet or sticky.

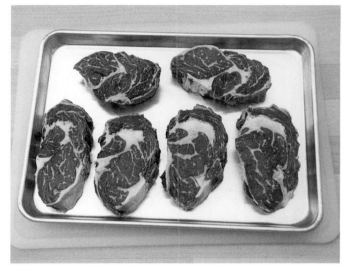

BROWN IS BETTER

Whichever cut of meat you choose, and whatever its grade might be, you'll get the most flavor from it when the surface is cooked to a deep brown color. When sugars and proteins in the meat are heated by the grill, they produce literally hundreds of flavors and aromas. That's why so many recipes in this book involve searing over direct heat. A lot of people will tell you that searing seals in moisture, but that theory has been debunked. Instead, searing develops a layer of incredible flavor and also some nice texture.

Wet meat doesn't sear, it steams, so be sure to pat the surface dry with paper towels before grilling. Salt can also affect searing. I recommend waiting to salt red meat until 20 to 30 minutes before grilling because, over a longer period of time, salt pulls blood and juices from inside the meat, making the surface wet. Salt does, however, need to go on before grilling. Salt added afterwards doesn't penetrate very well.

CUTS OF STEAK

RIB-EYE
A rib-eye steak's abundant internal fat melting into the meat creates one the juiciest steak-eating experiences imaginable. Do yourself a favor; before grilling, trim the fat around the perimeter to about ¼ inch. That will reduce the chance of flare-ups.

STRIP
Call it a New York strip, a Kansas City strip, a strip loin, a top loin, a shell steak, a club steak, an ambassador steak…it all depends on where you are and who's talking. Regardless of the name, it's a relatively lean cut with a firmer texture than a rib-eye or filet mignon, but the flavor is great.

FILET MIGNON
Pricey and velvety soft, filets mignons make a nice splurge for special guests, though it's really the tenderness you are buying. The flavor can be a little underwhelming unless you lightly char the outside with a blazing hot grill.

PORTERHOUSE
This is the classic steakhouse steak that features both a strip steak and filet mignon, separated by a bone. Start these steaks over high heat and finish them on a cooler section of the grill so you don't blacken the bone or the meat beside it.

T-BONE
It's just like a porterhouse except the piece of tenderloin is not as big, because this steak is cut a little farther forward on the animal.

TOP SIRLOIN
These flat, firmly grained steaks bring kabobs quickly to mind because it's so easy to cut them into solid cubes. Pick out the top sirloin steaks with visible marbling and don't take them beyond medium rare.

TRI-TIP
A tri-tip is taken from the sirloin area. It's not so much a steak as it is a skinny roast, but you can grill it like a thick steak. The meat is relatively affordable and very flavorful. Just don't overcook it.

FLANK
You can quickly spot this steak by its flat oval shape and its long, clearly defined grain. It used to be the steak of choice for London broil. Now the flank steak stars in all kinds of grilled recipes. Minimize the chewy effect of the grain by slicing across it.

SKIRT
Like the flank steak, the coarsely grained skirt steak is cut from the chest area of the animal, so chewiness is an issue. Even so, after grilling, it tends to be juicier and richer in flavor than flank steak, especially if you marinate it first.

FLATIRON
Normally you would expect a steak cut from the shoulder to be tough, but the flatiron, a.k.a. a top blade steak, is nestled into a tender pocket of the shoulder area, so it's a surprisingly soft exception to the rule. In some cases you'll need to remove a thin vein of gristle running down the center of a flatiron.

TYPES OF RED MEAT FOR THE GRILL

Tender cuts for grilling	Moderately tender cuts for grilling	Bigger cuts for searing and grill-roasting	Tougher cuts for barbecuing
Beef tenderloin (filet mignon) steak Beef rib steak/rib-eye steak Beef porterhouse steak Beef T-bone steak New York strip Lamb loin chop Lamb sirloin chop Veal loin chop	Beef top sirloin Beef flank steak Beef hanger steak Beef skirt steak Beef flatiron steak Veal shoulder blade chop Lamb shoulder blade chop Lamb sirloin chop	Beef whole tenderloin Beef tri-tip roast Beef standing rib roast (prime rib) Beef strip loin Rack of veal Rack of lamb Leg of lamb	Brisket Beef ribs

WAY TO FREEZE STEAKS

Cutting steaks from a big piece of meat like a strip loin or a boneless rib roast allows you to make steaks just the right thickness. Grill some of the steaks now and freeze the remaining ones for another day. Here's how: The key to freezing a steak properly is to prevent air from touching the surface of the meat. Wrap each steak individually with plastic wrap, not butcher paper or aluminum foil, and seal it as tightly as possible. Place the wrapped steaks in a resealable freezer bag and set the freezer as close to 0°F as it will go. The colder, the better. Steaks packaged this way will keep very well for about 3 months. Label them so that you don't forget when to grill them!

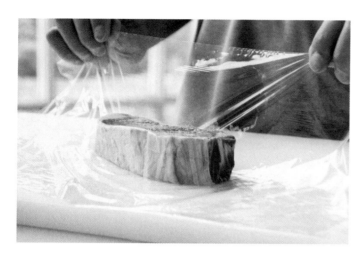

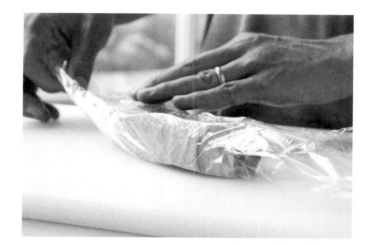

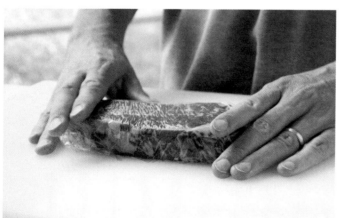

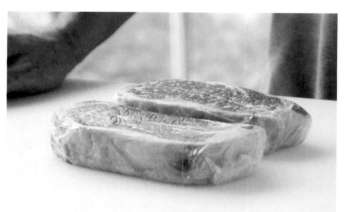

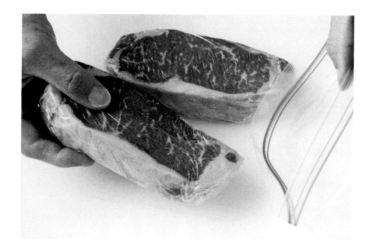

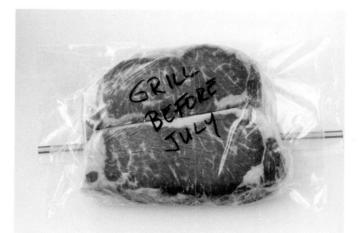

WHEN IS IT DONE?

Recognizing the moment when a big piece of red meat has reached the degree of doneness you want is actually quite simple. Stick the probe of an instant-read thermometer into the thickest part of the meat. When the internal temperature is 5 to 10 degrees below what you ultimately want to eat, take the meat off the grill. That's because larger pieces of meat, such as a beef strip loin or a leg of lamb, retain quite a bit of heat as they "rest" at room temperature. They continue to cook.

For optimal safety, the USDA recommends cooking red meat to 145°F (final temperature) and ground red meat to 160°F. The USDA believes that 145°F is medium rare, but virtually all chefs today believe medium rare is closer to 130°F. The chart below compares chef standards with USDA recommendations. Ultimately, it is up to you what doneness you choose.

Checking for the doneness of steaks and chops is a little more difficult with an instant-read thermometer because you need to position the sensing "dimple" of the probe right in the center of the meat. It's easy to miss the center and get an inaccurate reading, so I recommend learning to use the "touch test." Most raw steaks are as soft as the fleshiest part of your thumb when your hand is relaxed. As they cook, the steaks get firmer and firmer. If you press your index finger and thumb together and press the fleshiest part of your thumb again, the firmness is very close to that of a rare steak. If you press your middle finger and thumb together, the firmness on your thumb is very close to that of a medium-rare steak.

If you are still not sure of the doneness, take the steak off the grill and put the best-looking side (presentation side) facing down on a cutting board. With the tip of a sharp knife, make a little cut in the middle so you can see the color of the meat inside. If the color is still too red, put it back on the grill. Otherwise, get the rest of the meat off the grill and pat yourself on the back. Before you serve the steaks, feel their firmness and remember that for the next time you use the touch test.

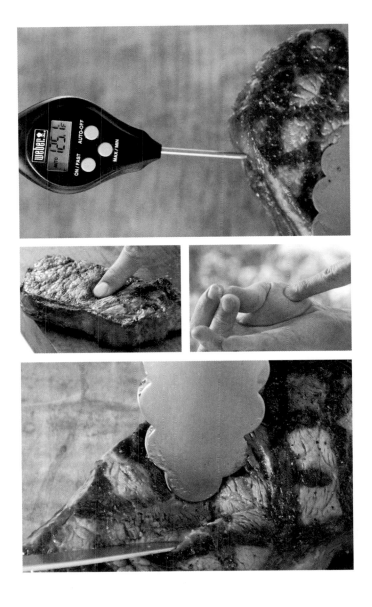

DONENESS	CHEF STANDARDS	USDA
Rare	120° to 125°F	n/a
Medium rare	125° to 135°F	145°F
Medium	135° to 145°F	160°F
Medium well	145° to 155°F	n/a
Well done	155°F +	170°F

BEEF GRILLING GUIDE

The following cuts, thicknesses, weights, and grilling times are meant to be guidelines rather than hard and fast rules. Cooking times are affected by such factors as altitude, wind, outside temperature, and desired doneness. Two rules of thumb: Grill steaks and kabobs using the direct method for the time given on the chart or to your desired doneness, turning once. Grill roasts and thicker cuts using the indirect method for the time given on the chart or until an instant-read thermometer reaches the desired internal temperature. Let roasts, larger cuts of meat, and thick steaks rest for 5 to 10 minutes before carving. The internal temperature of the meat will rise by 5 to 10 degrees during this time.

BEEF	THICKNESS/ WEIGHT	APPROXIMATE GRILLING TIME
Steak: New York strip, porterhouse, rib-eye, T-bone, and tenderloin	¾ inch thick	**4 to 6 minutes** direct high heat
	1 inch thick	**5 to 8 minutes:** sear 4 to 6 minutes direct high heat, grill 1 to 2 minutes indirect high heat
	1¼ inches thick	**8 to 10 minutes:** sear 6 minutes direct high heat, grill 2 to 4 minutes indirect high heat
	1½ inches thick	**10 to 14 minutes:** sear 6 to 8 minutes direct high heat, grill 4 to 6 minutes indirect high heat
	2 inches thick	**14 to 18 minutes:** sear 6 to 8 minutes direct high heat, grill 8 to 10 minutes indirect high heat
Skirt steak	¼ to ½ inch thick	**4 to 6 minutes** direct high heat
Flank steak	1½ to 2 pounds, ¾ inch thick	**8 to 10 minutes** direct high heat
Kabob	1 to 1½ inch cubes	**4 to 6 minutes** direct high heat
Tenderloin, whole	3½ to 4 pounds	**35 to 45 minutes:** sear 15 minutes direct medium heat, grill 20 to 30 minutes indirect medium heat
Ground beef patty	¾ inch thick	**8 to 10 minutes** direct high heat
Rib roast (prime rib), boneless	5 to 6 pounds	**1¼ to 1¾ hours** indirect medium heat
Rib roast (prime rib), with bone	8 pounds	**2½ to 3 hours:** sear 10 minutes direct medium heat, grill 2⅓ to 3 hours indirect low heat
Strip loin roast, boneless	4 to 5 pounds	**50 to 60 minutes:** sear 10 minutes direct medium heat, grill 40 to 50 minutes indirect medium heat
Tri-tip roast	2 to 2½ pounds	**30 to 40 minutes:** sear 10 minutes direct medium heat, grill 20 to 30 minutes indirect medium heat
Veal loin chop	1 inch thick	**5 to 8 minutes:** sear 4 to 6 minutes direct high heat, grill 1 to 2 minutes indirect high heat

Note: All cooking times are for medium-rare doneness, except ground beef (medium)

LAMB: THE OTHER RED MEAT

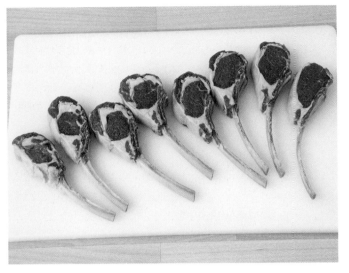

When buying lamb, ook for meat that is light red (not too dark) and f nely grained (not coarse). The fat should be white (nct yellow). Lamb chops cut from the rack are quite flavorful and tender. Be sure to trim the fat close to the meat so you don't face flare-ups. The lamb loin also produces very nice chops, with a little bone in the m ddle of each one, just like a miniature T-bone steak. Even chops from the sirloin and shou der areas are tender enough for grilling, because the animals are almost always younger than one-year-old when they are brought to market. A leg of lamb opens up lots of possibilities, too, including gril -roast ng it ove indirect heat or cutting the meat into cubes for kabobs.

LAMB GRILLING GUIDE

The following cuts, thicknesses, weights, and grilling times are meant to be guidelines rather than hard and fast rules. Cooking times are affected by such factors as altitude, wind, outside temperature and desired doneness. Two rules of thumb: Grill chops using the direct method for the time given on the chart or to your desired doneness, turning once. Grill roasts and thicker cuts using the indirect method for the time given on the chart o until an instant-read thermometer reaches the desired internal temperature. Let roasts, larger cuts of meat, and thick chops rest for 5 to 10 minutes before carving. The internal temperature of the meat will rise by 5 to 10 degrees during this time.

LAMB	THICKNESS/ WEIGHT	APPROXIMATE GRILLING TIME
Chop: loin, rib, shoulder, or sirloin	¾ to 1½ inches thick	**8 to 12 minutes** direct medium heat
Leg of lamb roast, boneless, rolled	2½ to 3 pounds	**30 to 45 minutes:** sear 10 to 15 minutes direct medium heat, grill 20 to 30 minutes indirect medium heat
Leg of lamb, butterflied	3 to 3½ pounds	**30 to 45 minutes:** sear 10 to 15 minutes direct medium heat, grill 20 to 30 minutes indirect medium heat
Rib crown roast	3 to 4 pounds	**1 to 1¼ hours** indirect medium heat
Ground lamb patty	¾ inch thick	**8 to 10 minutes** direct medium heat
Rack of lamb	1 to 1½ pounds	**15 to 20 minutes:** sear 5 minutes direct medium heat, grill 10 to 15 minutes indirect medium heat

Note: All cooking times are for medium-rare doneness, except ground lamb (medium).

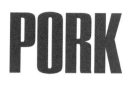

PORK

PORK GRILLING GUIDE

The following cuts, thicknesses, weights, and grilling times are meant to be guidelines rather than hard and fast rules. Cooking times are affected by such factors as altitude, wind, outside temperature, and desired doneness. Two rules of thumb: Grill chops and brats using the direct method for the time given on the chart or to your desired doneness, turning once. Grill roasts and thicker cuts using the indirect method for the time given on the chart or until an instant-read thermometer reaches the desired internal temperature. Let roasts, large cuts of meat, and thick chops rest for 5 to 10 minutes before carving. The internal temperature of the meat will rise by 5 to 10 degrees during this time.

PORK	THICKNESS/WEIGHT	APPROXIMATE GRILLING TIME
Bratwurst, fresh		**20 to 25 minutes** direct medium heat
Bratwurst, pre-cooked		**10 to 12 minutes** direct medium heat
Pork chop, boneless or bone-in	½ inch thick	**5 to 7 minutes** direct high heat
	¾ inch thick	**6 to 8 minutes** direct high heat
	1 inch thick	**8 to 10 minutes** direct medium heat
	1¼ to 1½ inches thick	**10 to 12 minutes:** sear 6 minutes direct high heat, grill 4 to 6 minutes indirect high heat
Tenderloin	1 pound	**15 to 20 minutes** direct medium heat
Loin roast, boneless	2½ pounds	**40 to 50 minutes** direct medium heat
Loin roast, bone-in	3 to 5 pounds	**1¼ to 1¾ hours** indirect medium heat
Pork shoulder (Boston butt), boneless	5 to 6 pounds	**5 to 7 hours** indirect low heat
Pork, ground	½ inch thick	**8 to 10 minutes** direct medium heat
Ribs, baby back	1½ to 2 pounds	**3 to 4 hours** indirect low heat
Ribs, spareribs	2½ to 3½ pounds	**3 to 4 hours** indirect low heat
Ribs, country-style, boneless	1½ to 2 pounds	**12 to 15 minutes** direct medium heat
Ribs, country-style, bone-in	3 to 4 pounds	**1½ to 2 hours** indirect medium heat

WHEN IS IT DONE?

Think pink! The USDA recommends that pork is cooked to well done (170°F), but most chefs today cook it to 150°F or 160°F, when it still has some pink in the center and all the juices haven't been driven out. Of course, the doneness you choose is entirely up to you.

The pork chop on the left, with raw meat in the center, is clearly undercooked. The chop on the right, with a dry, gray appearance, is overcooked. The chop in the middle, with a little bit of pink in the center, is cooked to 150°F (just right). See how the meat gives a little under pressure.

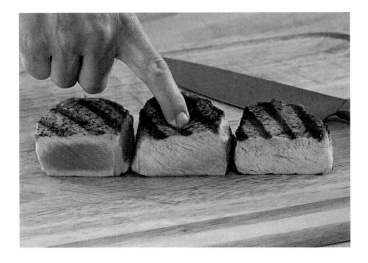

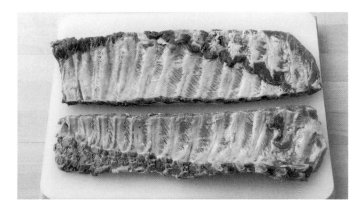

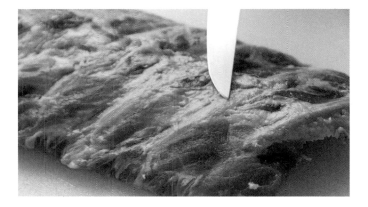

BABY BACK RIBS VERSUS SPARERIBS

Despite the big differences in the size of baby back ribs and spareribs, they are really just two pieces of the same slab of meat. Baby back ribs (bottom of photo) are cut from the top of the ribcage, near the backbone. Spareribs (top of photo) are cut from the bottom of the ribcage, and sometimes they include the brisket, which is a bony piece of meat that hangs from the bottom. The farther down the ribcage you go, the meatier the ribs get. That is essentially why spareribs take longer to cook.

WHAT IS A SHINER?

A shiner is an exposed bone on a rack of ribs. It is what unfortunately happens when a butcher cuts too close to the bone. Ribs should be meaty all over, so if you see a rack with shiners at the market, look for something better. Also avoid all ribs with dry edges or yellowish fat. And know that fresh ribs will almost always yield better results than previously frozen ribs.

TYPES OF PORK FOR THE GRILL

Tender cuts for grilling	Moderately tender cuts for grilling	Bigger cuts for searing and grill-roasting	Tougher cuts for barbecuing
Rib chop	Sirloin chop	Rack of pork	Baby back ribs
Loin chop	Shoulder blade steak	Sirloin loin roast	Spareribs
Center-cut chop	Ham steak	Center rib roast	Shoulder (Boston butt)
Tenderloin (whole or in medallions)		Center loin roast	
		Cured ham	
		Country-style ribs	

POULTRY

WHAT TO LOOK FOR IN CHICKEN

Chicken is chicken, right? Not exactly. Most supermarkets carry big national brands, or sometimes supermarkets put their own brands on these mass-produced birds raised in cages. They are low in fat, they cook quickly, and they are pretty tender, however, their flavor is pretty darn bland. Fortunately the grill provides just what they need. With a little oil, some seasonings, and maybe a sauce, they are very good on the grill.

Today we are seeing more and more premium chickens available, and usually they are worth their higher price, though not always. Typically, these chickens are from old-fashioned breeds known more for their flavor than their plump breasts and perfectly even shape. Often called "free-range" chickens, they have access to the outdoors, or at least the freedom to wander indoors. The exercise contributes to firmer, more flavorful meat. Check them out. Any chickens you buy should have skins that fit their bodies well, not spotty or shriveled or too far overlapping. The color of the skin says little about quality, but the smell of a chicken will tell everything you need to know about freshness. If it smells funny, don't buy it.

By law, the USDA insists that every chicken be chilled to at least 40°F within 4 hours of being slaughtered. Typically producers submerge their chickens in chlorinated ice water, which works quickly, but often the process means that the chickens absorb some water. Another process, which is not as common in the United States, involves spraying the chickens with chlorinated water and then sending them though long tunnels filled with cold air. The air-chilled chickens absorb less water, which is good. Who wants to pay extra for ice water?

Some chickens, even when they have been properly chilled, carry upsetting bacteria like salmonella. There is no sense in rinsing raw chickens prior to cooking. That would only raise the chances of spreading bacteria around your kitchen. Simply cook your chickens properly, and all the dangerous bacteria will be killed.

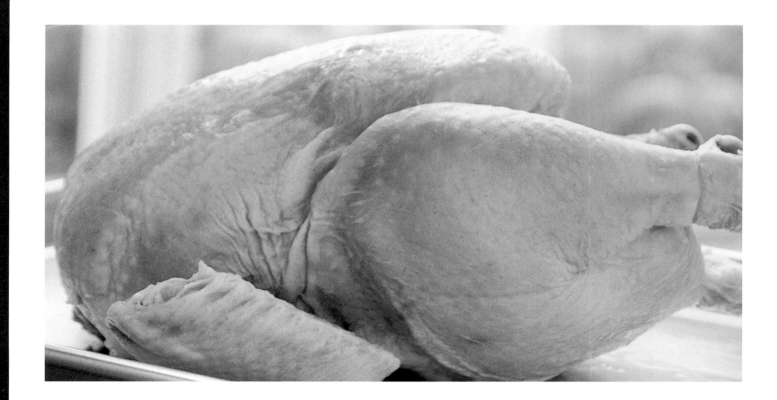

WHEN IS IT DONE?

The USDA recommends cooking poultry until the internal temperature reaches 165°F. Keep in mind that in whole birds the internal temperature will rise 5 to 10 degrees during resting.

Check the thigh meat by inserting the probe of a thermometer into the thickest part (but not touching the bone). If you don't have a thermometer, cut into the center of the meat. The juices should run clear and the meat should no longer be pink at the bone.

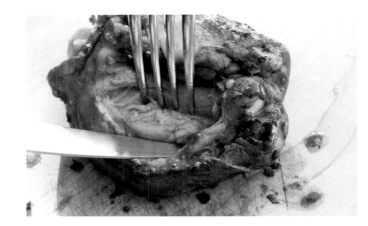

POULTRY GRILLING GUIDE

The following cuts, weights, and grilling times are meant to be guidelines rather than hard and fast rules. Cooking times are affected by such factors as altitude, wind, and outside temperature. Two rules of thumb: Grill boneless poultry pieces using the direct method for the time given on the chart, turning once. Grill whole poultry and bone-in poultry pieces using the indirect method for the time given on the chart or until an instant-read thermometer reaches the desired doneness. Cooking times are for the USDA's recommendation of 165°F. Let whole poultry rest for 5 to 10 minutes before carving. The internal temperature of the meat will rise by 5 to 10 degrees during this time.

POULTRY	WEIGHT	APPROXIMATE GRILLING TIME
Chicken breast, boneless, skinless	6 to 8 ounces	**8 to 12 minutes** direct medium heat
Chicken thigh, boneless, skinless	4 ounces	**8 to 10 minutes** direct high heat
Chicken breast, bone-in	10 to 12 ounces	**30 to 40 minutes** indirect medium heat
Chicken pieces, bone-in leg/thigh		**30 to 40 minutes** indirect medium heat
Chicken wing	2 to 3 ounces	**18 to 20 minutes** direct medium heat
Chicken, whole	3½ to 4½ pounds	**1 to 1½ hours** indirect medium heat
Cornish game hen	1½ to 2 pounds	**50 to 60 minutes** indirect high heat
Turkey breast, boneless	2½ pounds	**1 to 1¼ hours** indirect medium heat
Turkey, whole, unstuffed	10 to 12 pounds	**2½ to 3½ hours** indirect low heat
	13 to 15 pounds	**3½ to 4½ hours** indirect low heat
Duck breast, boneless	10 to 12 ounces	**9 to 12 minutes:** grill 3 to 4 minutes direct low heat, grill 6 to 8 minutes indirect high heat
Duck, whole	5½ to 6 pounds	**40 minutes** indirect high heat

SEAFOOD

TIPS TO PREVENT STICKING

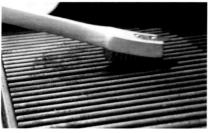

CLEAN COOKING GRATES
Use a stainless steel-bristle brush to get the grates really clean.

A LITTLE OIL
Coat the fish on all sides with a thin layer of oil, but don't oil the grates.

HIGH HEAT
Fish comes off the grate after a delicate crust of caramelization develops between the flesh and grate. That requires heat, usually high heat.

A LOT OF PATIENCE
Leave the fish alone. Caramelization happens faster when the fish stays in place on the hot grate. Keep the lid down as much as possible and turn the fish only once.

GOOD TIMING
The first side down on the grates will be the side that eventually faces you on the plate. Grill it a few minutes longer than the second side and it will release more easily and look fabulous on the plate, with picture-perfect grill marks.

WAY TO REMOVE FISH FROM THE COOKING GRATES
If the fillets have skin attached, grill the skin side last. When each fillet is ready to serve, slide a spatula between the skin and flesh, and then lift each fillet, leaving the skin behind.

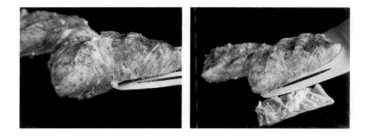

WHAT TO LOOK FOR IN FISH

The first thing to know is that firm fish and seafood are easiest to grill. The meatier they are, the better they hold together as they cook and as you turn them over. Many tender fish work nicely, too. Though they require a little more care. The chart below features many of your widely available choices. Feel free to substitute within the categories. If you f nd two fish with similar sizes and textures, just replace one for the other.

TYPES OF FISH FOR THE GRILL

Firm fillets and steaks	Medium-firm fillets and steaks	Tender fillets	Whole fish	Shellfish
Swordfish	Monkfish	Striped bass	Red snapper	Shrimp
Tuna	Halibut	Bluefish	Striped bass	Scallops
Salmon	Mahi-mahi	Trout	Grouper	Lobster
Grouper	Mackerel		Bluefish	Oysters
Squid	Chilean sea bass		Mackerel	Musse s
	Red snapper		Trout	Clams

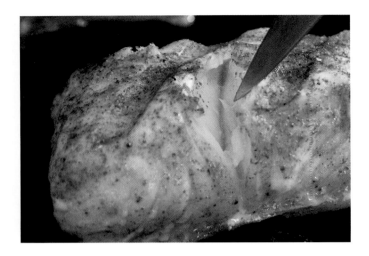

WHEN IS IT DONE?

Overcooking fish is a crime. With almost every kind of fish, you should get it off the grill before it flakes by itself. You are looking for an internal temperature of 125° to 130°F, but that's tough to measure with fillets or steaks, so rely on the internal appearance (the whitish color of the fish should be opaque all the way to the center), as well as the times given in the recipes and in the chart below.

SEAFOOD GRILLING GUIDE

The following types, thicknesses, weights, and grilling times are meant to be guidelines rather than hard and fast rules. Cooking times are affected by such factors as altitude, wind, outside temperature, and desired doneness. The general rule of thumb for grilling fish: 4 to 5 minutes per ½-inch thickness; 8 to 10 minutes per 1-inch thickness.

FISH	THICKNESS/ WEIGHT	APPROXIMATE GRILLING TIME
Fish, fillet or steak Includes halibut, red snapper, salmon, sea bass, swordfish, and tuna	¼ to ½ inch thick	**3 to 5 minutes** direct high heat
	½ to 1 inch thick	**5 to 10 minutes** direct high heat
	1 to 1¼ inches thick	**10 to 12 minutes** direct high heat
Fish, whole	1 pound	**15 to 20 minutes** indirect medium heat
	2 to 2½ pounds	**20 to 30 minutes** indirect medium heat
	3 pounds	**30 to 45 minutes** indirect medium heat
Shrimp	1½ ounces	**2 to 4 minutes** direct high heat
Scallop	1½ ounces	**4 to 6 minutes** direct high heat
Mussel (discard any that do not open)		**5 to 6 minutes** direct high heat
Clam (discard any that do not open)		**6 to 8 minutes** direct high heat
Oyster		**2 to 4 minutes** direct high heat
Lobster tail		**7 to 11 minutes** direct medium heat

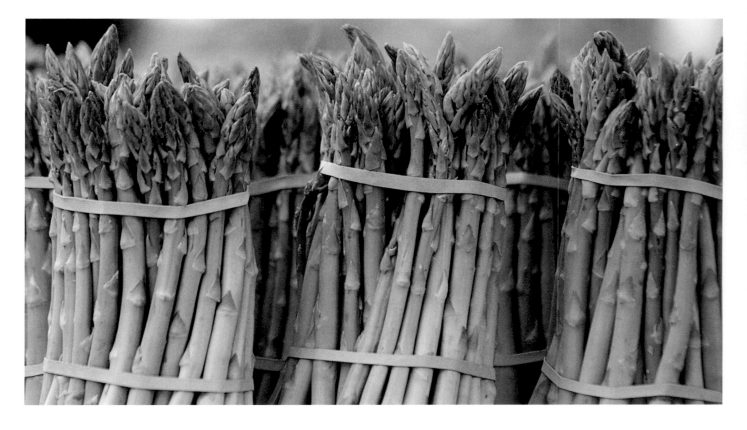

VEGETABLES

GRILL WHAT'S GROWING AT THE TIME

Vegetables in season locally have big advantages over whatever has been shipped from across the world. They are riper, so they taste better. That means you can grill them simply with great results.

EXPOSE AS MUCH SURFACE AREA AS POSSIBLE

Cut each vegetable to give you the biggest area to put in direct contact with the cooking grates. The more direct contact, the better the flavors will be. For example, choose peppers with flat sides that you can easily slice off the core. The flatter the sides, the more surface area will caramelize on the hot cooking grates.

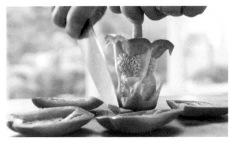

USE THE GOOD OIL

Vegetables need oil to prevent sticking and burning. Neutral oils like canola oil will do the job fine, but an extra-virgin olive oil provides the added benefit of improving the flavor of virtually every vegetable. Brush on just enough to coat each side thoroughly but not so much that the vegetables would drip oil and cause flare-ups. Season the vegetables generously with salt and pepper (some of it will fall off). For more flavors, marinate the vegetables at room temperature for 20 minutes to an hour in olive oil, vinegar, garlic, herbs, and spices.

WHEN IS IT DONE?

I like firm vegetables such as onions and fennel to be somewhere between crisp and tender. If you want them softer, grill them a few minutes longer, although watch them carefully for burning. The grill intensifies the sweetness of vegetables quickly and that can lead to burning. Cut the vegetables as evenly as you can. A ½-inch thickness is right for most of them.

VEGETABLE GRILLING GUIDE

Just about everything from artichokes to zucchini tends to cook best over direct medium heat. The temperature on the grill's thermometer should be somewhere between 350° and 450°F. If any parts get a little too dark, turn the vegetables over. Otherwise turn them as few times as possible.

VEGETABLES	THICKNESS/SIZE	APPROXIMATE GRILLING TIME
Artichoke (10 to 12 ounces)	whole	**14 to 18 minutes:** boil 10 to 12 minutes; cut in half and grill 4 to 6 minutes direct medium heat
Asparagus	½-inch diameter	**4 to 6 minutes** direct medium heat
Beet (6 ounces)		**1 to 1½ hours** indirect medium heat
Bell pepper	whole	**10 to 15 minutes** direct medium heat
Bell/Chile pepper	¼-inch slices	**6 to 8 minutes** direct medium heat
Carrot	1-inch diameter	**7 to 11 minutes:** boil 4 to 6 minutes, grill 3 to 5 minutes direct high heat
Corn, husked		**10 to 15 minutes** direct medium heat
Corn, in husk		**25 to 30 minutes** direct medium heat
Eggplant	½-inch slices	**8 to 10 minutes** direct medium heat
Fennel	¼-inch slices	**10 to 12 minutes** direct medium heat
Garlic	whole	**45 to 60 minutes** indirect medium heat
Mushroom, shiitake or button		**8 to 10 minutes** direct medium heat
Mushroom, portabello		**10 to 15 minutes** direct medium heat
Onion	halved	**35 to 40 minutes** indirect medium heat
	½-inch slices	**8 to 12 minutes** direct medium heat
Potato	whole	**45 to 60 minutes** indirect medium heat
	½-inch slices	**14 to 16 minutes** direct medium heat
Potato, new	halved	**15 to 20 minutes** direct medium heat
Scallion	whole	**3 to 4 minutes** direct medium heat
Squash, acorn (1½ pounds)	halved	**40 to 60 minutes** indirect medium heat
Sweet potato	whole	**50 to 60 minutes** indirect medium heat
	¼-inch slices	**8 to 10 minutes** direct medium heat
Tomato, garden or plum	halved	**6 to 8 minutes** direct medium heat
	whole	**8 to 10 minutes** direct medium heat
Zucchini	½-inch slices	**3 to 5 minutes** direct medium heat
	halved	**4 to 6 minutes** direct medium heat

FRUIT

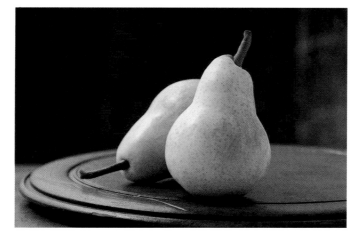

most fruits turns golden brown and delicious on the grill, but if left too long in one place, golden brown can turn to black and bitter. To check the color and doneness, slide a thin spatula gently under the fruit and slightly lift.

Warm fruit off the grill needs only a scoop of ice cream or frozen yogurt to seal a meal with style. Or use the grilled fruit to accompany a shortbread biscuit, a wedge of gingerbread, or a slice of pound

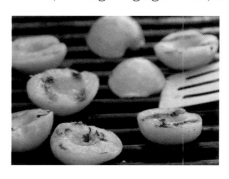

cake. Fruit served like this shows all your guests that you've developed the techniques to grill almost anything, from the appetizers through desserts.

Grilling fruit is much like grilling vegetables. Select fruit that's ripe (or almost ripe) and firm, because it will soften on the grill. Also, because of its texture, it's a good idea to watch fruit carefully while grilling and to turn it occasionally. The sweet succulence of

FRUIT GRILLING GUIDE

The following types, thicknesses, and grilling times are meant to be guidelines rather than hard and fast rules. Cooking times are affected by such factors as altitude, wind, and outside temperature. Grilling times for fruit will depend on ripeness.

FRUIT	THICKNESS/SIZE	APPROXIMATE GRILLING TIME
Apple	whole	**35 to 40 minutes** indirect medium heat
	½-inch slices	**4 to 6 minutes** direct medium heat
Apricot	halved, pit removed	**6 to 8 minutes** direct medium heat
Banana	halved lengthwise	**6 to 8 minutes** direct medium heat
Nectarine	halved lengthwise, pit removed	**8 to 10 minutes** direct medium heat
Peach	halved lengthwise, pit removed	**8 to 10 minutes** direct medium heat
Pear	halved lengthwise	**10 to 12 minutes** direct medium heat
Pineapple	peeled and cored, ½-inch slices or 1-inch wedges	**5 to 10 minutes** direct medium heat
Strawberry		**4 to 5 minutes** direct medium heat

GRILL MAINTENANCE

A little TLC is all it takes to ensure that you get years of use from your grill. Maintenance is the key (consult the owner's manual that came with your grill). Each time you use the grill, remember to clean the cooking grates. With the grill on high (either right before cooking or right after) brush the cooking grates with a long-handled, stainless steel brush. Be sure to get in between the grates with your brush, too.

MONTHLY MAINTENANCE PLAN FOR GAS GRILLS

1. When your grill is warm, but not hot, use a wet, soapy sponge or dishcloth to wipe the inside of the lid. This will help keep natural carbon build-up from accumulating inside the lid.

2. Remove the grates and brush the metal bars that shield the burners. A good brush, like the one you use to brush the cooking grates, will work well. This will help to eliminate flare-ups. (If you grill often, like I do, you may need to do this a little more frequently than once a month.)

3. Gently clean the burner tubes with a steel brush. Brush side-to-side along the burner tubes and take care not to damage the openings themselves by brushing too hard.

4. Use a plastic putty knife or spatula to scrape the grease from the bottom of the grill. If your grill has a collection tray, scrape the bits into it. Then dispose of the contents of the collection tray.

5. Wash the inside of the grill with warm, soapy water. Take care not to get water in the burner tubes.

6. Reassemble, wait a month, and repeat.

MONTHLY MAINTENANCE PLAN FOR CHARCOAL GRILLS

1. When the grill is cold, remove the ash from the bowl. Because the ash naturally contains a small amount of moisture, it is important to get the ash out of the bowl each time you use it and before storing your grill. If your grill has an ash catcher, empty after each use.

2. Wipe the inside of the bowl with a warm, wet sponge. This will help to keep natural carbon build-up from accumulating inside your grill.

MONTHLY MAINTENANCE PLAN FOR ELECTRIC GRILLS

1. When your grill is warm, but not hot, use a wet, soapy sponge or dishcloth to wipe the inside of the lid. This will help to keep natural carbon build-up from accumulating inside the lid of the grill.

2. Remove the grates. Use a plastic putty knife or spatula to scrape the grease from the bottom of the grill. If your grill has a collection tray, scrape the bits into it. Then dispose of the contents of the collection tray.

3. Wipe the inside of the grill with a warm, damp sponge, being very careful not to get the heating element wet.

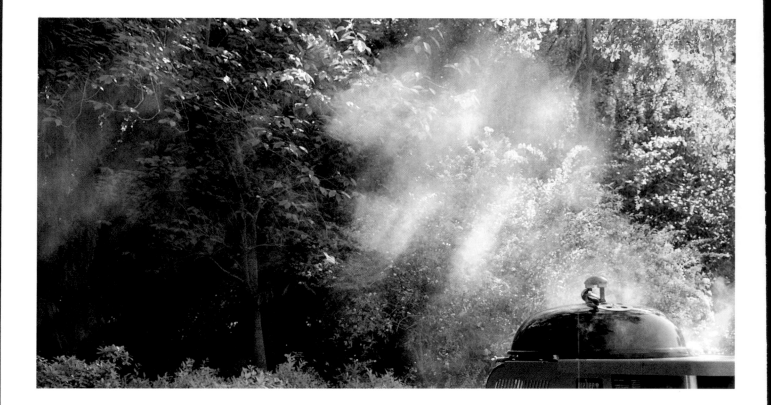

SELECTING THE RIGHT GRILL

One of the most valuable skills a good cook learns is the art of substitution. Tuna fillets, for instance, can substitute for mahi-mahi in a pinch, and a T-bone steak will work nicely in place of a porterhouse. However, when it comes to grills, there simply is no substitute for quality. After all, the one thing every meal you prepare from this book will have in common is your grill.

WHAT TO LOOK FOR IN A GAS GRILL

1. Check out the construction and durability. A grill is an important purchase and you will own it for years to come. Since most grills are kept outside and exposed to the elements, they need to be well made and durable. If you choose a stainless steel grill, look for heavy-gauge construction that will ensure the grill will last more than a season or two. A porcelain-enamel finish will also hold up well. Carefully check out the corners to make sure there are no sharp edges. Size up the fit and finish. If a grill's doors or frame are misaligned, it may be a reflection of poor design.

2. Lift the lid and kick the tires. The inner workings and construction of a grill are more important than how the grill looks on the outside. Lift the lid and see how the grill opens and closes. It should have a tight fit and the grill shouldn't feel wobbly when you open it. Look for heavy-duty cooking grates that will hold up to years of regular use.

3. Look at burner placement. Uneven heat is a griller's worst nightmare. A well-designed gas grill will have burners placed evenly across the cooking box. Angled metal bars will cover the burners, directing drippings away from the flames and minimizing flare-ups. These bars also serve to distribute the heat evenly across the entire grilling surface

4. Give yourself room. The cooking grate needs to be big enough to handle the amount food you like to grill, and remember, many recipes call for both direct and indirect heat. Be sure you have the room to move your food from direct to indirect heat any time.

5. Don't be blinded by BTUs. It's a common belief that more is better when it comes to BTUs. Not necessarily so. BTU stands for British Thermal Unit. It's a measure of how much heat it takes to raise one pound of water by one degree Fahrenheit. A gas grill burning 35,000 BTUs per hour should reach a searing temperature of around 550°F, no problem. Unless your grilling area is large, you should be fine with a grill with a BTU rating of 35,000 to 40,000 BTUs. More than that, and you may be wasting energy.

6. Don't overlook the basics. One of the most important things you should consider when buying a gas grill is where the grease and debris will go. Grease is combustible and if it is not channeled away from the inside of your grill, it could lead to some serious flare-ups. A well-designed system should include a removable grease tray that is accessible from the front of the grill. The drip pan itself should be at least a couple of inches deep and should come with disposable liners to make cleanup easier.

7. Be critical of the bells and whistles. These days, many grills come with nice added features such as a side burner or a rotisserie. These options can improve your grilling experience, if they are done well. Make sure the side burner has adequate power to do the job, or it may be a waste of money. It should also have a hinged cover so that you don't lose valuable grilling space when the burner is not in use. An added benefit of a hinged cover is that it can act as a windshield, improving the burner's performance. If you are buying a grill with a rotisserie, check out the motor. A wimpy motor will lead to wimpy performance. You will need a heavy-duty motor to turn larger items like turkey and leg of lamb. And check out the heft of the spit. Again, it needs to be strong enough to hold larger items and should have strong forks to hold the meat in place. Finally, look at the position of the rotisserie. Is the motor or the spit over the side burner? If so, you'll limit your ability to use it when you are rotisserie cooking.

WHAT TO LOOK FOR IN A CHARCOAL GRILL

1. Go for one with a lid. Open grills, such as hibachis, are fun to use but the design limits your flexibility. Buying a grill with a lid broadens your options. When you buy a charcoal grill, make sure it has a well-fitting lid, with top and bottom vents for airflow. The lid effectively turns the grill into an outdoor oven capable of both direct and indirect cooking. The vents allow you to control the temperature inside.

2. Make sure it's built to last. A good charcoal grill should last for years. Look for solid construction and a durable porcelain-enamel finish over thick gauge metal.

3. Look for great grates. Your charcoal grill should have thick, durable grates. Either heavy wire or stainless steel work well. For the serious griller, I recommend a hinged cooking grate that allows you to add more coals while cooking. My favorite way to prepare the Thanksgiving turkey is on my charcoal grill, and a hinged cooking grate allows me to easily add coals each hour to maintain even heat.

4. Make sure cleanup is easy. Charcoal is going to produce ash, which can be a mess to cleanup. Therefore, I recommend you choose a charcoal grill that is designed with a system to push ash from the bottom of your grill into a removable ash catcher. After all, the easier it is to clean your grill, the more you're going to use it.

ELECTRIC GRILLS

Until recently, if you lived in a condo or loft that didn't allow propane or charcoal grills, your only option was a less than stellar electric patio grill—or an indoor countertop grill. I'm happy to report that technology has improved and now there are new options with much improved performance. Like their gas and charcoal counterparts, electric grills should be solid, stable, and built to last.

SAFETY

GENERAL NOTES

1. Always read your owner's manual prior to use.

2. Grills radiate a lot of heat, so always keep the grill at least five feet away from any combustible materials, including the house, garage, deck rails, etc. Combustible materials include, but are not limited to, wood or treated wood decks, wood patios, or wood porches. Never use a grill indoors or under a covered patio.

3. Keep the grill in a level position at all times.

4. Use proper barbecuing tools with long, heat-resistant handles.

5. Don't wear loose or highly flammable clothing when grilling.

6. Do not leave infants, children, or pets unattended near a hot grill.

7. Use insulated barbecue mitts to protect hands while cooking or adjusting the vents.

GAS GRILL SAFETY

1. Always keep the bottom tray and grease catch pan of your gas grill clean and free of debris. This not only prevents dangerous grease fires, it deters visits from unwanted critters. A sprinkle of red pepper is another safe way to discourage animals.

2. If a flare-up should occur, turn off all burners and move food to another area of the cooking grate. Any flames will quickly subside. Then, light the grill again. Never use water to extinguish flames on a gas grill.

3. Do not line the funnel-shaped bottom tray with foil. This could prevent grease from flowing into the grease catch pan. Grease is also likely to catch in the tiny creases of the foil and start a fire.

4. Never store propane tanks or spares indoors (that means the garage, too).

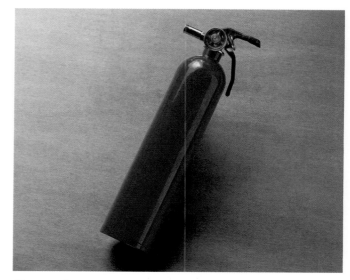

Keep a fire extinguisher handy in case of a mishap.

5. For the first few uses, the temperature of a new gas grill may run hotter than normal. Once your grill is seasoned and the inside of the cooking box is less reflective, the temperature will return to normal.

CHARCOAL GRILL SAFETY

1. Charcoal grills are designed for outdoor use only. If used indoors, toxic fumes will accumulate and cause serious bodily injury or death.

2. Do not add charcoal starter fluid or charcoal impregnated with charcoal starter fluid to hot or warm charcoal.

3. Do not use gasoline, alcohol, or other highly volatile fluids to ignite charcoal. If using charcoal starter fluid, remove any fluid that may have drained through the bottom vents before lighting the charcoal.

4. Do not use a grill unless all parts are in place. Make sure the ash catcher is properly attached to the legs underneath the bowl of the grill.

5. Remove the lid from the grill while lighting and getting the charcoal started.

6. Always put charcoal on top of the charcoal grate and not directly into the bottom of the bowl.

7. Do not place a chimney starter on or near any combustible surface.

8. Never touch the cooking or charcoal grate or the grill to see if they are hot.

9. Use the hook on the inside of the lid to hang the lid on the side of the bowl of the grill. Avoid placing a hot lid on carpet or grass. Do not hang the lid on the bowl handle.

10. To extinguish the coals, place the lid on the bowl and close all of the vents (dampers). Make sure that the vents/dampers on the lid and the bowl are completely closed. Do not use water as it will damage the porcelain finish.

11. To control flare-ups, place the lid on the grill and close the top vent about halfway. Do not use water.

12. Handle and store hot electric starters carefully. Do not place starters on or near any combustible surfaces.

13. Keep electrical cords away from the hot surfaces of the grill.

FOOD SAFETY TIPS

1. Wash your hands thoroughly with hot, soapy water before starting any meal preparation and after handling fresh meat, fish, and poultry.

2. Do not defrost meat, fish, or poultry at room temperature. Defrost in the refrigerator.

3. Use different utensils and preparation surfaces for raw and cooked foods.

4. Wash all plates and cooking utensils which have come into contact with raw meats or fish with hot, soapy water and rinse.

5. When resting meats at room temperature before grilling, note that room temperature is 65° to 70°F. Do not place raw food in direct sunlight or near any heat source.

6. Always grill ground meats to at least 160°F (170°F for poultry), the temperature for medium (well-done) doneness.

7. If a sauce will be brushed on meat during grilling, divide the sauce, using one part for brushing and the other for serving at the table. Vigorously boil marinades that were used for raw meat, fish, or poultry for at least 30 seconds before using as a baste or sauce.

PROPER GRILLING FORM

1. Trim excess fat from steaks and chops, leaving only a scant ¼-inch of fat, which is sufficient to flavor the meat. Less fat is a virtual guarantee against flare-ups and makes cleanup easier.

2. A light coating of oil will help brown your food evenly and keep it from sticking to the cooking grates. Always brush or spray oil on your food, not the cooking grates.

3. Keep a lid on it! A Weber® grill is designed to cook foods with the lid down. Keeping the lid on allows heat to circulate, cooking food evenly and without flare-ups. Every time you lift/open the lid, except when instructed to in a recipe, you add extra cooking time.

4. Take the guesswork out of grilling. Use a thermometer and a timer to let you know when it's time to take food off the grill. Checking meats for internal temperatures is the best way to determine when food is properly cooked or when done is about to become overdone.

5. Use the right utensils. Long-handled tools and long insulated barbecue mitts protect you from the heat. Use forks only to lift fully cooked foods from the grill and tongs or turners to turn them (forks pierce food and flavorful juices are lost).

6. Remember that cooking times in charts and recipes are approximate and based on 70°F (20°C) weather with little or no wind. Allow more cooking time on cold or windy days, or at higher altitudes, and less in extremely hot weather.

INDEX

TECHNIQUES

RECIPES

INDEX